THE AGE BEATERS and Their Universal Currency for

IMMORTALITY

Dr. Joel D. Wallach, BS, DVM, ND

and

Ma Lan, MD, MS, Lac

The Age Beaters and Their Universal Currency for

IMMORTALITY

Dr. Joel D.Wallach, BS, DVM, ND

And

Dr. Ma Lan, MD, MS, Lac

Library of Congress Cataloging in Publications Data

1. Longevity 2. Centenarians 3. Great Leap Forward
4. Vilcabamba 5. Titicaca 6. Chinese 7. Tibet
8. Hunza 9. Okinawa 10. Costa Rica 11. Nicoya
12. Wood ashes 13. Rice straw ash 14. Peat ash
15. Aging 16. Fire 17. Manufactured soil 18. Sardinia
19. Antioxidants 20. Calorie Restricted Diet
21. Essential Nutrients

The Age Beaters and Their Universal Currency for IMMORTALITY

First Edition, 2008

Second Edition, 2011

ISBN: 0974858161

Printed and Published by Wellness Publications LLC
P.O. Box 1222, Bonita, CA 91908
www.drjwallach.com

1-800-755-4656 USA and Canada
1-619-420-2435 local and international

Table of Contents

Part 3: The Age Beaters

Part 4: The Currency of the Age Beaters

Acknowledgements

Electronic research was critical to finding the necessary materials, old and new, to bring IMMORTALITY to life - to this end the efforts of Steve Wallach, John Taylor, Char Murphy, Margie Hatzinger were indispensable. Vince Merasigan, Vennessa Hunter, Michelle Wallach and Brian Davis were important in bringing life to the original cover design concept.

We are also greatful for the scientific reviews, comments and additions to Immortality by Dr. Gerhard Schrauzer, PhD and Dr. Edmond DeVroey, MD.

Dedication

To the centinarians of the world, past, current and future!

Additional Reading:

Let's Play Doctor - 1989

RARE EARTHS: forbidden cures* - 1994

Dead Doctors Don't Lie - 1997

Let's Play Herbal Doctor - 2000

God Bless America* - 2001

Hell's Kitchen* - 2005

Passport to Aromatherapy - 2005

Black Gene Lies - 2007

Energy Crisis - 2007

---

* longevity & immortality specific

Wellness Publications, LLC.
1-800-755-4656
1-619-420-2435

www.drjwallach

About the Authors

Dr. Joel D. Wallach, BS, DVM, ND

Dr. Wallach has been involved in biomedical research and clinical medicine for more than 50 years. He received his B.S. degree (agriculture) from the University of Missouri with a major in animal husbandry (nutrition) and a minor in field crops and soils; D.V.M. (doctorate in veterinary medicine) from the University of Missouri; three year post doctoral fellowship (comparative pathology/medicine) from Washington University, St. Louis, MO - The Center for the Biology of Natural Systems (the St. Louis Zoological Gardens, Shaw's Botanical Gardens, Botany Department, Washington University); Iowa State University (Department of Pathology and the State Diagnostic Laboratory), Ames, IA; Natal Parks Board, Umfolozi and Hluhluwe Game Parks, Natal, Republic of South Africa (Operation Rhino: Conservation of the Southern White Rhino - project veterinarian and capture officer); Southern Rhodesia (Zimbabwe), Wanke Game Park (Operation Elephant - consulting capture officer);St. Louis Zoological Gardens; The Chicago Zoological Gardens (Brookfield Zoo); Shedd Aquarium, Chicago, IL; Yerkes Regional Primate Research Center, Emory University, Atlanta, GA; N.D. (naturopathic physician)from the National College of Naturopathic Medicine, Portland, OR; Harbin Medical University, Harbin, Hei Long Jiang and the Shanghai Medical University, Peoples Republic of China.

He was a member of NIH site visit teams for facilities using exotic animal models for the study of human diseases for four years and was a member of the 1968 National

Science Foundation ad hoc committee that authored the 1968 Animal Welfare Act (humane housing, nutrition and care of laboratory and captive exotic species); a professor of nutrition at the National College of Naturopathic Medicine, Portland, OR; and a Consulting Professor of Medicine, Harbin Medical University, Harbin, Hei Long Jiang and the Shanghai Medical University, People's Republic of China.

Dr. Wallach has been the physician for university, amature, semiprofessional and professional athletes including those in the NBA, boxing, arena football, runners, cyclists, body builders and power lifters.

Dr. Wallach has appeared as an expert witness in State and Federal Courts as a comparative pathologist.

Dr. Wallach attained the rank of Lieutenant Colonel in the Missouri Air National Guard (131st Tactical Hospital), known as "Lindberg's Own," and the Alaska Air Reserve with responsibilities in public health and for the prevention and clean up of nuclear, biological and chemical attacks in North America and Europe.

Dr. Wallach was a recipient of the Wooster Beach Gold Medal Award (Association of Eclectic Physicians) for a significant breakthrough in the basic understanding of the cause and pathophysiology of Cystic Fibrosis. Dr. Wallach was nominated for the 1991 Nobel Prize in Medicine (Association of Eclectic Physicians) for his work in the understanding of the genesis and pathophysiology of Cystic Fibrosis.

Dr. Wallach received the 2004 Guardian of the Constitution Award (Emord & Assoc.) for his proactive and successful litigation efforts in obtaining nutrition claims from the FDA for Selenium and Omega 3 essential fatty acids. He also received the 2004 James Lind Scientific Achievement Award (Emord & Assoc.) for "brilliant discoveries that have paved the way for greater heath and longevity" for Americans.

Dr. Wallach has appeared frequently on local, national network and public radio and television (including a special on Cystic Fibrosis with ABC's 20/20), Fox News (The Morning

Show) regional and national talk radio programs (The Alan Combs Show) as an expert on health, longevity and trace mineral and rare earth deficiency diseases. Dr. Wallach is the host of his own syndicated talk radio show programs (Dead Doctors Don't Lie and Let's Play Doctor) on more than 100 stations since 1996. Because of his freewheeling style of humor and ability to zero in on the basic truth in health problems and medical politics, he is widely known as the "Rush Limbaugh" of alternative health.

Dr. Wallach has given an average of 300 free health lectures per year for more than 17 years, literally reaching millions of enthusiastic fans. His audio cassette tape (now CD), Dead Doctors Don't Lie (translated into eight languages) has sold more than 83 million copies world wide.

Dr. Wallach has more than 70 peer reviewed/referreed publications to his credit including a major reference, The Diseases of Exotic Animals - published by W.B.Saunders. This 1,000 page illustrated text is listed by the Smithsonian Institute as, "A recommended reference for all professional zoological parks and aquariums."

Dr. Ma Lan, MD, MS, Lac

Dr. Ma Lan was educated in the Peoples Republic of China. Dr. Ma Lan received her MD (medical degree)from the Beijing Medical University; took her residency at the People's Hospital, Beijing and was staff surgeon at the Canton Air Force Hospital; she received her MS (Master of Science) in transplantation immunology from Zhongshan Medical University, Canton, Peoples Republic of China; as with all Chinese doctors, Dr. Ma Lan was trained in Traditional Chinese Medicine (i.e.- acupuncture, herbs, manipulation, food medicine, massage and hydrotherapy) prior to entering the Western-style medical schools.

Dr. Ma Lan has been involved in biomedical research and clinical medicine for more than 44 years, her research credits include being an exchange scholar in microsurgery at Harvard School of Medicine, Boston, MA; a research fellow in laser microsurgery at St. Joseph Hospital, Houston, TX; the Department of orthopedic Surgery, the Medical College of Wisconsin, Milwaukee, WI; and the Department of Pharmacology, University of California, San Diego, CA.

Dr. Ma Lan has ten peer review publications to her credit in the fields of transplant immunology, pathology and laser vascular surgery and has co-authored nine best-selling books on the subjects of alternative health with Dr. Wallach.

Dr. Ma Lan attained the rank of Lieutenant in the Chinese Air Force with primary responsibilities as a general surgeon in the Canton Air Force Hospital, People's Republic of China.

Introduction

In the great scheme of things, the quest for a long and healthful life is a relatively new goal for humans. In the beginning, humans didn't know how long they could live, there were no bench marks or records or living examples - getting food, satisfying a salt hunger and survival itself were the universal drives of life.

We do know now, without a doubt, that humans can and do live well beyond 100 years of age - centenarians - the old ones; and super-centenarians older than 110 years are not that uncommon.

While in fact, we all have the genetic equipment to live healthfully well beyond 100 - consciously getting there today for the majority, however, requires a profound commitment to a time proven system, and a daily call to focused action - becoming a centenarian is a matter of proven, universal, proactive, yet simple choices and actions.

Most centenarians in the "Blue Zones" throughout the world get there without any conscious effort - in effect they get into the centenarian club by simply "falling off the turnip truck." They become centenarians because of where they live and because of successful cultural practices that have been developed and perfected by trial and error over the millennium.

When centenarians or super-centenarians are asked for their sage wisdom on how they got to be 100 years of age, it is quite obvious they themselves don't know - they will answer the ultimate, scientific, deep and thoughtful question with a quaint response such as, "have a good sense of humor," or "think good thoughts every day," or "love everyone," or "keep moving."

Becoming a centenarian is not related to "having a good sense of humor" or to an accident of "good genes" - we now know, reaching 100 years of age is a by-product of something else - a collection of four simple, universal, repeatable, daily habits and endeavors, many of which on the surface, are seemingly meaningless and unrelated to each other, our health and longevity, and yet they hold the unforgiving key to IMMORTALITY.

Unfortunately, we Americans and people of other industrialized nations, with an almost religious fervor, believe that their doctors, "break through" pharmaceuticals and comprehensive health plans will get us healthfully into the centenarian club - yet, despite spending three quarters of the world's annual expenditure for health care, according to the CDC and the WHO, we Americans ranked a dismal 48th in the world for health and longevity in 2008 - hardly a testimony of support for the continuation of this level of financial commitment or to our current medical beliefs. Albert Einstein said many things, however, one of his most profound observations says, "Insanity is doing the same thing over and over and expecting a different outcome."

This blind, and unjustified faith in the "medical system" has cost us untold misery, early death, and unspeakable amounts of money and in the end, our very way of life - Americans are universally sick with cardiovascular disease, obesity, diabetes, and arthritis; and the "American Dream" (millions of our manufacturing, assembly and "IT" jobs have left the country because of the outrageous cost of health care benefits for employees) of owning your own home, now seems beyond the average persons grasp - many of those who did get variable mortgages and subprime loans during the housing boom of the early 21st century have become perfect victims in a "perfect storm."

It is ironic that the people of Andora, a small western European country, are the longest lived people of the industrialized world in 2008 and that some third world countries have as many as 1:500 centenarians without access to healthcare, while we Americans and other high-tech industrialized nations with health care programs running out of our ears, have only 1:5,000-10,000 centenarians - why do they have up to 20 times the number of centenarians that we do, after all we are dedicated to following the instructions of our highly trained primary care physicians and specialists, and the use of pharmaceuticals and surgery - aren't we!

On the surface and to the casual observer, the countries, cultures and subcultures with a high average life span and high rates of centenarians seem vastly different from one another - what on earth can the Okinawans have in common with the Sardinians, Yao people, Hunzas, Georgians, Symiots, Campodimelani, Costa Ricans, Vilcabamba, Titicaca, Seventh Day Adventists and Mormons?

The secret of becoming a centenarian is "hidden" in plain view! The epiphany revealed in IMMORTALITY, is a compilation of the life's work (94 years between the two of us) of two physicians from separate worlds - China and America.

Between us we have traveled and studied the cultures, diets, health practices, diseases (20,000 autopsies - 17,500 on more than 400 species of captive wild zoo species and 3,000 humans) and the daily lives of the Chinese, Americans (all 50 states and the territories of Guam, the American Virgin Islands and Puerto Rico), Canadians, Australians, New Zealanders, Japanese, Okinawa, Mexico, Peru, Italy, Greece, South Africa, East Africa, Central Africa, Israelis, England, Switzerland, Denmark, Holland, Germany, Eastern Europe and the Balkan states.

In IMMORTALITY, the two of us view health, life, longevity, disease and death through the eyes and understanding of a farmer, animal and human nutrition, soil and plant nutrition and chemistry, veterinarian, primary care physician, surgeon,

Chinese Traditional Medicine and pathologist - this is the first time in history and human endeavor that these crafts, trades and professions have come together under one roof to solve the mysteries of the "centenarian club" and uncover the universal currency of the age beaters.

Although markedly different in culture, tradition, diet and dress, every human society from the simple primitive band of a few dozen members to the great populations of millions in large city states and vast countries share a common thread that predictably, as predictable as gravity, produces age beaters and centenarians - in effect IMMORTALITY!

This humble stuff, required by all who would become a centenarian, was first employed by humans in a conscious proactive way between 50,000 and 200,000 years ago. The use of this byproduct of daily living changed the paths of human culture so profoundly, so dramatically, that Jared Diamond, a professor at the University of California describes this period as "The Great Leap Forward."

What makes "The Great Leap Forward" interesting is that Professor Diamond, himself, never identified the stuff that created the "Great Leap" - he theorized that the Great Leap was produced by a perfection of the vocal cords "that resulted in the ability to communicate better and pass on information to the next generation."

The universal stuff that brought humans the ability to fulfill their genetic potential for living to be 100 years of age was not that glamorous - no, it wasn't a new and improved larynx, nor was it the steam engine or electricity - it was the humble plant minerals that were derived the ashes of carbon fuel (wood, peat, rice straw, kelp, manure, etc.).

Ashes from carbon fuels, in their purist form are not carbon, but rather they are a snow white collection of minerals that the plant sucked up from the soil and sea water and were the minerals that were left behind as heating and cooking fires consumed the stored carbon or "solar currency" in the fuel.

Technology, starting with the Industrial Revolution,

commercial use of fossil fuels, steam power and eventually the universal employment of electricity, natural gas and propane has been on one hand a plus for the greater human good and the advancement of technology. However - there are always unintended consequences!

Niether during the switch from wood as the universal fuel to electricity, nor after words did anyone (doctor or politician) say, "we no longer have easy or unconscious access to traditional sources of plant minerals required for healthy human and animal life and as a result we must supplement with all of the known essential minerals."

As a result of this historical failing to warn us, we moved almost instantly from our historic and deep relationship with the Earth and plant ashes (plant minerals) as a rich source of nutritional minerals to a nutritional mineral vacuum.

In the case of health and longevity, we Americans have been thrown under the bus by medical dogma (i.e.- "you can get everything you need just by eating the four food groups" and following "the principals of the seven food group pyramid").

The epiphany is that today's apple, bread and vegetable are not the same as your grandfather's apple, bread and vegetable! Yes, in our industrialized world we produce more tons and bushels of food than ever before, we feed billions of people around the world with empty calories, however, a basic ingredient in the modern process of farming, food production and preparation - minerals - are no longer available in either the proper spectrum or in optimal quantities - they are not a self renewing resource and are today universally missing from the human diet in the industrialized world!

The missing ingredient, plant minerals, was at one time in history a universal and basic by-product of daily life. We burned wood and other carbon fuels for heat, cooking and light. We know specifically, that at 3:00 p.m. in the afternoon on Monday September 4, 1882, that hundreds of thousands of years of basking in and improving in the benefits of "The Great Leap Forward" slowed, stalled and came to an end as the source of our "Great Leap" dried up.

This moment in September 1882, is the time and date on which Thomas Edison and his chief electrical technician, Johnathan Liebs, pulled the switch to start up the world's first commercial electric generating plant. It was located on Pearl Street, on a bluff, in New York City overlooking the construction of the Brooklyn Bridge - wood, peat, kelp, straw, manure, etc., the historic universal sources of fuel, our historical source of the essential plant minerals for garden fertilizer and human and animal nutrition (culinary ashes) from the beginning of time, in the form of wood and plant ash for all humans was now on the path to oblivion - the period we've come to call "The Great Slide Backwards" began.

According to Dan Buettner, author of *The Blue Zone*, demographer S. Jay Olshansky, University of Illinois at Chicago, and his band of "50 of the world's top longevity experts" released a position paper in 2002 to be "as blunt as they could fashion it…to squash charlatans forever."

The self-anointed Olshansky group stated, "Our language on this matter must be unambiguous. There are no lifestyle changes, surgical procedures, vitamins, antioxidants, hormones, or techniques of genetic engineering available today that have been demonstrated to influence the processes of aging."

If you take the Olshansky position paper literally, they, were quite correct, however, they left out Calorie Restricted diets and plant minerals. You cannot effectively use any nutrients, phytonutrients or raw materials physiologically without mineral cofactors - even oxygen and water are unavailable to you at the cellular level without mineral cofactors!

The people found in most of the "Blue Zones" of the world live in remote and poor environments, they unconsciously subsist on environmentally imposed Calorie Restricted diets of about 1,200 to 1,500 calories per day, consume large quantities of antioxidant foods and drink (coffee, green tea, chocolate, wines, fruit, sweet potatoes, kelp and vegetables) and consciously and proactively use multiple sources of minerals, including flood silt, dust compost, "Glacial Milk," plant mineral supplements (wood ash, kelp ash, peat ash, rice straw ash, manure ash, etc.) in their food as culinary ashes and in their gardens and terraces as fertilizer from wood, peat, kelp, rice straw and manure ash!

Wood ashes, peat moss ash, rice straw ash, kelp ash and animal manure ash were the universal historic sources of fertilizer and nutritional plant minerals for humans and animals - and they still are employed in what Buettner calls the "Blue Zones!"

In countries where cultural cooking with wood, peat, rice straw, kelp and manure, the environmentally imposed and common use of Calorie Restricted diets is common and the daily consumption of serious levels of antioxidants still prevails, the greater concentrations and numbers of centenarians are found.

To maximize your chances of reaching the status of a centenarian in our modern high-tech world YOU are now obligated to consume a Calorie Restricted diet, consciously supplement with plant minerals, as wood ash *per se* is no longer commonly available to fertilize our gardens or add to our food as "culinary ashes" and consume large quantities of high grade antioxidants each day.

Read on! The wood ash/plant mineral epiphany, the CR diet and the consumption of antioxidants as the path to being in the centenarian club is so clear, that if you can read the fifth grade reading level and you can bake perfect oatmeal cookies from a recipe, you will personally begin to supplement with plant minerals, cut your caloric intake and guzzle antioxidants before you finish the pages of this book!

Dr. Joel D. Wallach & Dr. Ma Lan

Part 1

The Aging Process

"Everything that will happen to you today is the result of every choice you have made in the past."

Dr. Albert Schweitzer

Chapter 1

"In a sense the human species is immortal. We as individuals are not. We age and die. But some of the cells in our body are part of a stream of cells we call the germ line, or the reproductive lineage itself, and they have been proliferating since life began on the planet. They don't know what death is."

Dr. Michael West, 2008
Biology visionary

Aging

In 1914, there was enough knowledge regarding the need for vitamins and minerals for optimal health, maximum production and maximum longevity, that dozens of nutritional companies sprang up that produced nutrient enriched feeds for livestock. One such company was Purina Mills of St. Louis, MO.

The use of vitamins and minerals in livestock feeds became commonplace to increase survival, fertility, production (more babies, meat, milk and eggs per pound of feed) and to prevent and reverse diseases. Vitamins, minerals, amino acids and essential fatty acids were added as a complete package or "pre-mix" to pellets comprised of alfalfa, corn, soybeans, wheat, oats and beet pulp.

To improve the efficiency of the enriched feeds and to prevent the animals from sorting through the feed mix and eating only what they preferred, the ration, the mix of grain, hay, beans and vitamin-mineral premix was compressed into uniform sized and nutritionally homogenous pellets. Today, there are pelletized rations for laboratory animals of all species, for pet animals of all species and for farm animals of every species.

Over the years, this pelletized ration system was perfected and became so universally successful, that their use resulted in the elimination of (the prevention and cure of) as many as 900 different diseases in animals that still plague humans in 2008, and these dietary formulas have doubled and quadrupled the life spans of all animal species in the home, the farm, the laboratory and the zoological park!

This miraculous health and longevity benefit was not due to the use of wonder drugs, genetically engineered proteins, stem cells or organ transplants - these health and longevity benefits were simply the result of the application of nutritional science - complete nutrition in a pellet - what a concept! Agricultural scientists were not going to let the chicken's food choices or cow's food choices affect their own health or the farmer's production or income.

Sixty years ago, an "old dog" was ten years old, today an "old dog" is 25 years of age; 100 years ago an old rat was three to four years old, today an old rat is five to six years of age. These gerontological miracles of more than doubling the life spans of dogs, rats and other species was not engineered with good organically grown food, exercise, genetically engineered proteins, stem cell injections, pharmaceuticals, organ transplants or bionic implants - this gerontological miracle of eliminating disease and more than doubling life spans in animals was brought about by simply adding vitamins, minerals, trace minerals, rare earths, essential fatty acids, amino acids and antioxidants to a commercially prepared diet of alfalfa pellets or dog food - simply described as "lab chow" or "dog food."

Dog food and lab animal chow formulations, for the cost of only a few billion dollars over a period of 75 years, solved the longevity riddle in two ways:

1) providing all known essential nutrients in every mouthful consumed, at every meal, every day.

2) providing all known essential nutrients at levels sufficient to eliminate or significantly reduce the risks of disabling, chronic, degenerative diseases and fatal birth defects.

Since 1964, we have been on a quest to translate this longevity miracle produced by nutrient enhanced "lab chow" and "dog food," into an identical plan for humans.

After 44 years of implementation of our beliefs with human patients, we have become quite adept at accomplishing this science-based goal in practical every day life situations for literally millions of people every day.

Gilgamesh

The oldest known story relating to the active search for the secrets of longevity is the 5,000 year old saga of Gilgamesh, the Sumarian King from Uruk, who along with Enkidu, a good friend and the general of his armies, decided they would live forever.

When Enkidu, the king's friend and general died suddenly of disease in the mid-years of his life, Gilgamesh panicked and decided to put all of his fortune and energies into a "do or die search for eternal youth and immortality."

Gilgamesh climbed to the tops of the highest mountains,

searched the dense forests and dove deep into the depths of rivers and oceans in his legendary, frantic and fanatical search for youth, longevity and immortality.

Gilgamesh was originally regarded as a gerontological myth until the discovery of 12 ancient clay tablets that archeologists determined to be 5,000 years old. Pieced together after their discovery in the ancient city of Sumar, the tablets confirmed that Gilgamesh was in fact a king, adventurer and hero of his times who led a great quest for the "key to immortality" - he called for a "revolt against death itself!!"

As the legend goes, Gilgamesh eventually and heroically found a wise old man in the high mountains, who spoke of a fragrant flower that "looked like a buckthorn and prickled like a rose."

The wise prophet shared with Gilgamesh that the plant could be found at the floor of the world's deepest sea, and by coming into possession of this plant and tasting it, one could regain their youth.

Gilgamesh located the life preserving and longevity promoting plant, however, before he could eat sufficient quantities of it to rejuvenate himself, it was stolen from him by a serpent seeking a new skin.

Was this anti-aging plant a form of kelp or sea vegetable that contained significant amounts of plant minerals and antioxidants?

Chronological Age

Certainly each of us appreciates the reality of chronological age, the period of existence of a person or age arranged according to irreversible sequences of time.

Chronological aging is as predictable as gravity. When you are 75 years old you are in fact 75 years old. There are 365 days per year X 75 years which equals 27,375 days. When you are 100 years old you are in fact 36,500 days old, etc.

Chronological numbers cannot be altered, they are irreversible, when you are 75 years old you are 27,375 days old; when you are 100 years old you are 36,500 days old - the math works!

Cosmetics, face lifts, derm-abrasion, Botox injections, breast enhancement, tummy-tucks and liposuction can make people look ten to 25 years younger, you will feel better about yourself, however, none of these procedures will add ten years of chronological time to your life, help you attain your genetic potential for longevity, prevent or cure chronic and degenerative diseases - essentially, cosmetics and "plastic Surgery" procedures alone, without a complete fitness and nutrition program, are the equivalent of putting a classy new paint job on a 50 year old rusted out and poorly maintained worn out car - why not have it all, why not do both - go for it, do the non-toxic and non-invassive beauty practices and the nutrition program?

From experience, personal observation and the accumulation of data from sources ranging from the Census Bureau, Centers for Disease Control, to medical journals, we know that with the passing of time and without conscious effort and intervention, the risk and probability of falling victim to disease, disability and death increases unless you intervene as early and as proactively as possible!

Biological Aging

Biological aging, when compared to chronological aging is another matter. Biological aging, uninterrupted, is a progressive time-related breakdown in an organism's ability to respond, alter and adapt to its internal and external environment.

The result of uninterrupted biological aging is as predictable as gravity - you will die long before your genetic capacity for longevity and that your last months and years will be miserable, painful and in industrialized societies very, very costly!

Just having "good genes" and a grandmother who lived to be 103 years of age is not enough - it only tells you that you have the possibility of getting there - but only if you do everything right!

Theories of Biological Aging

There are two basic theories that attempt to explain the process of biological aging - 1) genetic and 2) stochastic.

Genetic Theory

All human beings have the genetic equipment and therefore the capacity to live well past 100 years of age - it doesn't matter if everyone in your family died at age 35 years of age, you, as an individual, with conscious effort, can still live beyond 100 years of age.

Conversely, if all your relatives lived to be older than 110 years of age, you are not quaranteed to get there yourself, unless YOU do everything right!

In general, genetics give no guarantee or warrantee that one will live to be 100 years of age, run a hundred meters in nine seconds, reach seven feet in height if you don't do your part! You as a human being are given a "genetic potential" for health, performance and longevity that can only be completely achieved with an extraordinary and proactive effort.

The genetic potential in all cases imposes an upper limit - While many biblical prophets are credited with life spans of almost 1,000 years, it is highly improbable, however, that humans can live to be 5,000 years of age.

Age of the Biblical Patriarchs at Their Time of Death

Before the Flood	
Adam	930
Seth	912
Enos	905
Cainan	910
Makalaleel	895
Jared	962
Methuselah	969
Lamech	777
Noah	950

After the Flood	
Shem	600
Arphaxad	436
Salah	433
Eber	464
Peleg	239
Reu	239
Serug	230

Nahor	148
Terah	205
Abram	175
Isaac	180
Jacob	147

To maximize the fulfillment of your genetic potential for health and longevity, you must avoid the land mines (don't smoke, don't participate in destructive behavior, don't eat fried foods, etc.), and you must ensure that you will provide your spiritual self, your physiological self, and your physical self with all the raw materials (with an emphasis on plant minerals and antioxidants) necessary to maximize and fulfill your genetic potentials for health, height, performance and longevity, you must embrace a Calorie Restricted diet - You and You alone are the gate keeper to this potential!

Given the knowledge of health and longevity, the average age of peoples in the industrialized world should be somewhere between 95 and 100 years of age. However, the average age of those living in the industrialized world is somewhere around 75 years of age (give or take five years), in fact 20 to 25 years short of our genetic potential for longevity.

In a CDC (Atlantha, GA) and WHO survey in 1990, Americans ranked 17th in the world in longevity; in the year 2000 Americans dropped in ranking to 24th in longevity; and in 2005, Americans dropped in ranking again to a pitiful 46th, and in 2008 Americans again dropped to 48th in the world when it comes to health and longevity.

With a population of 300 million, Americans are the third largest population in the world behind only number one, China with a population of 1.8 billion and number two, India with a population of 1 billion.

Americans spend three quarters ($2.3 trillion) of the world's (193 nations) annual expenditure for health care ($2.7 trillion) and it is obvious, even to the casual observer, that whatever we're doing isn't working - we are leaving out essential ingredients of the recipe!

In June 2008, four months of longevity was added to the American average as a result of a dramatic drop in new cases of life threatening diseases (not better treatments after diagnosis)! This health and longevity benefit was not the result of anything that doctors or pharmaceutical companies had done, on the contrary, the unexpected benefit was the result of a general and self prescribed increase in the use of vitamins, minerals and antioxidants by the American public - Americans had finally revolted, against the advice of their doctors, they had decided to intervene on their own behalf and supplement with two of the three longevity factors!

Studies employing identical (monozygotic-one egg/ one sperm) twins show that, their life spans are on average within three years of each other. Fraternal twins (dizygotic-two eggs/two sperm) have a much wider disparity in genetic make up and life spans.

Experts of genetics and human aging estimate, however, that less than 0.5% of the informational content of the human genome is responsible for the increase in human life span potential.

Life Span Potentials

Animal	Maximum recorded Life span (years)
Bristle cone pine	2,000
Gingko biloba tree	1,000
Galapagos tortoise	200
Human	122
Parrot	100
Asian elephant	60
Orangutan	58
Gorilla	55
Chimpanzee	50
Whale	50
Horse	40
Grizzly bear	35
Hyena	32
Domestic cat	30
American bison	26
African lion	25
Rhesus monkey	24
Dolphin	23
Dog	20
Domestic goat	20

Moose	17
Kangaroo	16
Rabbit	15
Vampire bat	13
Skunk	8
Rat	6
Mouse	3
Shrew	2

The "Stochastic" Nature of Aging

Gerontologists and doctors, in their ignorance, pontificate and perpetuate the dogma that there is nothing that you can do to ensure that you will reach the centenarian club. They preach endlessly that there are no common threads that can be used by all, to successfully reach 100 - they preach that aging is "stochastic" or uncontrollable or a gamble that only a few lucky ones from the "Blue Zones" will randomly attain.

We know for an irrefutable fact that aging or longevity has a genetic upper limit or genetic potential in all species, including man, yet, our input, either conscious or unconscious is required to consistently achieve or reach the upper limit of our genetic potential for longevity.

Having "good genes" alone will certainly not get you to 100 years of age in a healthful way without you doing everything else right! Just having "good genes" is not a guarantee.

As organism's age, their capacity to survive environmental and physiological challenges declines and often fails. Any significant challenge or bump in the road of health and lifespan can result in death to both young and old individuals, survival statistics, however, are in general in favor of the younger individual.

A plethora of factors, including nutritional competency and deficiencies, affect the course of events in an individual's ability to avoid disability and the relative ability of a human to reach their maximum potential for longevity.

Aging is not an all or nothing process - aging is like a puzzle, a few pieces cannot give you the full and complete picture, as the pieces of the puzzle are put into the structure of the puzzle, the greater the ability to see the complete and full picture.

Cellular Immortality

In 1912, Dr. Alexis Carrel, who had won the Nobel Prize for developing the original technique for "end to end anastomosis (joining) of blood vessels with fine suture," began to grow undifferentiated fibroblasts (connective tissue cells *aka* "stem cells") from chicken hearts in flasks in his laboratory at the Rockefeller Institute.

He fed these isolated and undifferentiated fibroblast or "stem cells" with filtered extracts of blended chicken embryos and the "stem cells" kept multiplying and growing for 34 years (including 2 years after Carrel's own death).

These early "cell cultures" were so successful that, excessive numbers were shared with other investigators or discarded "to prevent them from performing one of those 2n multiplication feats ("Andromatous Strain") and cover the earth."

Carrel's work led to the theory that, "Cells are inherently immortal if given an ideal environment, and the aging of organisms we see in the laboratory and in the mirror must be due to interactions between cells, or to some central mechanism, hormonal perhaps, whose influence reaches everywhere."

Two years after his death, Carrel's colleagues got bored with the experiment and threw the 34 year old fibroblast cultures out. However, Carrel's experiment resulted in the theory that "cells are inherently immortal if they are fed a perfect diet and kept in a perfect environment."

In 1961, Dr. Leonard Hayflick and Paul Moorhead at the Wistar Institute in Philadelphia challenged Carrel's findings. Hayflick, currently at the School of Medicine at the University of California, San Francisco, is a highly regarded biogerontologist.

In his experiment, Hayflick, using his own growth media, human embryonic lung fibroblasts could only "double" 50 times with a predictable intracellular accumulation of ceroid lipofuscin (pigments of aging that indicate a selenium deficiency) that eventually disabled and killed the cells.

Hayflick's definition of "doubling" was that the culture flask became filled with new cells and he would dump 50% of the cells to make living space for continuation of the cultures. How many, individual duplications, of Carrel's chicken embryo heart fibroblast cells, did it take to fill the flask with the new cells - hundreds, thousands, millions?

Fibroblasts begin looking old as they near the "doubling" limit. When viewed under the microscope they become larger and accumulate an increased quantity of the golden "pigment of aging" - ceroid lipofuscin.

Hayflick attributed Carrel's chicken heart fibroblast longevity success to "contamination" by new embryonic fibroblasts from the chick embryo media.

Hayflick's 50 "doubling" limit in normal human lung cells has come to be known as the "Hayflick limit."

When old nuclei are inserted into young cells and young nuclei are inserted into old cells, the data indicates that the physiological age of the cell, the number of "doublings" they have left, is controlled by the nucleus. It suggests that there is a programmed synthesis of a "senescence factor" in old cells and that this factor inhibits DNA replication when the music stops - suggesting that the "Hayflick limit" may in fact may be alterable and is not set in concrete!

Using the same growth media, the Hayflick limit varies from species to species and appears to be related to the maximum known life span of the species.

Hayflick Limit by Species

Species	Hayflick Limit
Man (normal cells)	50
Man (HeLa cancer cells)	indefinitely
Mice	15
Chicken	25
Galapagos tortoise	110

Hayflick learned that when he froze his cell culture after 20 doublings, they could "remember" that they had a maximum of 30 doublings left when they were thawed and re-fed.

HeLa cells were the first human cells to be successfully propagated outside the body in significant numbers. HeLa cells, which came from a biopsy of a cervical cancer, "ignore the Hayflick limit for human cells. In a sense they are immortal." They will continue to grow and divide as long as they have nutrients, oxygen, space and means of getting rid of their waste.

The human donor for the original HeLa cells was Henrietta Lacks, a poor black woman from Baltimore, whose identity was only revealed years after her cells were being proliferated around the world and long after she had died.

Chapter 2

"We are now at the threshold of the Superlongevity Revolution, the radical extension of the human lifespan that will shake society to its very foundation. Its impact will be felt by every person, institution, and organization."

- Michael G. Zey, Ph.D.
Ageless Nation

Regulating Life Span

According to Dr. Michael West, a professor and biology visionary from the University of California, Berkeley, "In a sense the human species is immortal. We as individuals are not. We age and die. But some of the cells in our body are part of a stream of cells we call the germ line, or the reproductive lineage itself, they have been proliferating since life began on the planet. They don't know what death is."

James Hilton made the legendary city of Shangri-La famous, through his 1934 novel, *Lost Horizon*, where people lived healthful, loving, productive and long lives beyond 200 years of age.

The novel was made into a classic black and white movie of the same name in 1937 and then remade in the 1960s as a color film entitled, Shangri-La.

In the original novel and movie, the people of Shangri-La attributed their youthfulness, health and longevity to a Spartan diet (McKay's well publicized Calorie Restricted diet), peaceful low stress attitude, a work ethic devoted to gardening and farming (wood ash, plant mineral enriched compost),and a rich Christian faith and lifestyle.

The remake film version portrayed an eastern type meditation as the basis of their health and longevity which contributed to the passion for Eastern Meditation by the "hippy" movement of the 1960s and 1970s.

Regulating Life Span

Numerous methods have been developed for estimating physiological age. The most commonly employed measure, especially in population studies, is blood pressure levels, blood sugar levels and age at death. Statistical analysis of mortality data can be employed to separate age-related deaths (chronic disease and sudden death) from age-unrelated deaths (car accidents and house fires).

Any complete understanding of aging will necessarily and eventually explain conditions and treatments that increase the maximum life span. At least three methods of increasing maximum life span in laboratory animals (that are fed perfect diets) are known:

1) lower metabolic rate (hypothermia)

2) Calorie Restricted intake (without malnutrition)

3) enhance antioxidant protection (genetic engineering and supplements)

The observation that life span can be predictably increased demonstrates that "aging" and the ability to maximize life span in fact, is not immutable or stochastic. Understanding the mechanisms by which experimental treatments extend life span has revealed many of the processes that control aging.

Humans must come to grips with the fact that if we are to reach our "genetic potential" for health and longevity we must become independent of our mineral deficient soils, the limited and unpredictable nutritional value of our anemic food through supplementation, consume Calorie Restricted diets and load up on the antioxidants!

We must not bet our health and our lives on - or ignorantly depend on the random distribution of essential minerals in our food or maybe not in our food at all or we will surely fail in our quest for health and longevity no matter how much money and effort we spend on medical care.

We constantly need oxygen, we constantly need water and we constantly need "essential macro and micro nutrients."

We pay an enormous amount of redundant attention, to detail, when we send humans into space and yet we continue to leave the essential nutrient intake of our cells and the building blocks of our enzymatic and physiological life on earth to blind chance.

Lowering Metabolic Rate

Decreasing the rate of metabolism either by lowering the ambient temperature of cold-blooded animals or by restricting movement, can significantly extend the life spans of many invertebrate species. These facts point to the fact that the rate of metabolic output can affect longevity.

The "old ones" (those over age 75) in all Blue Zones spend a lot of time sunning themselves, gleaning large doses of vitamin D_3 from the sun (by sitting in the sun or gardening) and lowering their metabolic rate each day by consciously devoting time to "siesta time" or meditation.

Sohal reported that 200 houseflies maintained in a one cubic foot cage (to stimulate flight activity) resulted in a mean lifespan of 14 days.

Housing smaller numbers of houseflies in a large cage resulted in an average life span of about 35 days.

Placing the flies in small bottles with a cardboard maze, that permitted them to walk, but eliminated their flight activity, extended mean life span to 70 days.

Further decreasing the metabolic activity of the flies by placing them in small vials at a decreased temperature (18 degrees C) extended their life span to 120 days.

The total amount of oxygen consumed during life by each group of flies (per unit weight) was identical.

The maximum survival rate or longevity for fish has been extended by 300% in the UCLA laboratory of Dr. Roy Walford by maximizing the micronutrients (minerals) fed to the fish as well as lowering the water temperature by just a few degrees.

Within individual species, the metabolic rate of individuals clearly affects life span. Dr. Thomas Perls has produced the clearest description of this relationship in *"The Rate of Living Theory."*

According to Perls' hypothesis, all species exhibit a genetically determined metabolic potential and species' specific life span is therefore dependent on the rate of metabolism. Many studies have confirmed the validity of this observation in cold-blooded animals.

Calorie Restriction without Malnutrition

Gerontologists theorize that our prehistoric ancestors clung to life through long periods of time without food - the human body's amazing survival mechanisms would then come into play - slow metabolism and slow aging. This mechanism allowed humans to survive through times of drought and famine.

The profile of people who actively pursued longevity is found in the writings of authors on longevity who, living by their beliefs, lived to at least their tenth decade. Five of the most famous of this group are Luigi Cornaro, Sir Hermann Weber, Sir James Crichton-Browne, Dr. Alexandre Gueniot, and Scott Nearing.

The most well known and famous of these five longevity icons is Luigi Cornaro. Luigi Cornaro, wrote *The Art of Living Long,* one of the four most famous autobiographies of the Renaissance (the piece was translated into every European language and later endorsed by George Washington). Cornaro was born in Venice in 1464 and died in Padua at the age of 103 years in 1567.

Cornaro was born into Italian nobility, he practiced "a dissolute, gluttonous life," which lead to a disabling ill-health by the age of 37. Cornaro was morbidly obese, suffered from gout, "stomach fever," cold temperatures (hypothyroidism) and generalized pain (arthritis, fibromyalgia, etc.).

Cornaro's physicians gave him little hope for survival for one year so he decided to become his own physician; he asked the old women working in the fields what they ate.

After these interviews, Cornaro became aware of the peasant's Calorie Restricted diet (imposed by access only to small plots of land and heavy taxation) and became convinced that his maladies, as with most diseases of the human species, were due to a life of intemperance, homage to the "belly gods" and the "nervous" life they commanded.

Cornaro consciously changed course and "he voluntarily practiced a severe, rigid, temperate and dietarily restrictive routine."

Cornaro's diet was the same every day and some meals consisted of a single egg yolk. He faithfully ate "12 ounces of solids, a little meat, one egg yolk, a slice of bread, vegetable soup and 14 ounces of young wine," which provided a total of 1,000 calories or less" per day.

The part that wine, "the milk of the old," played in Cornaro's diet is considered a historical "fluke" by gerontologists. Cornaro liked young local wines.

Cornaro faithfully practiced this Calorie Restricted dietary routine for the rest of his life (he never retired, rather he worked his estate from horseback, counseled members of the Paduan society as a revered elder and wrote books on health until the end) - he became lean and his health prospered. Despite his sinful younger years, Cornaro lived to be 103 years of age and reported in his autobiography that, "he was high for his remaining sixty-six years."

Four hundred years after the time of Cornaro, three European physicians of some great fame made longevity one of their main interests. Each of the three doctors had many long-lived patients; all three wrote books or essays on longevity when they were in their 90s.

Sir Hermann Weber (1823-1918) stressed exercise as well as a Calorie Restricted lactovegetarian diet - he recommended one to three hours of walking each day and vacations that included climbing, hiking and hunting.

Sir James Crichton-Browne (1840-1938) commented on Cardinal de Satis, who lived to be 110, cited a mix of a Calorie Restricted diet, walking and riding daily and to "continuing projects throughout one's life."

Dr. Alexandre Guenoit (1832-1935) of Paris, and president of the Paris Medical Academy, followed a somewhat less restrictive Cornaro-type diet as a lactovegetarian, walked up 56 steps to his apartment even until age 99 years to gather his notes, write his book and died in 1935 at the age of 102 years.

Today, it is a well established fact that consuming fewer calories (Calorie Restricted diets) can and does extend life.

Scott Nearing (1883-1983), like Cornaro became a legend in his own lifetime. Alone or with his wife Helen, Nearing wrote on the subjects of pacifism, socialism and lactovegetarian beliefs.

In 1932, the Nearings bought a farm in Vermont and began to live out Scott's alternative culture beliefs. They farmed with hand tools and implements for more than 50 years. Their work included digging, hoeing, weeding, composting (wood ashes) and hauling. In addition, Scott did his own sawing and chopping of wood for their wood-burning stove. They have constructed 15 stone buildings on their two homesteads. Scott calls them "one-man/one-woman" projects, and Helen admits that, "she became so involved in the (construction of the) Maine house, that she personally selected and placed every stone." That home was finished in 1977, when Scott was 94 years of age and Helen was 73.

The Nearings rarely if ever used doctors, pills, or hospitals, yet Scott lived to a "hale and hearty 100 and died when he decided to by fasting for a month and a half at the very end."

Nearing had always been physically active, in the woods, in the garden, and in building construction. He was also active mentally, having written 40 books, including an autobiography - *The Making of a Radical*.

A month or two before he died, Scott was sitting at the dinner table and said, "I think I won't eat anymore."

On his last day, Helen and Scott were together at home; no interruptions; no doctors or hospitals. They were quiet together and Helen said, "It's alright Scott. Go right along. You've lived a good life and are finished with things here. We love you and let you go. It's alright."

In 1935, Clive McKay, a professor of physiology at

Cornell University observed that a Calorie Restricted diet, or "under nutrition without malnutrition" could extend life. With a 60% reduction of free choice calories at weaning age, came a doubling of the 50% survival rate and doubled the known maximum life span of laboratory rats!

The McKay Calorie Restricted diet was super-supplemented with extra vitamins and minerals. On this 60% regimen, the animal's growth rate was significantly reduced, however, in all other ways they were super healthy.

The CR diet fed rats could be held in this growth retarded condition for up to 1,000 days, by which time all of the traditionally fed rats had died. When the CR diet rats were allowed a full diet, growth started again. The rats were also more sexually active and reproduced normally at a more advanced age than the rats fed the traditional diet.

In the 1960s and 1970s, Morris Ross of the Institute for Cancer Research in Philadelphia, conducted a series of experiments that produced a maximum life span of 1,000 to 1,099 days in fully fed rats and 1,600 to 1,699 days in CR fed rats - a 60% increase. These studies pitted the standard lab diets for rats against the reduced amounts of the enriched diets - the classic "under nutrition without malnutrition."

These experiments have been repeated successfully many times in many species of animals. In fact, a Calorie Restricted (CR) diet "without malnutrition" is the only intervention that has ever consistently, predictably and successfully increased both the mean and maximal life span of mammals.

The positive effects of Calorie Restriction without malnutrition have been observed in diverse vertebrate and invertebrate species. Diet-restricted mammals retain youthful characteristics, including immune function, vitality, long after their higher calorie fed litter mates are dead.

Calorie Restricted diets have been studied in the rhesus monkey by gerontologist Richard Weindruch, at the University of Wisconsin at Madison. Only four of his CR monkeys have died, half the death rate of the standard fed monkeys. The CR monkeys have not developed diabetes, while 50% of the standard diet monkeys have developed the disease.

Because most investigators of CR diets forget the "without malnutrition" piece it is not surprising that the lab animals on unsupplemented CR diets develop diseases of malnutrition including a significant drop in bone density, reduced libido, dysmenorrhea, infertility and wide fluctuations in body temperature.

Calorie Restricted diets consistently produce biological effects that are directly linked, in laboratory animals, to longer life. Understanding the mechanisms of these biological effects helps to translate theory into practical application.

Some of the obvious CR effects were quickly identified in the early studies, additional long term effects have been identified as the studies have continued; we also realize that we can enhance or modify these CR effects by conscious choices:

1) lowers circulating glucose levels

2) lowers circulating insulin levels

3) lowers percentage of body fat

4) lowers blood & tissue levels of growth stimulators

5) reduces cell loss from the aging process

6) decreases body load of "inflammation" or "free radical injury."

7) encourages a youthful physiology Under nutrition (Caloric Restricted diet) without malnutrition (diet contains elevated levels of vitamins and minerals above the RDA) experiments are most effective in laboratory animals when started in infancy, however,

they also show dramatic longevity benefit even when the low calorie/nutrient dense diet is begun in mid-adulthood.

In Luigi Cornaro's example, he intervened at age 37 and lived to be 103. This observation should give all individuals encouragement to change their habits for the better and intensely supplement - it's never too late!

Low calorie/nutrient dense diets may not be for all human children as there is a relatively high mortality rate on the front end of this type of program. Children can flourish and do well on optimal caloric intake/nutrient dense nutritional programs.

In the 1940s, professors A.H. Carlson and F. Holzol added a creative twist to the concept of the CR diet by studying the effects of intermittent periods of fasting on the life span of rats. They free choice fed rats a high-quality diet rich in vitamins and minerals in unlimited amounts, but fasted them completely every other day; another group was fasted every third day and another group fasted every fourth day.

The maximum life span in the un-fasted animals was 800 days, however, in all three intermittently fasted groups the maximum life span was extended to 1,000 to 1,100 days - a 20 to 30% increase in maximum life span.

Dr. Charles Goodrick of the National Institute on Aging (Gerontology Research Unit) studied intermittent fasting by feeding the control a perfect diet while the study group was fasted every other day. Maximum life span was increased from the 875 days of the normally fed rats to 1,295 in the restricted rats, from 630 days 50% survival to 980 days.

Nelson Mandela, the first black president of South Africa turned 90 years of age on July 18, 2008. During an interview with reporters on the occasion of his birthday, Mandela was quite lucid mentally and physically animated as he answered questions.

What makes Mandela's high energy 90th birthday

remarkable was that he had spent 27 years in a South African prison on Robin Island. He was fed a very low calorie and protein restricted diet (small servings of fish each week). He worked every day in a limestone quarry and was allowed to have a vegetable garden which was fertilized with limestone dust (mineral fertilizer).

Immediately upon release from prison Mandela began to drink South African wine (a significant source of resveratrol and polyphenols - antioxidants) and supplement with a liquid form of plant derived minerals shipped to him from Atlanta, Georgia by former UN Ambassador Andrew Young.

Art Linkletter of "People Are Funny" television fame, sent Dr. Allen Banik, an eye doctor, to Hunza to learn their secret of health and longevity.

Dr. Banik learned that Hunzakuts were forced to consume a high protein (i.e. goat, lamb, yak, beef, chicken, eggs, milk, cheese, yogurt, etc.) Calorie Restricted diet (1,500-1,800 calories) because they lived in a relatively poor place, they consumed minerals from Glacial Milk, directly as drinking water and indirectly as fertilizer; they also fertilized their gardens with wood ash (plant minerals) enriched compost; the Hunzakut used red wine and green tea daily as antioxidants.

In 2008 Art Linkletter turned 96 years of age; he continues to give 75 two hour lectures each year. Linkletter followed the Hunza diet by consuming a Calorie Restricted diet, eating appropriately and supplementing heavily with vitamins, minerals and antioxidants (resveratrol, etc.).

On July 2, 2008, Frank Calloway of Tusccaloosa, Alabama, turned 112 years old. He works seven to nine hours each day using pencils and crayons, creating 30 foot long murals of the agricultural South from the early 20th century. Many of his crayon drawings, created on simple butcher paper, sell for more than $1,000. In a recent interview, Calloway said, "I couldn't get time to go to school much, stopped in the third grade reader, that's all I could get, third grade reader."

Diagnosed with schizophrenia, Frank Calloway has lived in an Alabama mental institution since 1952 on a typical, calorie and protein restricted diet of a state operated chronic care facility.

The Calorie Restricted Diet

To initiate your personal journey into a CR diet lifestyle requires a conscious decision. It can be as simple as reducing your total daily caloric intake by five percent.

Daily Calorie Requirements for Humans

Gender	Age (years)	Activity Level		
		Sedentary	Moderate	Active
Child	2-3	1,000	1,000-1,400	1,000-1,400
Female	4-8	1,200	1,400-1,600	1,400-1,800
	9-13	1,600	1,600-2,000	1,800-2,200
	14-18	1,800	2,000	2,400
	19-30	2,000	2,000-2,200	2,400
	31-50	1,800	2,000	2,200
	51+	1,600	1,800	2,000-2,200
Male	4-8	1,400	1,400-1,600	1,600-2,000
	9-13	1,800	1,800-2,200	2,000-2,600
	14-18	2,200	2,400-2,800	2,800-3,200
	19-30	2,400	2,600-2,800	3,000
	31-50	2,200	2,400-2,600	2,800-3,000
	51+	2,000	2,200-2,400	2,400-2,800

5% Calorie Reduction

A drop of as little as 5% of your typical daily calorie intake will certainly improve your health.

At this level of caloric reduction, a woman will reduce her daily calorie total by 100 calories, which means give up the slice of toast for breakfast or only eat one half of that hamburger bun for lunch; a man will give up 125 calories at a 5% calorie reduction.

A 5% calorie reduction could be as simple as giving up the 3:00 pm two scoop ice cream snack for a one scoop portion.

10% to 15% Calorie Reduction

A reduction of 10% to 15% of your typical caloric intake will trigger a metabolic event, known as "hormesis." Hormesis refers to limiting your caloric intake in an intelligent manner, so that you challenge your body with a beneficial physiological or metabolic stress or "hormesis."

With fewer easy fuel calories available for energy production, your body shifts from the command to store fat to the command to preferentially burn fat as fuel for energy production.

Eventually (usually within a week) your body becomes more efficient in its ability to produce energy from fat and your stamina improves. The need for an increased rate of cell reproduction and replacement is reduced, allowing the body to direct more effort towards defenses against free radical damage and extended life!

To maximize the positive CR effect, reduce your daily protein intake to between 45 to 60 grams for men and 40 to 50 grams for women.

A 10% caloric reduction for women translates to reducing the total daily caloric intake by 200 and 250 for men. A 15% reduction would translate to a reduced daily caloric intake for women by 300 and 475 for men.

In practical terms, this means giving up the daily ration of potatoes and eating more green vegetables; give up the pancakes or waffles for breakfast and eat a veggie omelette.

20% Calorie Reduction

A 20% reduction in daily caloric intake will translate to women giving up 400 calories and men giving up 500 calories.

Giving up 20% of your daily calories will translate to giving up lunch and replacing it with an 80 to 100 calorie protein shake, an egg or our favorite, a pre-bagged handful of mixed salted nuts.

It is not unusual for a slight hunger awareness to creep into your life at this point. The way to eliminate the hunger sensation is to increase your daily dose of certified organic plant minerals and have a small snack consisting of one handful (remember, its only one) of mixed salted nuts.

Fat vs Thin

Do naturally thin or skinny people live longer than those individuals of "normal" weight? To answer this question, a large study of mortality versus body weight was conducted among 750,000 men and women by Drs. Lew and Garfinkel of the American Cancer Society.

The overall mortality of people who were more than

10% lighter than average, was actually increased - an apparent paradox. McKay found that the degree of body fat in later life was more important than such variables as percent protein intake or even exercise. Overtly fat rats lived shorter lives.

It is of interest to note here that Sir Winston Churchill was obese, spent most of his adult life in bed until noon, smoked a whole box of Cuban cigars daily and drank a quart of brandy per day and died at 89 years of age - being thin by itself is not the "secret ingredient" for a long healthy life.

McKay's rats that were unable to gain weight and fatten on a totally permissive diet, and tended, despite the diet, to remain at a weight less than average, also lived considerably shorter lives. Therefore, being "naturally thin" and unable to gain weight in spite of excessive food intake is not the same health-wise as thinness induced by dietary restriction.

People, who remain underweight, despite increased food intake, display a slightly increased metabolic rate and increased body temperature, both of which reduce maximum life span.

If you are the type of individual who gains weight easily by overeating, but you elect to lose weight by CR diets, then you have an increased survival advantage!

Naturally thin individuals can live longer by becoming even thinner, so long as there is no malnutrition - you too must get into the CR lifestyle and ramp up on the your intake of essential nutrients (plant minerals) and antioxidants!

Numerous biochemical measurements show that CR animals are considerably bio-chemically younger than their chronological age.

Antioxidant Defenses

A third laboratory method used to increase life span is to genetically engineer animals to over express genes tied to oxidant or free radical removal. Oxygen free radicals and other reactive oxygen species (ROS) are thought to be important factors in a large number of disease processes and aging.

Because of the very toxic affects of ROS, aerobic survival depends on the prevention of the associated oxidative impact. Antioxidant enzyme systems are normally present in all healthy aerobic cells - remember, antioxidants also need raw materials and mineral cofactors to operate at their optimum capacity (glutathione requires selenium, etc.).

The superoxide dismutases (SOD) quench or neutralize superoxide radicals (O^-_2) but create H_2O_2 as a byproduct. Cells also have high levels of non-enzymatic, low molecular weight antioxidants. These non-enzymatic anti-oxidants remove the potent hydroxyl radical (-HO·), a very potent byproduct of the O_2 and H_2O_2 free radical reactions.

Fruit flies genetically engineered to over express only SOD or catalase show little or no change in longevity. However, when the fruit flies are genetically engineered to over express both SOD and catalase, they are able to increase the mean and maximum life span by as much as 40%.

These studies suggest that the quenching of O_2 and H_2O_2 free radicals can positively affect the basic processes that control aging.

Free Radical Theory of Aging

Free radicals are a diverse and destructive group of agents which can be brought into the body transdermally and by breathing, eating and drinking; they can also be produced in significant numbers internally during normal metabolism and as a byproduct of a fat-burning weight loss program.

These highly reactive substances differ from other less harmful molecules in that they possess an extra electrical charge - a free unpaired radical or a "free" electron.

Free radicals set off abnormal reactions at the cellular level that are typically "once-only," irreversible, and energetically wasteful.

Most free radicals that the human body is exposed to are oxidants, "their free electron whirling around a super-activated oxygen atom (i.e. - hydroxyl free radical, singlet oxygen, and hydrogen peroxide).

Dr. Roy Walford referred to free radicals as the "Great white sharks in the biochemical sea" - these short-lived but voracious chemicals oxidize and damage tissue, particularly cell membranes and mitochondrial membranes.

Free radical "shark attacks" on polyunsaturated fats and cholesterol found in tissue membranes, produce lipid peroxides, which in turn decompose to yield chemicals known as aldehydes, which cross-link proteins, lipids and DNA.

Walford described oxygen based free radicals very well, "Not everybody realizes that the oxygen of our atmosphere is a highly poisonous gas. Alien entities arriving from a methane planet would choke and die on the stuff we breathe so casually. It rusts iron, is involved in the decay and crumbling of granite boulders, and participates in every fire in town…yet we live in it (require it) and love it."

Lipids become "peroxidized" or damaged as a result of interactions with ROS or free radicals. This damage results in structural, geometrical or "steric" physical changes that decrease membrane fluidity.

Aging decreases membrane fluidity because of oxidant-induced depletion of unsaturated lipids. As a result, aging membranes become more rigid (nutrition and oxygen can't go in and wastes can't get out), significant negative changes are then recorded in membrane-bound proteins. Membrane-bound enzymes and mitochondrial enzymes are regularly found to display age-related changes in activity.

Peroxidized lipid molecules undergo several rearrangements to form highly reactive cross-linking agents, such as malondialdehyde (MDA). MDA reacts with amino groups of proteins and amino acids, further increasing the negative effects of free radical oxidation on cell wall lipids.

The end byproduct of MDA activity and damage is a fluorescent pigment called ceroid lipofuscin. This pigment, a product of oxidized cell wall and mitochondrial wall lipids will accumulate in the cell cytoplasm itself over time.

Percent of Ceroid Lipofuscin in Aging Human Brain Cells

Age	% intracellular volume occupied
30 - 40	35
50 - 60	41
70 - 80	55
90 - 100	78

(Adelman, et al., 1988)

The medical "dogma" goes like this: as these ceroid lipofuscin pigments accumulate in the cell over time, they interfere with the internal physiological functioning of the cell and mitochondria. Medical doctors, and most gerontologists, falsely believe the accumulated aging pigments are not preventable, removable or reversible and as they reach significant levels, the lipofuscin-gorged and disrupted cells and mitochondria "age," become dysfunctional, diseased and die.

Ceroid lipofuscin shows up in humans as "age spots" or "liver spots" on the skin of the hands or face. If you have one liver spot or age spot on the outside you have millions of them on the inside!

The number and intensity of pigment levels in age spots are directly related to the level of free radical damage and can be a predictive barometer of sinister things to come - i.e. - cataracts, macular degeneration, coronary artery disease, diabetes, senile dementia, Alzheimer's disease, cancer, etc.

Fortunately, the accumulation of ceroid lipofuscin in the brain, heart, liver, lungs, bone marrow, eyes, etc. can easily be prevented and quickly reversed. Cell culture studies, animal studies and human studies demonstrate very clearly that the accumulation of ceroid lipofuscin, the "pigment of aging," is not set in concrete and in fact can be prevented and reversed.

Preventing and reversing the accumulation of ceroid lipofuscin pigments is well documented in many animal species and humans - to accomplish this "antiaging" feat requires a significant reduction of the intake of free radicals (fried foods, trans fats, burnt fats, heterocyclic amines, super-heated carbohydrates, acrylamides, nitrites, alcohol, sugar, etc.) and a significant increase in the intake of all known essential nutrients and an extraordinary increased intake of antioxidants (20,000 to 25,000 ORAC points/day).

The obvious question is, if free radicals cause aging and contribute to the infirmities of aging, then shouldn't a reduction of free radical damage slow the rate of aging and extend longevity ever closer to the individual's genetic potential for longevity and even beyond the generally accepted maximum life span for humans. Such studies have shown that increases in antioxidant intakes alone will increase the mean life span of a population but not the maximum life span.

Considerable evidence has been collected to support the idea that the 50% survival rate of a population can be extended significantly by the consumption of combinations of antioxidants, including vitamins A, C, E, selenium, sulfur bearing amino acids (methionine, cysteine, cystine, etc.) and phytochemicals such as catechens (green tea, coffee, red wine, dark berries, exotic fruit, etc.), resveratrol (red wine, red grape juice, giant Japanese knotweed, etc.), proanthocyanins (red grape skins and seeds), leutines (green leafy vegetables), lycopenes (tomatoes), flavonols and polyphenols (dark chocolate, red wine, green tea, etc.).

Aging is chronological and progressive and is typically the normal course of events in all biological systems, however, decreased metabolic rate, Caloric Restriction (without malnutrition) and an increase in the levels of antioxidant protection will all significantly increase longevity.

To fulfill one's genetic potential for longevity they must consume large amounts of antioxidants, consciously supplement daily with all known essential nutrients (with a special focus on minerals) and eat a Calorie Restricted diet and equally as important, they must avoid as many land mines as possible.

Chapter 3

"What's it worth to you to live five or 10 years longer? Research shows that some health-related extras have a real impact on longevity."

Angie C. Marek
Smart Money, June 2008

Without Malnutrition

Most investigators and practitioners of Calorie Restricted (CR) diets overlook and discount the importance of the "without malnutrition" (WM) part of Clive McKay's original equation:

CR Diet + WM = 30% to 100% longevity increase

"Without malnutrition" means considerably more than sufficient calories to survive. The concept of "without malnutrition" refers to the unwavering provision of every known essential nutrient in at least optimal levels (which are considerably higher than the RDI) - to be consumed with every mouthful - every meal - every day.

When we look at the lofty professional and political positions in the industrialized world, the wealthy, the people who have access to the best of everything, the fit and the educated, we are continuously disappointed with their sad and unfulfilled paths of life, production records and lack of a good result for personal health and longevity.

Billionaires: According to *Forbes Magazine*, the average life span of billionaires is 78 years of age; and there has never been a billionaire ever live to be 100 years of age.

The longevity statistics, or rather, the lack of longevity statistics in the billionaire community, is a profound red flag, a scream for change - a change from the medical dogma, that "you can get everything you need by eating from the four food groups" and "following the dietary principals of the seven food group pyramid."

If there is any group of people in the world who has access to "good food," and the money to buy it, it has got to be the members of the billionaire club! Billionaires, have access to the finest quality and variety of food, high priced chefs, personal trainers, the best primary care physicians who have graduated from the finest schools and have good golf scores, the best specialists from anywhere in the world, the greatest health plans - and if need be they can spend unlimited amounts of money to get access to cutting edge health information, drugs, procedures and the entire staff of Harvard Medical School.

In the June 2008 issue of *Smart Money (THE WALL STREET JOURNAL MAGAZINE)*, a cover article says, "Yes! $100,000 can add 10 years to your life." Even if that claim were true and not just a theory or a "pipe dream," ten years added to the average billionaire life span of 78 comes to 88 years - still, 12 years short of the magic number of 100! And the cost comes to a whopping $10,000 per additional year of life.

We calculate that a 150 - 175 pound person can add 25 to 50 additional healthful years to their life with a net savings in their cost of living by practicing a CR diet and by faithfully employing a modified supplement program - the reduced cost of food more than compensates for the cost of the supplement program which comes to less than a cup of Starbucks' espresso late' per day!

Executive Physicals: These physicals (a classic example of closing the barn door after the horse is out) are geared toward early detection of cancer, heart disease and diabetes; and include CT scans, MRIs, Alzheimer's screens (smell test), monitoring of the biological age of DNA and batteries of blood test. ($33,500)

Yoga Retreats: Many experts credit an individual's ability to live to be 100 years of age to their ability to cope with stress. ($15,300)

Personal Chef: Learn to prepare, cook and eat healthy and control portion size. (Healthy, Chef-cooked meals for one year - $24,700).

Personal Trainer: Get drill sargeant supervision three times per week. (two year program $26,500)

Billionaires: Despite these high priced "early detection" programs and life style changes, billionaires don't fair very well at an average age of 78 years - this is because medical doctors are disconnected from the soil and from the human body's need for raw materials other than calories and great attention to ratios of carbohydrates, fats and protein, pharmaceuticals and surgery.

Jerry Zucker, (April 22, 2008) philanthropist and billionaire (owner of the Hudson Bay Company) made pacemakers and surgical instruments and held 350 inventions and patents, died of cancer at home at age 58.

Sydney Craig, (July 21, 2008) co-founder of the Jenny Craig, weight-loss empire. He sold the business to Nestle in 2006 for $600 million. He died of cancer at age 76.

Hyman Golden, (September 14, 2008) Co-founder and chairman of Snapple beverages, died of a stroke in Great Neck, New York at the age of 85. The company was sold to Quaker Oats Co. for $1.5 billion. Snapple ended up with Cadbury Schweppes and is known as the Dr. Pepper Snapple Group.

Nina Wang, (April 4, 2007) Asia's richest woman and billionaire, and Chairwomen of ChinaChem (a recycling company) died of cancer at age 69.

Nobel Prize Winners: There has never been a Nobel Prize winner live to be 100 years of age. Despite complete access to information, advanced technology and people on the cutting edge of science, Nobel Prize winners die of simple diseases that even a turkey wouldn't die from!

Albert Einstein, (76), Famous for his unimpeachable "Theories of Relativity" died April 18, 1955 of a ruptured aortic aneurysm, a simple copper deficiency.

Francis Crick, (88), died of colon cancer - July 2004. Nobel Prize-winning scientist, who, with James Watson elucidated and unraveled the double-helix structure of DNA in 1953. He was a long-time faculty member of at the Salk Institute for Biological Studies in La Jolla, CA.

Medical Doctors: According to their own surveys and published research, the average life span of a primary care physician and family doctor in 1999 was 56 years of age.

The main causes of death reported in medical doctors - at the top of the list - are cancer, diabetes, heart disease and stroke.

If doctors were to live to be 150 years of age we should hang on every word they spoke, however, doctors are definitely not the "go to" people for health and longevity - living to an average age of 56 shows that they can't even help themselves, why on earth could you ever believe that they could help you live to be 100?

Dr. Gail L. Clark (47), a cardiologist and head of the cardiac rehabilitation unit at St. Luke's Hospital, St. Louis, MO., died of a heart attack July 26, 1993.

Dr. Stuart Berger, (40), best selling author of diet and health books including, *Dr. Berger's Immune Power Diet* and *Forever Young - 20 Years Younger in 20 Weeks*, died suddenly February 23, 1994. Dr. Berger had dropped from 420 pounds, down to 210 pounds.

Dr. Stewart Cartwright (38), a family practice physician who worked for Kaiser Permanente Out Patient Clinics, died suddenly (January 20, 1993) of a ruptured coronary artery aneurysm (a simple copper deficiency). Dr. Cartwright was "an avid athlete."

Dr. W. Thomas Nessa, (48), a cardiologist, a member of the "dream team" of cardiologists, who treated the Boston Celtic's captain, Reggie Lewis, died of a heart attack in January of 1995, one and one half years after Lewis collapsed and died of a cardiomyopathy heart attack (a selenium deficiency). Nessa had regularly run the Boston Marathon, had been a member of the Celtic's medical team and helped to create the standards for the cardiological evaluation of professional athletes.

Dr. Jeffrey M. Isner, (53), research cardiologist, who developed a procedure to stimulate the growth of blood vessels in the heart. Isner's team, at St. Elizabeth's Medical Center in Boston, and Tufts University School of Medicine, worked with cardiac patients who were "too sick" for bypass surgery; they injected genes that were taken up by the heart and then stimulated the production of "growth factor." He died October 30, 2001 from a heart attack.

Dr. Roy Walford, (79), a gerontologist and best selling author of books on longevity including, *Maximum Lifespan* and *The 120 Year Diet*; and he himself stayed on a Calorie Restricted diet for 30 years, died of complications of Lou Gehrig's disease April 2004.

Athletes: With the exception of three black athletes from the old "Negro Baseball League" days in the 20s and 30s, there has never been a professional athlete ever live to 100 years of age.

The average professional athlete lives to be 62 years of age, while the average professional couch potato lives to be 78 years of age - if you take a simple view of these statistics you could believe that exercise can shorten your life by 16 years.

Athletes sweat, not only water, but a "soup" of all the known essential nutrients. If one continuously sweats out essential nutrients (particularly minerals) and then only drinks water, ice tea, soft drinks or Gator-Aid (contains only two minerals) to replace fluids and nutrients, disaster is inevitable.

In fact, "exercise without supplementation is suicide." According to the Centers for Disease Control, some 75,000 to 100,000 young Americans under the age of 35 years, who work out or train regularly, die suddenly each year.

Jim Fixx (52), author of the 1977 best seller, *The Complete Book of Running,* was considered the "guru" of the concept of personal fitness through running, died in July 20, 1984 from a heart attack shortly after his daily run in rural Hardwick, VT. Jim Fixx had dropped from 240 pounds to 165 pounds by running, he believed that exercise alone, totally exclusive of supplements, was the only true path to health and longevity - and to that end he consciously avoided consuming vitamin and mineral supplements, banking his life on the medical dogma that "you can get everything you need by eating the four food groups."

Dr. George Sheehan (74) a cardiologist, author, self-proclaimed expert on physical fitness and runner, died of prostate cancer on November 1, 1993.

He was the medical editor of *Runner's World* magazine, authored the best selling books on running, *Medical Advice for Runners* and *Dr. Sheehan on Running* - his most famous remarks on diet and supplementation were, "Well, I don't care much about diet. I don't talk about it. But there is one demand, an extremely practical one that I make of a diet (and supplement): that it doesn't interfere directly with my running." Oops, he forgot the selenium!

Brian Maxwell (51), multi-millionaire apostle of Jim Fixx, co-creator of PowerBars™ (the Maxwell's sold the PowerBar™ business to Nestle four years before his March 2004 death for $375 million) with wife Jennifer. Maxwell, who had earned 14 gold medals for marathon wins in the Olympics, World Games and Iron Man competitions, died of a heart attack following a jog, while standing in line, in a post office in northern California while waiting to cash a money order.

Reggie Lewis (27) Captain of the Boston Celtics, died of a cardiomyopathy heart attack, a simple selenium deficiency (July 27, 1993) while shooting baskets at the Celtic's training center at Brandeis University, Waltham, MA. Lewis had collapsed earlier in the year during a playoff game against the Charlotte Hornets April 29, 1993.

Ryan Shay (28),(November 3, 2007) iconic long distance runner who trained by running 145 miles per week and won the NCAA 10,000 meter race in 2001 for Notre Dame, died of a heart attack at the 5.5 mile marker during final trials in the New York City Marathon event for the 2008 Beijing Olympic trials.

Vegans: There are several sub-cultures of "vegetarians." Most individuals who call themselves "vegetarians" are truly "omnivores" who choose not to eat "red meat," yet eat some combination of dairy, eggs, fish, poultry, etc.:

Vegans - true vegetarians, who strictly, with a religious fervor, eat only grains, vegetables, fruit and nuts and do not supplement - very dangerous!

Lacto-vegetarians - omnivores, who, eat dairy, in addition to grains, vegetables, fruit and nuts.

Ovo-vegetarians - omnivores, who, eat eggs, in addition to grains, vegetables, fruit and nuts.

Ovo-lacto-vegetarians - omnivores, who, eat eggs and dairy in addition to grains, vegetables, fruit and nuts.

Pisco-vegetarians - omnivores, who, eat fish in addition to grains, vegetables, fruit and nuts.

Pollo-vegetarians - omnivores, who, eat poultry in addition to grains vegetables, fruit and nuts.

Ovo - lacto - pollo - pisco - vegetarians - omnivores, who, eat eggs, dairy, poultry and fish in addition to grains, vegetables, fruit and nuts.

There has never been a vegan live to be 100 years of age; there are no flourishing colonies of vegans with dozens of rosy-cheeked kids running around. The vegan lifestyle without a serious and complete supplementation program tends to be more of a political statement than a healthful dietary regime.

Most vegans do not seriously supplement heavily and correctly with a special emphasis on minerals, and as a result strict vegans develop grey hair, receding gums, periodontal disease, blood sugar problems, arthritis, osteoporosis, anemia, hypertension, fibromyalgia, chronic fatigue syndrome, cancer, liver cirrhosis, cognitive, memory and emotional problems before five years has elapsed.

Certainly not all, but most vegans direct their energies and attentions to concocting "complete" amino acid mixes from combinations of grains and legumes to assure adequate intakes of plant proteins; they assume because they are "eating correctly" and because they consider themselves "spiritually elevated" they believe they can get optimal amounts of all essential nutrients (including amino acids, essential fatty acids, vitamins, minerals, trace minerals, rare earths, etc.) without supplementation.

Vegans as a group tend to lie to themselves and convince themselves (and try to convince others) that all of the long-lived people on earth do not eat animal products. In fact all long lived peoples on earth eat red meat (including pork, beef, goat, lamb, etc.), poultry, fish, eggs and dairy.

Plants only require 16 essential nutrients, only nine of which are minerals, to be healthy and reproduce themselves; we believe human beings require 90 essential nutrients (of which 60 are minerals) to be healthy and reproduce themselves.

Those vegans who eat an organic diet, un-supplemented with plant minerals are anywhere from 51 to 57 minerals short - plants can not manufacture minerals and nutritional minerals do not occur in a uniform blanket throughout the crust of the earth.

Nutritional minerals do not occur in a uniform blanket over the crust of the earth, minerals occur in veins like chocolate in chocolate ripple ice cream and plants can not manufacture minerals - plants can manufacture vitamins, amino acids, essential fatty acids and carbohydrates (all carbon compounds) but plants can not manufacture minerals.

> **Linda McCartney**,(56), died April 17, 1998), high profile wife of Beatles star Paul McCartney, animal rights activist, authored, *Linda McCartney's Home Cooking* (biggest selling vegetarian cookbook in the UK and best selling in the USA at 250,000 copies) and international crusader for the vegan lifestyle died of complications of breast cancer.

> **Ramchandra Gandhi**, (70), died June 14, 2007, grandson of Mohandas Gandhi (brought an end to the British colonial rule of India following his legendary "Salt March"), died of "natural causes."

> **Rita Gara** (55), a psychiatric nurse, was the director of The Himalayan Institute in Schaumberg, IL, where she taught meditation, yoga and stress management. She died at home from complications of breast cancer August 2, 1993.

Without a doubt, as predictable as gravity, the concept "Without Malnutrition" applies to all humans. Regardless of one's financial, educational or professional station in life, location on earth, race, gender or age, we humans require all essential nutrients in our food, not only in optimal amounts, but also, we require these essential nutrients in every mouthful of food, in every meal every day without fail if you want to live to be 100 years of age.

"Taking a multiple vitamin-mineral supplement to fill in the blanks as insurance" won't cut it - we must be more intense, more serious, more accurate and more professional about providing redundant sources of raw materials to every one of our cells, our metabolism, our physiology, our enzymatic systems and our spiritual, mental and physical performance if we are to be successful.

By contrast to the human health care industry that has failed us in providing us a guaranteed healthful life span of more than 100 years, the animal industry has been very successful in increasing longevity, production, performance, fertility, survivability of offspring, eliminating birth defects and increase resistance to disease simply by designing and creating complete rations that were species and function specific, that were guaranteed to be nutritionally perfect in every mouthful, every meal and every day without compromise.

Chapter 4

"Every animal and every human being that dies of natural causes dies of a nutritional deficiency disease."

Dr. Joel D. Wallach
The Center for the Biology of Natural Systems. 1968.

Essential Nutrients

Essential nutrients are referred to as "essential nutrients" for two reasons:

1) We as humans can't manufacture certain nutrients that are required for health, reproduction and optimal longevity - in fact, because we can't manufacture them, we must consume them in optimal amounts each and every day, every meal and every mouthful either as food or as supplements.

2) Failing to consume the essential nutrients in optimal amounts with every mouthful of food, with every meal, every day, we will, with the predictability of gravity, fall ill, become infertile, bear children with birth defects and produce lives that are unnecessarily short, expensive and miserable!

The Center for the Biology of Natural Systems

When I (Wallach) was a kid of nine, Marlin Perkins, the director of the Lincoln Park Zoo, appeared on "Zoo Parade," a weekly Saturday morning black and white, TV program that featured visits to animal cages in the Chicago Lincoln Park Zoo.

Marlin would, like magic, drive up to the cage in a golf cart, hop out and begin a learned discussion on the featured endangered animal - then, as if by another miracle, the viewer was transported to Africa, Asia, South America, the Arctic, the Antarctic, North America or Europe to observe the "endangered species" in its natural environment.

Perkins went on to become the director of the St. Louis Zoological Gardens and the host of the Mutual of Omaha's "Wild Kingdom" TV show, an upscale color version of the original Zoo Parade.

I wanted a job like Perkins had. I wanted to work with wild animals, be like Frank Buck and "Bring Them Back Alive." I wanted to save endangered wild species.

I got in line and applied for a summer job in the St. Louis Zoo - I told the interviewer, I was willing to do anything, anything to work with and for Perkins - it became an obsession.

My intensity paid off and I was picked out of literally thousands of kids to work in the elephant house through several summer breaks.

My first job with the elephants was to manually remove a bushel basket of grapefruit-sized manure balls from the rectums of each of seven show elephants just before their daily stage appearance in the world famous St. Louis Zoo's circus style elephant show - three times daily Monday through Friday and four times each day on Saturday and Sunday.

To perform this manure removal duty, I was instructed to strip to the waist, apply a liquid dish washing detergent to my ungloved right hand and arm and go at it. To complete the job properly and totally empty their rectum required that I plunge to a depth armpit deep. To prevent dislocation of my shoulder and prevent me from being thrown around like a rag doll by movements of the elephant to be emptied, they were chained to the floor by all four legs.

I went on to enter and graduate from the School of Agriculture, at the University of Missouri. My major was in animal husbandry and nutrition - the general theme was to learn how to formulate rations for animals that would extend life, reduce disease, increase fertility and production; my minor was in the subjects of field crops and soils, which gave me a solid base of soil and plant chemistry and soil and plant nutrition.

Two years into agricultural school I applied for and was accepted into veterinary school at the University of Missouri. During the last two years of agricultural school I also took the full load of courses to get me through the first two years of veterinary school.

At this juncture, I was eligible to take graduate courses, which I did. While in my sophomore year of veterinary school I had developed a fascination for the specialty of pathology, so I loaded up on graduate level animal and human pathology courses.

Upon graduation from veterinary school I took a position at the Iowa State University School of Veterinary Medicine and State Veterinary Diagnostic Laboratories, Ames Iowa with responsibilities for diagnostic pathology and teaching graduate level gross and microscopic pathology to graduate students.

After one year of teaching and doing service pathology, an opportunity came up to go to South Africa and participate in conservation and nutritional study projects in wild animal reserves.

Marlin Perkins gave me high recommendations which went a long way in helping me get the position. After two years of working on "Operation Rhino" in South Africa and several months in "Operation Elephant" in Southern Rhodesia (now Zimbabwe), Perkins sent me a telegram and invited me back to the states to work on a large project of great "national and world importance."

Perkins and Dr. Barry Commoner, a professor of Botany at Washington University, had gotten a $7.5 million grant from the National Institutes of Health, to perform autopsies on zoo animals and urban dwelling humans who had died of "natural causes" to determine whether or not pollution might be a factor in their causes of death.

As a comparative pathologist, I (Wallach) performed more than 20,000 autopsies of over 17,500 captive wild animals, laboratory species and domestic animals, of over 454 species and 3,000 humans for a comparison.

These autopsies included the review of clinical records, microscopic and electron microscopic examinations of histopathology, microbiology culture investigations for fungi, bacteria and viruses and chemical and biochemical profiles.

The original purpose of this huge multidisciplinary project (funded by the NIH, multiple zoos, Yerke's Regional Primate Research Center and multiple universities), known as The Center for the Biology of Natural Systems, was to investigate the possibility of environmental pollution and food contamination contributing to causes of illness and death.

What was found was that, "every animal and every human being that dies of natural causes dies of a nutritional deficiency disease!"

Diets were formulated, supplemented and corrected for species that until then were considered "too sensitive to reproduce in captivity." Fertility levels, pregnancies and reproduction records skyrocketed in species that had historically displayed little or no inclination to reproduce in captivity.

The principals of nutrition that had become successful

The sugar and carbohydrates manufactured in the leaves will be used for energy to support the physiological and biochemical activities and the growth of the plant or tree - excess production above the plants immediate needs will be stored as energy or "solar income" in the plants leaves, stems, roots, seeds, pods and fruits - ultimately the sun provides the energy to support all living systems on earth. To draw on this "solar currency" stored in the plant, the carbohydrate or sugar is "burned" in the human body producing chemical energy and the byproducts of carbon dioxide and water.

Glucose and complex carbohydrates can provide fuel for energy that is required for human movement, mechanical work and life itself. Grains furnish a major source of carbohydrates for humans and have the highest yield of stored solar energy per acre of land when compared with other foods.

The level of carbohydrate consumption varies significantly between countries and regions within countries. In America, approximately 45% of the diet is carbohydrates (in poorer section of big cities the percent of carbohydrates in the diet rises to 65% or more); in Asia, a high rice diet, carbohydrates can make up 65% or more; in the tropics as much as 90% of dietary energy comes from carbohydrates.

Carbohydrates are classified as monosaccharides, disaccharides, oligosaccharides and polysaccharides. The monosaccharides or simple sugars cannot be hydrolyzed to a simpler form. Disaccharides can be hydrolyzed to give two molecules of the same or different monosacchraides. Oligosaccharides yield three to ten monosaccharides and polysaccharides yield more than ten simple sugars, up to 10,000 or more.

Carbohydrates of all kinds (sugars and starches) provide a protein-sparing effect. If little or no sugar or carbohydrate is in a meal, the body, will breakdown protein into glucose via a process known as gluconeogenesis.

Monosaccharides

Glucose: (dextrose, grape sugar) is found in abundance in fruit, sweet corn, corn syrup, sugar beets and honey. Glucose is the principal sugar produced by the breakdown of the more complex carbohydrates in the process of digestion. Glucose is the "blood sugar" found in the blood stream (10 gm in an average size adult).

Glucose is burned in the cells as fuel to produce energy and is stored in the liver and muscles as glycogen, a complex carbohydrate called "animal starch."

Approximately 110 gm of glycogen is stored in the liver and 225 gm is stored in the skeletal muscles. Typically the brain uses glucose as its primary energy fuel.

Fructose: (levulose, fruit sugar) is found together with glucose and sucrose in honey and fruit. It is the sweetest of the natural sugars. Sweeteners containing glucose and levulose can be made from grains (corn) as well as from the sugar beet and sugar cane to make high-fructose corn syrup.

Sorbitol: a hexahydric alcohol derived from glucose, it has the sweetening power similar to glucose. Sorbitol is absorbed slowly and it serves to keep blood sugar levels high following a meal. It is commonly used in weight loss products as an aid to delay the onset of hunger pangs. Sorbitol has the same energy value as glucose and is naturally found in many fruits, vegetables and diet aids.

Galactose: is not found by itself in nature but is part of the lactose or milk sugar molecule. It is found naturally in nerve tissue.

Mannitol: is a hexahydric alcohol derived from

mannose and is found in a wide variety of foods. It is poorly digested and thus yields about half as many calories per gram as glucose. Dried pineapple, olives, asparagus, sweet potatoes, carrots and "sugarless" gum often contain mannitol.

Xylitol: a sugar alcohol of xylose with the sweetness of sucrose, it is absorbed at only one fifth the rate of glucose; for this reason xylitol is commonly used in sweeteners and foods for diabetics; it is also used in "sugar free" chewing gum and high quality weightloss chocolates. Xylitol is found naturally in fruit and vegetables.

Disaccharides

Disaccharides, or double sugars, include sucrose (cane or beet sugar), maltose (malt sugar) and lactose (milk sugar):

Sucrose = glucose + Fructose

Maltose = glucose + glucose

Lactose = glucose + galactose

Disaccharides are broken apart into the single monosaccharides before being absorbed through the intestine.

Polysaccharides

The primary polysaccharides commonly found in human nutrition including starch, dextrin, cellulose and glycogen are simply chains of glucose molecules.

Dietary fiber is different than simple crude fiber. In addition to lignin and cellulose, dietary fiber contains hemicellulose, gums, pectin, and other carbohydrates that are indigestible by humans.

Mucopolysaccharides occur mixed with protein in body secretions and physical structural units and are necessary for the natural viscosity of body mucus secretions.

Mucopolysaccharides are found in significant quantities in food. Some of the more common mucopolysaccharides include hyaluronic acids (HA) found in intercellular tissues including cartilage; chondroitin sulfate, typically found in the cornea of the eye, cartilage, tendons, ligaments, intervertebral discs, skin, aorta and heart valves; heparin, a naturally occurring anticoagulant found in blood, [illegible] sulfates witch are associated with blood groups; and dermatan sulfate found in skin.

Proteins

Protein, is derived from the Greek, "of first importance" was isolated almost 200 years ago. Proteins, the key organic compounds of all living tissue and organisms are nitrogen containing carbon compounds that will yield amino acids when broken down into the basic building blocks.

Proteins are the fundamental structural compounds in the cell; they are essential components of the nucleus and protoplasm of every cell. Proteins are the most abundant of the organic compounds in the body.

Most of the protein in the human body is found in skeletal muscle; the balance is distributed in soft tissue, internal organs, bones, teeth, blood and other body fluids.

Hormones and enzymes are proteins that do work. As proteins are required for essential functions in the body, and since many indispensable protein components can't be manufactured by the body and must be obtained solely through dietary sources, it is obvious that the amounts and quality of the protein sources are matters of considerable importance.

Composition and functions of Protein

Proteins, like fats and carbohydrates, contain carbon, hydrogen and oxygen, however, they also contain 16% nitrogen along with sulfur, and can contain phosphorus, iron and cobalt. The building blocks of proteins are the amino acids. They are found in chains in a number of geometric and chemical combinations to form unique proteins, all of which are very large and complex molecules, each having its own physiological function.

Even though they are structurally complex, proteins are easily broken apart by enzymatic action or boiling in acid or alkaline solutions.

Plants obtain their nitrogen from the nitrates and ammonia in the soil, and with them are able to synthesize protein. Animals and humans obtain their nitrogen by eating plants and other animals. The byproduct of animal metabolism (feces, urine), excretion and death returns the nitrogen to the soil - this continuing cycle is termed the "nitrogen cycle."

Essential Amino Acids

There are 12 amino acids that are required by the body as protein building blocks, and because the body is unable to manufacture them, they are termed "essential amino acids." If any of these "essential" amino acids are missing, from the diet for any length of time, a specific, sometimes reversible disease will occur.

Valine	**methionine***
Tyrosine	**histidine**
Tryptophan	**Phenylalanine**
Lysine	**arginine**
Isoleucine	**Taurine**
Threonine	**Leucine**

Proteins can be broken down and used as a source of heat and energy. Proteins supply four kcalories per gm, the same as using carbohydrate for fuel; however, the process is more biologically "expensive" than burning carbohydrates for fuel (five percent of calories required to burn carbohydrates and fat versus 30% calories to burn an equal amount of protein).

* Selenium researcher, Dr. Gerhard Schrauzer, considers selenomethionine, the selenium analog of methionine the 13th essential amino acid.

Lipids

Lipids (fats) are a large heterogeneous group of compounds made up of fatty acids. This group of organic compounds includes ordinary fats and oils, waxes and related compounds. They all have the common features of being insoluble in water; soluble in organic solvents such as ether and chloroform; and they are utilizable and required by all living organisms.

The majority (98%) of the fats found in the human body, are triglycerides, and the greater majority of these are long chain triglycerides. The balance of lipids found in the body, are comprised of monoglycerides and diglycerides, free fatty acids, phospholipids and sterols.

Fatty acids are described by three characteristics: 1) chain length; 2) degree of "saturation" with hydrogen; and 3) the location of the first "double bond" on the carbon chain.

The length of a fatty acid is determined by the number of carbon atoms in the chain - C16 refers to 16 carbons in the chain. The chains can be further described by "short" (six or fewer carbons); "medium" (seven to 11 carbons); and "long" (12 or more carbons).

The degree of hydrogen "saturation" is defined by the number of double bonds between the carbon atoms in the chains. A chain may contain all of the hydrogen it can hold and have no double bonds, in this instance it is referred to as a "saturated fatty acid." The chain may contain one double bond and be called a monounsaturated fatty acid, or it can be a polyunsaturated fatty acid and contain several double bonds. The location of the first double bond as counted from the tail of the fatty acid is the omega number (i.e. - omega-3, omega-4, etc.).

Fats supply a concentrated source of energy. Each gram of fat supplies 9 kcalories, which is more than twice the amount of energy supplied by each gram of carbohydrate. Because of the high energy density and low solubility of fats, they are used as a storage form of energy. Up to two thirds of the total energy of the cells may be supplied by triglycerides rather than carbohydrate. Fat spares protein for tissue synthesis.

Fats aid in the transport and absorption of the fat-soluble vitamins A, D, E and K. Fats spare thiamin since they can be metabolized for energy without the need for thiamin, whereas, the metabolism of carbohydrate requires thiamine.

Triglycerides: (the primary component of fats and oils) are similar to carbohydrates in that they are composed of carbon, hydrogen and oxygen. One hundred grams of fat from triglycerides will contain 95 grams of fatty acids.

Cholesterol: Cholesterol is a member of a large group of compounds known as sterols. They all have the same complex ring structure. The "ol" ending of the cholesterol indicates that it is an organic alcohol.

Cholesterol is an essential nutrient and an essential component of the structural membranes of all cells, all steroid hormones and is a major component of brain (myelin) and nerve cells.

Cholesterol is found only in animal tissues, however, some similar sterols are found in plants. Ergosterol, a yeast sterol, is converted to vitamin D_2 when exposed to ultraviolet light. Cholesterol is converted by the intestinal mucosa to 7-dehydrocholesterol, the provitamin of vitamin D_3, cholecalciferol. This process is also carried out by the skin and other tissues, when exposed to ultraviolet light and sunlight.

Essential Fatty Acids (EFA): Three polyunsaturated fatty acids, linoleic, linolenic and arachidonic acids, have essential fatty acid activity. Only linoleic and linolenic fatty acids have been designated as essential fatty acids, as arachidonic acid can be synthesized from linoleic acid.

The essential fatty acids have important roles in fat transport and metabolism and in maintaining the function and integrity of cellular membranes.

The essential fatty acids are the building blocks and raw materials for a group of hormone-like compounds including prostaglandins, thromboxanes and prostacyclins, that participate in the regulation of blood pressure, heart rate, vascular dilation, blood clotting, lipolysis, the central nervous system and airway dilation.

The daily requirement for the essential fatty acids is two to three percent of the total calories consumed. A daily diet containing 1,500 calories would dictate an essential fatty acid requirement of 45 calories or five grams of EFA.

The EFA Health Claim Story

It had been known for more than 65 years that there were in fact essential fatty acids that were required in the human diet for optimal health, disease prevention and longevity, however, because the FDA ruled that the information was "inconclusive" it was deemed illegal to inform people that they could reduce their risk of stroke and coronary thrombosis sudden death by supplementing with omega-3 essential fatty acids.

To make a long story short, Wellness Lifestyles, Inc (Wallach) filed a petition for an Amended Health Claim: Omega-3 Fatty Acids and Coronary Heart Disease (Co-Petitioner); Docket No. 03Q-0401; filed on 6/23/2003; qualified claim allowed by FDA on 9/8/2004. Claim approval from the FDA was hard fought and won so that the world would have access to the benefits of supplementing with omega-3 essential fatty acids to reduce their risks of stroke and sudden death from heart attacks.

Vitamins

Vitamins are an essential group of unrelated organic carbon compounds needed only in minute quantities in the diet. They are essential for metabolic processes within the cell and necessary for normal growth, maintenance and longevity. Deficiencies of many vitamins during pregnancy can result in catastrophic birth defects (neural tube defects, mental retardation, muscular dystrophy, cycstic fibrosis, cleft lip, cleft palate, heart defects, etc.).

Many vitamins act as coenzymes or a prosthetic group of enzymes responsible for facilitating essential physiological reactions.

Vitamins are often called "accessory food factors" in view of the fact that they do not in of themselves supply calories or contribute to building body mass.

Vitamins regulate metabolism, participate in the citric acid cycle and converting fat, sugar, carbohydrates and proteins into energy.

There are three categories of vitamins:

1) Water soluble vitamins: B complex and vitamin C

The B complex consists of 10 separate water soluble vitamins. In general they function as essential nutrients in the metabolic processes of all living cells by acting as cofactors in multiple enzyme systems that drive the oxidation or "burning" of food and the production of energy.

Thiamine or B_1 is essential throughout life for tissue respiration and energy production. Thiamine combines with phosphorus to form the coenzyme thiamine pyrophosphate (TPP), which functions as a cocarboxylase enzyme. TPP is required for the oxidative decarboxylation of pyruvate to form active acetate and acetyl coenzyme A, the central compound of the Krebs cycle.

Clinical signs of thiamine deficiency (beri-beri), primarily involves the nervous system and cardiovascular systems.

Mild deficiencies produce mental confusion, muscular weakness, peripheral paralysis, calf muscle tenderness, muscle fatigue, emotional instability, loss of appetite, loss of interest in daily tasks and general lethargy.

Chronic deficiencies of thiamine result in a polyneuritis and congestive heart failure with edema and life-threatening pulmonary edema.

Central nervous system manifestations include stiffness while walking and Wernicke-Korsakoff syndrome, an encephalopathy that is expressed as a loss of short term memory (looks like early Alzheimer's disease), disorientation, nystagmus (rhythmic side to side movements of the eyes) and ataxia (a type of staggering gait).

Simple consumption of thiamine and elimination of sugar from the diet oftentimes will produce a rapid cure.

Riboflavin or vitamin B_2 was recognized in 1879 as a yellow-green fluorescent pigment in milk whey. The biological significance of this yellow pigment was not understood until 1932 when a team of German investigators isolated "Warburg's yellow enzyme" from yeast and demonstrated that the substance was necessary for the functioning of an intracellular enzyme. The substance was synthesized in 1935 by Kuhn and named riboflavin.

Riboflavin is present in small amounts in milk, cheddar and cottage cheese, organ meats (liver, heart, kidney, etc.), eggs and green leafy vegetables.

Deficiency symptoms begin with soreness and burning of the lips, mouth and tongue (glossitis); photophobia; lacrimation; burning and itching of the eyes; and loss of visual acuity.

Chronic deficiency of riboflavin results in the development of cheilosis (fissuring of the lips) and angular stomatitis (cracks in the skin at the corner of the mouth).

Niacin (nicotinic acid) or vitamin B_3, its deficiency or pellagra has been recognized for centuries where people used corn as a staple diet - it was described by Casal of Spain in the early 18th century and in Italy soon afterwards.

Pellagra was first described in the United States in the early 1900s. It was initially thought to be an infectious disease and the federal government built "retardation centers" across the old Confederate states and treated pellagra patients in much the same manner as tuberculosis patients. The United States Bureau of Public Health eventually identified the root cause of pellagra to malnutrition and a corn-based diet resulting in a niacin deficiency.

Niacin functions in the body as a component of the coenzymes nicotinamide adenine dinucleotide (NAD) and nicotinamide adenine dinucleotide phosphate (NADP), known as the pyridine nucleotides. The coenzymes are necessary for the function of subcellular respiratory enzymes. NAD is also used in glycogen synthesis.

The early stages of niacin deficiency show up as muscular weakness, anorexia, indigestion and skin eruptions. Severe deficiency of niacin produces classic pellagra which is characterized by the "3 D's" of pellagra (dermatitis, dementia and diarrhea), tremors and sore tongue or "beef tongue."

The role of corn based diets in the precipitation of pellagra is well known. There is very little niacin in corn and the tryptophan in the corn is unavailable and can't be absorbed from the intestine, as a result there is no available tryptophan to be converted into niacin.

In successful corn consuming societies such as in Mexico, Central America and South America the corn is soaked in lye and wood ashes overnight before it is consumed - the alkali in the lye and wood ashes allows the tryptophan to be absorbed and pellagra is rare; in India where sorghum or millet is a common food, high levels of leucine in the grains produce an increased requirement for vitamin B_6 and several of the enzymes in the tryptophan-niacin pathway are B_6 dependent, therefore a diet high in sorghum or millet can produce pellagra.

Pantothenic acid or vitamin B_5 is part of coenzyme A, which functions in two-carbon unit metabolism. Pantothenic acid is required for the metabolism of carbohydrates, lipids and proteins.

Deficiencies of pantothenic acid appear as dermatitis, burning sensations of the feet, pain in the arms and legs, loss of appetite, nausea and indigestion -many become quarrelsome, sullen and depressed, fainting attacks and tachycardia (rapid pulse rate) are common.

Pyridoxine or vitamin B_6 was identified in 1938 as a fraction or separate entity of the vitamin "B-complex." Vitamin B_6 is a functional complex of three closely related chemical compounds - pyridoxine, pyridoxamine and pyridoxal.

Deficiency of B_6 produces depression, nausea, vomiting, seborrheic dermatitis, mucus membrane lesions, peripheral neuritis, ataxia, hyperacusis, hyperirritability, altered mobility and alertness, abnormal head movements and convulsions.

Treatment of tuberculosis patients with Isonazid produces an antagonistic reaction against pyridoxine function which then results in the classical symptoms of deficiency.

"Morning sickness" commonly observed in the first trimester of pregnancy is thought to be due to pyridoxine deficiency.

Fifteen to 20 percent of women taking oral contraceptives show the symptoms of pyridoxine deficiency manifested by malaise, depression and glucose intolerance.

A deficiency syndrome for pyridoxine has been identified in mentally retarded children that also have convulsions due to an inborn error of B_6 metabolism. It is thought that these children are unable to synthesize GABA; correction of this syndrome requires daily ingestion of large amounts of B_6 to prevent permanent retardation.

Children with cryptogenic epilepsy that appears at several years of age will require large oral doses of vitamin B_6 to improve the EEG and control the seizures.

Folacin or folic acid was identified as one of many growth factors in bacteria and laboratory animals and in the prevention and treatment of anemia. It was synthesized in 1946 and quickly established as an essential nutrient for humans.

Folic acid deficiencies may be the most common

vitamin deficiency in humans. The deficiency of folic acid produces poor growth, megablastic anemia, multiple blood disorders, glossitis and gastrointestinal tract disturbances.

Protein malnutrition can impair the utilization and function of folicin and conditions in which the requirements are unusually great, such as pregnancy, hemolytic anemia, leukemia, Hodgkin's disease and drugs (methotrexate).

In pernicious anemia (B_{12} deficiency), folic acid will produce a marked improvement in the anemia, however, the gastrointestinal symptoms and neurologic lesions will continue to progress - this is referred to as the "masking effect" of folic acid.

Untreatedandunmanagedgluten-sensitive enteropathy (celiac disease) can result in folic acid deficiency.

Neural tube defects (hydroencephaloceole, spina bifida, etc.) are extremely common in babies born to women who have folic acid deficiency during the first trimester of pregnancy.

Cobalamin or vitamin B_{12} was isolated from a liver extract in 1948 and shown to prevent and reverse pernicious anemia. The vitamin B_{12} structure contains the heavy metal cobalt, chelated in a large tetrapyrrole ring very similar in structure to the porphyrin ring structure of hemoglobin and chlorophyll.

The form of vitamin B_{12} originally isolated contained cyanide (cyanocobalamin). Several cobalamin compounds have vitamin B_{12} activity including cyanocobalamin and hydroxycobalamin.

Cobalamin is poorly absorbed from the intestinal tract unless the "intrinsic factor" (a mucoprotein enzyme called "Castle's intrinsic factor") is present in the gastric secretions.

The presence of hydrochloric acid is necessary to split vitamin B_{12} from its peptide bonds. The intrinsic factor combines with vitamin B_{12} in the food and in the bound form becomes adsorbed to a receptor in the membranes of the ileum, through which it is actively transported to the cells in pinocytic vesicles and calcium is a required cofactor for this transfer to take place.

There is an enterohepatic circulation of B_{12} that recycles the vitamin from the bile and other intestinal secretions - this conservation pathway is the reason why vitamin B_{12} deficiency can take so long to develop in vegans.

Vitamin B_{12} is present in significant levels in animal proteins. Vitamin B_{12} is found in liver, kidney, fresh whole milk, eggs, cheese and muscle meats are rich sources. Pasteurized and evaporated milk have lost 40 to 90% of vitamin B_{12}. While a small amount of bacterial synthesis of vitamin B_{12} occurs in the colon, distal to the terminal ileum, it can't be absorbed.

Deficiencies of vitamin B_{12} can occur when the stomach pH (acid level) rises toward neutral or alkaline levels and/or when insufficient amounts of intrinsic factor are produced. Surgical resection of or the by-passing of the intrinsic factor-secreting portions of the stomach (fundus and cardia) or of the ileum (celiac disease, Crohn's disease, etc.) can produce vitamin B_{12} deficiency.

Vegans (vegetarians who consume only grains, fruit, vegetables and nuts to the complete exclusion of animal products and supplements) have an extremely low intake of vitamin B_{12} and are very likely to develop a vitamin B_{12} deficiency and a classic megaloblastic anemia and a classic and progressive demyelinating neuropathy unless they supplement.

Biotin or vitamin H (coenzyme R) was first isolated in 1936 and synthesized in 1943. Originally biotin deficiency was observed in chicks and rats that were fed raw egg whites, which it was learned later, contained an "egg-white-injury" factor.

Avidin, a material found in egg white, combines with biotin in the intestine making it unavailable for absorption. It takes 24 raw egg whites to contribute enough avidin to create a biotin deficiency in humans. Avidin is denatured and rendered harmless by normal cooking temperatures.

Symptoms of biotin deficiency in humans include skin lesions over the nose and mouth, depression, hyperesthesia and paresthesia particularly over the extremities, muscle pain, conjunctivitis, blepharitis and a progressive loss of hair and hair color.

Choline has been known for more than 100 years as being essential and it has a vitamin-like coenzyme function. Man can synthesize choline from the amino acids methionine or serine in the presence of vitamin B_{12} and folacin. The rate at which choline can be synthesized is insufficient to meet daily requirements and for this reason it is considered an essential nutrient.

The function of choline in humans is part of the metabolism of and in the transport of fat from the liver. A deficiency of choline can result in a fatty liver. As a component of phospholipids, choline functions in triglyceride transport and in cell membrane structure. In the liver, choline forms lecithin (phosphatidyl choline). During this process, fatty acids are removed from the glycerides of the liver, thus reducing the triglyceride level.

Choline is also a component of another phospholipid, sphingomyelin, which is an important component of the brain and peripheral nerves. As a precursor for acetylcholine, choline is involved in the transmission of nerve impulses.

Deficiencies of choline result in a "fatty liver," which in a severe, form can land you on a liver transplant list. Large doses of choline have proved to be beneficial for managing and alleviating the symptoms of tardive dyskinesia and Huntington's disease in humans.

Inositol was identified as a vitamin in 1940. It occurs abundantly in diets containing whole grains and raw vegetables as inositol phospholipids and as phytic acid (inositol hexaphosphate or "phytates").

Phytic acid interferes with the absorption of calcium, iron, zinc and other nutrients - on one hand a required nutrient and on the other a negative in the diet.

Myoinositol, "muscle sugar," has a chemical structure that resembles glucose and is concentrated in the brain, cerebrospinal fluid, skeletal muscle, heart muscle and other tissues. Free inositol is found in especially high levels in the organs of the male reproductive tract, particularly in semen.

Inositol has been shown to have a therapeutic role in diabetic neuropathy.

Deficiencies of inositol will produce pathological fatty liver disease.

Ascorbic acid or vitamin C is known to prevent and cure scurvy. Scurvy was first described during the Crusades and was common among soldiers and sailors until the Dutch discovered that the consumption of citrus fruit and fresh vegetables could prevent and cure the disease. British sailors were oftentimes referred to as "limeys" because they carried lemons (not limes) on their ships to prevent and cure scurvy.

The identification of ascorbic acid as the specific agent that prevented and cured scurvy did not occur until the 20th century. Pure ascorbic acid was isolated in 1928 by Albert Szent-Gyorgyi, who discovered it in adrenal tissue, orange and cabbage and identified it as hexuronic acid. It was not until 1932 that C. Glenn King at the University of Pittsburgh reisolated ascorbic acid from lemons that it was identified as vitamin C and had the properties of preventing and curing scurvy in guinea pigs.

After much fanfare, vitamin C supplementation has been shown to reduce the rate, severity and duration of a cold on the average by 20%.

A deficiency of vitamin C is characterized by general weakness, poor appetite and growth, anemia, tenderness, swollen and inflamed gums, bleeding gums, loose teeth, osteoporosis, swollen wrist and ankle joints, shortness of breath, small pin-head hemorrhages (petechial), fractures, wounds heal slowly, scars break open, secondary infections are common, depression and neurotic disturbances including hysteria.

Cigarette smoking increases the need for ascorbic acid to about twice the normal requirement.

2) Fat soluble vitamins: A, D, E, and K

Fat soluble vitamins are related primarily as a result of their being soluble in lipids and insoluble in water and they are stored primarily in the bodies fat stores - this simple fact is where their similarities end.

The fat soluble vitamins are absorbed along with other common and essential dietary lipids and any health challenge or health practice that interferes with the absorption of fats (antibiotic use, gall bladder disease, celiac disease, dietary fat deficiencies, extremely high fiber diets, mineral oil consumption during meals and overt deficiencies) interferes with fat soluble vitamin absorption and function.

Retinol or vitamin A was the first fat soluble vitamin to be recognized. McCollum and Davis at the University of Wisconsin and Osborne and Mendel at Yale University reported their discoveries almost simultaneously in 1913. They observed that young weanling animals became unhealthy, failed to thrive and grow when fed fat free diets.

Investigators also noted that those animals that lived longer on fat free diets developed inflammation and infections of the eyes - these conditions were quickly reversed when fats from butter or cod liver oil were added to the diet.

In 1924, Bloch, a Danish investigator, showed that xerophthalmia in children was the same disease described in 1913 in laboratory rats, and that the disease could be prevented or cured by adding liver, butter or cod liver oil to their diet.

Vegetables were later found to contain vitamin A activity in relation to their carotenoid content - carotene, cryptoxanthin and other yellow, red or orange pigments that were oftentimes hidden by the green pigment of chlorophyll.

*Vitamin A Content of Food**

Food	I.U.
Liver, beef, 100 gm	43,900
Carrots, raw, 1 medium	11,000
Sweet potato, baked, 1 sm	8,100
Spinach, cooked, 1/2 cup	7,300
Apricots, dried, 8 halves	5,500
Squash, winter, 1/2 cup	4,200
Cantaloupe, 1/4 melon	3,400
Broccoli, 1 stalk	2,500
Crab, 100 gm	2,170
Peach, 1 medium	1,330
Halibut, 125 gm	850
Egg yolk, 1 medium	580
Milk, whole, 1 cup	370
Cheese, cheddar, 1 oz.	370
Orange, 1 medium	300
Butter, 1 tsp	165
Margarine, fortified, 1 tsp	165
Apple, 1 medium	140
Peanuts, raw, 100 gm	16

** USDA 1984*

Vitamin A Functions:

Vision

Growth and bone development

Epithelial tissue development and maintenance

Immune system support

Anti-cancer function

Calciferol or vitamin D was recognized, in the Middle Ages, as a prevention and cure for rickets, however, it was not until WW I that the cause and effect of vitamin D deficiency was recognized as the specific cause of rickets.

Vitamin D was separated from vitamin A in 1922 by McCullum. In 1924 Steenbock and Hess discovered that irradiation with ultraviolet light produced antirachitic properties to certain foods. In 1936, Windaus demonstrated that the natural prehormone found in the skin which converts to calciferol when irradiated by UV light was 7-dehydrocholesterol.

In 1968, Blunt, De Luca and Schnoes discovered that the metabolically active form of vitamin D was not calciferol but rather 25-hydroxycholecalciferol (vitamin D_3), which was synthesized in the body from calciferol when the skin was exposed to ultraviolet light or sun light.

In 2006 Dr. Michael Holick, a professor of medicine, physiology and biophysics at Boston University said, "The bottom line is, we now recognize that vitamin D_3 is important for health for both children and adults and may help prevent many serious chronic diseases."

Holick's studies have shown that deficiencies of vitamin D_3 in adults results in an increase in risk of heart attacks, increased mortality in breast and colon cancer victims, increased risk of mortality in dialysis patients and an increased risk of developing type II diabetes in children.

A large study reported in the June 8, 2007 issue of the *American Journal of Clinical Nutrition*, is the first study in which researchers significantly boosted - and measured - blood levels of vitamin D_3 and then followed identical groups of patients from start to finish.

"The findings, which show a reduction in the risk of several types of cancer by 60%, are a breakthrough of great medical and public health importance," said Cedric Garland, a prominent vitamin D researcher at the University of California, San Diego. "No other method to prevent cancer has been identified that has such a powerful impact," Garland continued.

The danger of vitamin D_3 deficiency is very high in the 21st century as people have been directed by their doctor and the government to avoid the sun, spend little or no time in the sun and when they do they are instructed cover themselves with sun blockers, long sleeves, gloves and hats.

Vitamin D Functions:

Stimulates the active, energy requiring intestinal absorption of calcium.

Stimulates the active phosphate-transport system in the intestine.

With the parathyroid hormone, it mobilizes calcium from bone to maintain normal blood levels of calcium.

It mobilizes phosphate from the bone to maintain proper serum phosphate levels.

It supports reabsorption of calcium from urine by the kidney.

It increases reabsorption of phosphate from urine by the kidney.

Tocopherol or vitamin E was first identified by Evans and Bishop in 1922, when they observed infertility in rats could be reversed when they were fed a substance isolated from vegetable oils. Vitamin E was chemically identified in 1938 and named tocopherol after *tokos* from the Greek which translates to "offspring."

Deficiency of vitamin E can produce a hemolytic anemia (rupture of red blood cells), especially when diets are too high in unsaturated fatty acids and iron. Deficiency also produces muscle weakness, accumulation of ceroid lipofuscin in smooth muscle, liver spots in the skin and creatinuria as seen in muscular dystrophy and patients with celiac disease, cystic fibrosis, sprue, etc.

Additional symptoms of vitamin E deficiency include miscarriage, fetal reabsorption, testicular atrophy, birth defects, muscular dystrophy, hemolytic anemia, myocardial degeneration, encephalomalacia and liver necrosis.

Vitamin E Function:

Antioxidant activity which prevents the formation of peroxides.

Prevents oxidation damage of polyunsaturated fatty acids.

Enhances the activity of vitamin A by preventing its oxidation.

Protects cellular and mitochondrial membranes from oxidation.

The ability of vitamin E to protect membrane lipids from peroxidation has been related to its anti-aging properties.

A relationship between vitamin E, selenium, glutathione peroxidase, cystine and polyunsaturated fats in the cell membrane has been clearly demonstrated.
Selenium, which activates glutathione peroxidase, destroys peroxides after they are produced but before they can cause cell membrane damage.

Sulfur-containing amino acids, such as cystine, maintain optimal tissue glutathione levels.

Phylloquinone or vitamin K is the naturally occurring form of the synthetic fat soluble vitamin menadione (K_3). In 1935, Dam in Copenhagen observed a fatal hemorrhagic disease in newly hatched chickens fed a laboratory diet that contained all of the known essential nutrients. When hog liver fat extract or alfalfa was added to the diet normal clotting time was restored.

In the liver, vitamin K is required as an essential cofactor for an enzyme (carboxylase) that converts specific glutamic acid residues of certain proteins to a new amino acid, alpha-carboxyglutamic acid (Gla) in the completed proteins. These proteins include the vitamin K-dependent blood clotting factors prothrombin (factor II) and factors VII, IX and X.

Several Gla-containing proteins are found as well. The vitamin K-dependent Gla-containing protein called "osteocalcin" is now known to modulate calcium deposition into bone matrix - vitamin K is as essential to healthy bone maintenance as vitamin D. It is this calcium-binding action of Gla that gives prothrombin its unique place in coagulation.

The coumarin anticoagulant drugs (warfarin and dicumarol) act to prevent coagulation by antagonizing the action of vitamin K.

The deficiency of vitamin K is uncommon except when an individuals diet is low in green leafy vegetables and the growth of intestinal flora has been inhibited by the use of antibiotics or there is a fat absorption problem.

3) Flavanols (Bioflavonoids): Epicatechins and polyphenols.

Flavonoids or vitamin P commonly found in cocoa, tea and wine are now considered to be the third category of vitamins and are officially added to the water soluble and fat soluble groups by Harvard Medical School.

Norman Hollenberg from Harvard Medical School and Brigham and Women's Hospital reports, "that the island-dwelling Kuna people who drink the flavanol-rich cocoa, have a 10% lower risk of four of the five most common killer diseases: stroke, heart failure, cancer and diabetes."

"If these observations predict the future, then we can say without blushing that they are among the most important observations in the history of medicine," said Hollenberg.

Flavonoids were first used clinically in 1936 by Szent-Gyorgyi to treat patients with diseases characterized by increased permeability and fragility of the capillary wall that resulted in hemorrhages.

The flavonoids found in "dark chocolate have been found to lower blood pressure," says Dr. Dirk Taubert from the University of Cologne, Germany - an extensive report was published in the August 27, 2003 issue of The *Journal of the American Medical Association*.

Minerals

Minerals refer to elements in their simple inorganic form. Unlike the carbon-based essential nutrients, which plants can manufacture, plants can not manufacture elemental and mineral nutrients and therefore man and animals must either serendipitously or consciously consume them.

The Hunzas are legendary for long healthful lives. Their health and longevity has been attributed to several things including the minerals found in the "glacial milk" produced by the Ultar Glacier grinding up rock and the resultant rock silt being placed in their terraces through irrigation and the compost (wood ashes, manure, kitchen wastes, etc.) regularly used to fertilize their gardens.

After much consideration we realized that the people of Hunza had a very unique combination of sources of minerals and that only 0.00001% of humans on earth live near glaciers and only 0.0001% of humans on earth live on flood plains that are inundated with flood water every year with the resultant silt (mineral dust) deposits revitalizing the soil - these facts begged the question, "Where and how were the greater masses of humans on earth getting their daily source of minerals."

A determined search revealed that humans universally used wood ashes (plant minerals - not carbon), peat moss ash, rice straw ash, manure ash, kelp ash and kelp ash and sea salt mixes as their basic and daily source of minerals. World wide, humans used plant minerals from various and oftentimes multiple sources (Hunzas - glacial milk and wood ashes; Okinawa - wood ashes, rice straw ashes, kelp ash; etc.) for fertilizing their gardens, thereby getting minerals indirectly that were taken up by the fruits, vegetables and grains and adding plant minerals directly into their food as "culinary ashes."

There are three major categories of minerals known in human and animal nutrition:

Major minerals

Trace minerals

Rare earths

Chapter 5

Minerals - The Staff of Life

Minerals were used proactively as nutritional supplements some 50,000 to 200,000 years ago. Originally the source of minerals were the minerals in plant and animal food sources and then at the start of "the Great Leap Forward" humans began to proactively put plant minerals derived from wood, grass, kelp and manure ashes onto and into their food ("culinary ashes").

The ancient civilizations of China, India and Egypt learned to use pure elements and ground up jewel dust (minerals) as medicines 6,000 to 10,000 B.C. to treat and cure specific deficiency diseases.

Nutritional minerals never occurred in a uniform blanket over the crust of the earth. These essential elements occurred in veins like chocolate in chocolate ripple ice cream or veins of gold and silver. Neighboring farms will often have different varieties and amounts of minerals in their soil - therefore the farmers and their families on one property containing many minerals in large quantities could have few diseases and live to the age of 103 years, while their neighbor might have few minerals on their property with the result they would be sickly and only lived to be 48 years of age - not genetcs, but rather a mineral deficient microenvironment.

As a result of the wide regional variation in mineral

content of the soil, diseases of deficiency appeared in regional patterns. Iodine deficiency (goiter) occurred in communities living at a distance from the sea; Keshan disease (cardiomyopathy) caused by a selenium deficiency occurred in Keshan Province, China; phosphate deficiency (pica) was common in South Africa; copper deficiency (enzootic ataxia) was common in Australia, etc.

Dr. Willhelm Heinrich Schuessler (1821 - 1898) of Oldenburg, Germany, cremated the remains of indigent patients in his hospital. He performed an analysis of the resulting ashes using the limited techniques of the day. He was able to identify 12 mineral elements which he called "Tissue Salts"("cell salts") in the human ashes, and by relating the mineral content of each body to the disease the patient had suffered and died from he identified and created 12 "Biochemic Tissue Salts" or "cell salts" with which he then successfully treated live patients who suffered from the same diseases.

Schuessler published his findings in his classic book, *Shortened Therapeutics*, in 1873.

Only when one looks at a USDA data base that compares the level of vitamins and minerals in certain common foods between 1975 and 2004, do we truly understand how depleted our foods have become since we gave up the back yard gardens and wood ashes (plant minerals).

USDA Nutrient Data Base

Food	1975	2004	% change
Iron (mg per 100 grams)			
Apples	0.3	0.12	-60%
Blueberries	1.0	0.28	-72%
Onions	0.5	0.19	-62%
Tomatoes	0.5	0.45	-10%
Carrots	0.7	0.30	-57%
Spinach	3.1	2.71	-13%
Corn	0.7	0.52	-26%
Peas	1.9	1.47	-23%
Broccoli	1.1	0.73	-33%
Kale	2.7	1.70	-37%
Strawberries	1.0	0.42	-58%
Calcium (mg per 100 grams)			
Apples	7.0	6.0	-14%
Blueberries	15.0	6.0	-60%
Onions	27.0	22.0	-18%
Tomatoes	37.0	33.0	-11%
Green beans	56.0	37.0	-33%
Corn	3.0	2.0	-33%
Peas	26.0	25.0	-4%
Broccoli	103.0	47.0	-54%
Kale	249.0	135.0	-46%
Strawberries	21.0	16.0	-24%

Vitamin A (Int. units per 100 grams)

Apples	90	54	-40%
Blueberries	100	54	-46%
Onions	40	2	-95%
Tomatoes	900	623	-31%
Corn	400	1.0	-400%
Broccoli	2,500	660.0	-74%
Strawberries	60	12.0	-80%

Vitamin C (mg per 100 grams)

Blueberries	14.0	9.7	-31%
Onions	10.0	6.4	-36%
Carrots	8.0	5.9	-26%
Potatoes	20.0	11.4	-43%
Green beans	19.0	16.3	-14%
Spinach	51.0	28.1	-45%
Corn	12.0	6.8	-44%
Broccoli	113.0	89.2	-21%
Kale	186.0	120.0	-35%
Strawberries	59.0	59.0	-0%

A simple barometer of the nutritional value of our diet is to look at the health of immigrants. We can look at what happens to people who leave their third world birth place and come to the U.S. for a new life. In a study published in the *Journal of the American Medical Association*, December 15, 2004, it was reported that, "The longer you live in America, the more likely you are to be obese." (Remember - obesity is a mineral deficiency disease - not a disease of excess)

The study examined the obesity rates among

immigrants compared with native born Americans. It found that immigrants, regardless of race or country of origin, living in the USA for more than 15 years resulted in an average of a 10 pound weight gain. These events are the result of being placed in the mineral deficient "Feedlot Syndrome" fostered by the American "four food group" mentality, combined with the loss of their historical "culinary" and garden ashes (plant minerals) without any conscious effort to take responsibility and supplement with plant minerals to replace the loss.

The most significant development in the trace element field of study in the last 50 years of the 20th century was the recognition that trace mineral elements have a fundamental role in health maintenance for humans and that optimal intakes from food sources can no longer be taken for granted.

Linus Pauling, two time Nobel laureate, and author of the great work, *The Nature of the Chemical Bond*, relegated minerals to secondary importance to vitamins, recommending only eight to eleven minerals (calcium, magnesium, phosphorous, iron, zinc, copper, manganese, chromium, molybdenum, iodine and selenium) and then only at minimal doses - an example was selenium for which he insisted the upper safe limit was 15 mcg (today the recommended safe limit for selenium is 200 to 1,000 mcg for an adult). Pauling died of prostate cancer at age 94 - a common result of a selenium deficiency.

The essential role of trace elements in the support and maintenance of the human immune system in its fight against bacteria, viruses, fungi and cancer, degenerative diseases and birth defects are well documented. The mode of action and the tissue concentrations of trace elements vary considerably. The only common denominator of trace minerals is that they are all found in exceedingly low levels in healthy tissue. They are usually present in levels of parts per million (ppm); micrograms/gram (u/g); or as low as parts per billion (ppb) or nanograms per gram (ng/g).

The concentration of trace elements in tissue or requirement levels does not represent their relative importance as an essential nutrient. The concentration of trace elements and their functional concentration must be continuously maintained within narrow physiological limits if the functional and structural fabric of the tissues and organs of the animal and human body are to be maintained for optimal fertility, development, growth, health, energy and longevity.

Higher species such as birds, mammals, and humans have a "homeostatic" mechanism that maintains tissue concentrations of trace minerals at optimal levels at their physiological sites at the cost of trace mineral reservoirs.

Almost all trace elements function as catalysts for a cellular or sub-cellular enzyme system. Enzymes are simply proteins that do work and in their role as catalysts their function ranges from that of a weak ionic (pH affects) modulator to highly specific metalloenzyme ("metallic finger") functions for DNA and RNA.

In metalloenzymes, the metal atom cannot normally be substituted by any other trace element. Although Vallee demonstrated that cobalt and cadmium can replace zinc in certain enzymes with some change in substrate specificity but the enzyme is not deactivated!

Because of the frequent wide disparity between the absolute and the dietary requirements (results from different intestinal absorption efficiencies for individuals and individual elements) the most efficient form of trace mineral supplement, such as plant derived colloidal minerals should be consciously and proactively consumed.

For the metallic form of iodine the ratio of absorption is almost 1:1; for iron its 1:10 and for chromium its 1:100.

The RDA (Recommended Daily Allowance) and RDI (Recommended Daily Intake) and other dietary recommendations for trace elements are conceived by the National Science Foundation to "meet the needs of practically all healthy people" - they are in reality not applicable for people with increased energy requirements, "health challenges" or full blown disease states.

More than 79 elements and minerals have been detected in animal and human tissue (i.e.- blood, liver, muscle, brain, bones, connective tissue, etc.) in the 20th and 21st centuries. Their presence in human tissue fulfills the first criteria for designating an element or mineral an "essential nutrient." Literally thousands of additional studies provide support for designating 60 of these 79 elemental nutrients to be essential nutrients.

These studies were performed on animals at every stage of life: pregnant, newborn, suckling, weanling, mature and aged. These studies were carried out on animals of virtually every description: laboratory mice, rats, rabbits, hamsters, guinea pigs, dogs cats, pigs, sheep, cattle, horses, primates, chickens, turkeys, ducks, hundreds of species of captive wild animals, etc.

Minerals are required by humans for building and maintaining structural components and enzymatic and biochemical cofactors that facilitate the physiological workings of the human cell, tissue, organ, system and body - nothing in the body can function without mineral cofactors.

On the average there are ten deficiency diseases that can occur in the absence of each essential mineral, others, like calcium can produce as many as 147 different diseases when the body is deficient.

Initial Depletion Phase

Initial depletion of trace elements in animals and humans is characterized by changes only in the metabolism of the element itself in response to a suboptimal intake, the individual target tissue compensating so that no disturbance of biological structure or function are detectable by means of a test. However, the individual usually complains of "lack of energy."

Increased intestinal absorption efficiency, and/or reduction in excretion; and gradual diminishment of body reserves occur. Pica, or the "munchies" appear in a mild form in this early stage of deficiency. This phase of trace mineral deficiency returns to normal (including the elimination of the "munchies") quickly following the return of an optimal intake.

Compensated Metabolic Phase

The compensated metabolic phase is characterized by a reduction of certain specific biochemical functions, such as trace mineral dependent enzyme reactions or receptor sites. The "homeostatic" mechanism becomes ineffective in maintaining the normal trace mineral concentrations at receptor sites causing a reduction in biochemical function (i.e. - low blood sugar, irregular heart beat, loss of hair color, weight gain, mild obesity, etc.). The "munchies" become consciously evident in the individuals everyday life - they become "chocoholics" or "cola addicts." Supplementation with minerals will, quickly reverse the symptoms, behavior changes, including pica, and the more extreme "munchies."

Decompensated Metabolic Phase

The decompensated phase of trace element deficiency is characterized by the appearance of serious clinical symptoms or defects in the metabolic (i.e. - pre-diabetes, significant weight gain, obesity), cognitive (i.e. - learning disabilities, ADD, ADHD, autism, etc.), emotional (i.e. - DR. Jykell/Mr. Hyde, "Bad Seeds," depression, manic depression, bipolar, anger, rage, anxiety attacks, panic attacks, etc.), developmental (i.e. - dyslexia, gay orientation, spina bifida, neural tube defects, cleft lip, cleft palate, heart defects, cerebral palsy, Downs Syndrome, etc.), structural (i.e. - muscular dystrophy, morbid obesity, etc.), fatigue and loss of work stamina and reduction of the longevity of a species (i.e. - average lifespan of an M.D. in the U.S. is 56 years of age).

Obsessive pica and the "munchies" are obvious, even to the casual observer - the affected individual is aware that they can not help themselves in curbing their cravings and appetites by means of conscious will alone.

Clinical Phase

The clinical phase of trace mineral deficiency is characterized by the onset of full blown disease states and even death (i.e. - cardiomyopathy, diabetes, aneurysm, arthritis, periodontal disease, degenerative disc disease, cataracts, goiter, morbid obesity, etc.). For most trace mineral deficiencies in the clinical phase, correct diagnosis by the "orthodox" physician is almost nonexistent; the cure, however, is accomplished simply by the replacement of the specific trace element.

A correct diagnosis can lead to a remarkably rapid positive clinical response ranging from 48 hours to 30 days for recognizable results; including the loss of one pound of excess weight per day on a proper mineral supplement program; others do not reach full return to normal after permanent biochemical (i.e. - gout), chromosomal (Downs Syndrome) or gross physical damage (i.e. - cataracts) has occurred.

Metallic Minerals

Metallic minerals include egg shell, oyster shell, calcium carbonate, limestone, coral calcium, dolomite, bentinite, inorganic mineral salts, sea water, Great Salt Lake minerals, mineral oxides (i.e. - iron oxide, copper oxide, zinc oxide, etc.), vortex waters, sea bed minerals, "soils" (which are usually clay), sea bed clay, clay, "rock flour," and various antacids such as Rollaids and Tums.

Typically, metallic minerals are found in tablets, powders, capsules and a few are found as liquids (i.e. - calcium gluconate solutions, zinc gluconate solutions, etc.), lactates, sulphates, carbonates, oxides, sea water, etc.

Metallic minerals, despite wild claims to the contrary are only 8 to 12% biologically available to younger animals and humans; after attaining the age of 35 to 40 years, the availability of metallic minerals for humans plummets to 3 to 5%.

A typical metallic mineral supplement, either alone or part of a multiple is calcium carbonate. Calcium carbonate can be purchased in 1,000 mg tablets or capsules, which breaks down to 400 mg of metallic calcium and 600 mg of carbonate. Two 1,000 mg calcium carbonate capsules or tablets do not give you 2,000 mg of calcium - they only supply 800 mg of elemental calcium and at a 10% availability rate you will net only 80 mg of available calcium. Therefore, to get 2,000 mg of usable calcium from a 1,000 mg capsule or tablet of calcium carbonate, you would have to take 25 capsules each day! A 100 capsule bottle of calcium carbonate will therefore only last 4 days.

Amounts of Metallic Calcium in a 1,000 mg Tablet

Calcium Source	Mg Available
Calcium gluconate	90
Calcium carbonate	400
Calcium acetate	230
Calcium citrate	210
Calcium lactate	140
Cow's milk (1,000 mg fluid)	10

Chelated Minerals

Chelated (Key-lay-ted) minerals were an invention of the livestock industry. In the 1940s, the livestock industry, to ensure maximum availability of dietary and supplemental minerals fed to livestock being fattened for market, created a new form of minerals.

The original chelating agent use was calcium EDTA, a man-made amino acid that was created by the Germans just prior to WWII to antidote arsenic and lead exposure in chemical warfare attacks (calcium EDTA is used today for intravenous chelation therapy to open up obstructed arteries).

The term chelated, from the Latin, literally means "claw," but in more modern times it is used to describe the process by which an amino acid, protein or enzyme (enzymes are proteins that do work) is wrapped around the mineral molecule which enhances the bioavailability of the metallic mineral.

Chelated minerals are approximately 40 to 65% bioavailable, a 400% increase over the availability of metallic minerals - certainly, a significant improvement over the amounts elemental minerals that are absorbed.

Chelated minerals are easily recognized on the label of a multiple vitamin/mineral supplements or free standing single supplement such as selenomethionine, chromium picolinate, or sometimes as an "amino acid chelate."

Colloidal Minerals

Colloidal (Koal-oid-ul) chemistry, while not a new concept, is not widely known about or understood by the general public. Simply said, a colloid refers to a substance that exists as ultra fine particles (Angstrom unit) that are suspended in a medium of different matter. The colloidal state is the state of a solute (mineral or other substance such as a paint pigment) in a solution when its molecules do not separate into atoms as with a true solution (sodium chloride or salt separates into separate sodium and chloride atoms while in solution), but rather the colloidal particle remains grouped together to form solute particles.

The presence of these inorganic colloidal particles, which are approximately one hundred-thousandth to one ten-millionth of a centimeter in diameter (about 400 thousandths to four millionths of an inch), can often be detected by means of an electron microscope. As a result of the grouping of the molecules, a solute in the colloidal state cannot passively pass through a suitable semi-permeable membrane and gives rise to a negligible osmotic pressure (they will pass through filter paper), depression of freezing point and elevation of boiling point effects.

These ultra-fine particles of the colloid are just barely larger than most molecules and are so small that they cannot be seen with the naked eye-about one billion of these colloid particles would fit into 0.01 cubic inch.

The "solution" part of a colloid provides a solid, gas or liquid medium in which the colloid particles are suspended. The suspended particles in a colloid can also be a solid, gas or liquid.

In 1925, H. Freudlich classified solutions into three categories:

1. True solutions

2. Colloidal solutions

3. Emulsions and suspensions

The four part method of classifying solutions is as follows:

1. Identify particle size

2. Determine the presence of Brownian movement (random movement of particles suspended in liquids or gases resulting from the impact of molecules of the fluid surrounding the particles).

3. Ability to pass through filter paper

4. Level of solubility

In 1975, S.S. Voyutsky (a Russian) wrote the classic text on colloidal chemistry. Voyutsky referred to solutions as "molecular dispersion systems" and "heterogeneous highly dispersed colloid systems."

The exact point between molecular and the colloidal degrees of dispersion cannot be established because the transition from molecularly dispersed systems to coarsely dispersed systems is a continuum.

A colloidal system must have three basic characteristics:

1. It must be heterogeneous (consists of dissimilar ingredients or constituents).

2. The system must be multi-phasic (i.e. - solid/liquid; gas/liquid, etc.)

3. The particles must be insoluble (do not dissolve in the solution).

Each one of these classifications interacts with the others to give colloids their unique qualities. The interesting thing about colloids is that they remain heterogeneous, multi-phasic and insoluble at different concentrations as long as a larger number if not all of the particles are within a range of sizes of colloids (1n to 100n) known as "nano-technology."

The molecular groups or particles of the colloid solute carry a resultant electrical charge, generally the same sign (negative) for all of the particles. A small percentage of these inorganic colloids will pass through the intestine of a living animal or human because a natural chelating process takes place in the gut in the presence of protein-containing food.

Inorganic colloidal material which readily passes through filter paper may be separated from dissolved substances, such as starch, sugar or salt, by placing the mixture of mineral colloid and non-colloid in a parchment shell surrounded by distilled water. The inorganic colloids are "too large" to pass through the membrane, but the molecules of salt, starch and sugar or any other dissolved substances pass readily through the semi-permeable membrane (they separate into individual atoms or very small molecules). This kind of separation process is referred to as "dialysis."

In the process of digestion, the inorganic minerals in food or supplements soon become inorganic colloids and as an inorganic colloid they cannot penetrate the intestinal wall to enter the blood stream. In the presence of amino acids, a small percentage of the inorganic colloids form chelated minerals and organic colloids which are able to be dialyzed through the mucus membranes of the intestinal walls into the blood stream - this bio-available mineral state is known as a "crystalloid."

Crystalloids or organic colloids readily pass through cell walls, while inorganic colloids are "too large." Additionally, we must remember that in the living organism there are other physiological forces at work, notably "active transport," which interferes with or modifies the expected osmotic phenomenon.

Active-transport, refers to the physical act of the intestinal mucosal cell reaching out with a pseudopodium, engulfing and transporting the particle into itself and then transported into the adjacent blood stream. In fact almost all absorbed food and nutrients are absorbed into the human body by active transport rather than by a passive trip through a semi-permeable membrane.

Colloidal mineral supplements and commercial colloids are found in four different forms:

1. Unprotected colloids are made of bare "rock flour," this is the form of inorganic colloids found in the sea bed minerals, clays, "soils," and "glacial milk." This form of inorganic colloid is in fact a metallic mineral and is only efficiently available to plants when there is a healthy soil population of bacteria and fungi.

2. The second type of mineral colloid is found in living systems of bacteria, fungi, green plants (food crops), animals and humans and is coated with a water-loving (hydrophyllic) substance such as gelatin, albuminoids or collagen. This coating protects the now "organic mineral colloid" and allows it to be a crystalloid for absorption, storage and physiological uses and thus maximizing its bioavailability up to 98%.

3. The third type of organic mineral colloids has a

protective coating of carbon with a molecular chain length of 10 to 12 carbon atoms. This type of colloid is also found in bacteria, fungi, plants (including some forms of petrified wood), animals and humans and is thought to be the most stable form of natural organic mineral colloid.

4. The fourth type of mineral colloid is not found in nature, but rather is manufactured industrially by coating the metallic colloid with sulfated castor oil (lipophyllic or fat or oil loving) to form commercial detergents.

The following list of elements and minerals is presented in alphabetical order according to the chemical symbols of each:

Ac- Actinium originates in igneous rocks and is usually found at extremely low concentrations of 5.5 x $10^{(-16)}$ ppm. Actinium is readily absorbed by plant roots, however, very little is transported to the stem, leaves, and shoots of the plant.

Actinium is a metal and like radium it glows in the dark. Its name is taken from the Greek word *aktinos,* which translates to "ray" or "beam."

There are 26 known isotopes of actinium and all are radioactive to some degree. Its chemical properties resemble those of the rare earth element lanthanum.

Actinium accumulates in and presumably has metabolic functions in the bones and liver.

Ag-Silver originates from igneous rocks and sedimentary rocks. It's found at the rate of 0.07 ppm in rocks, 0.01 ppm in soils, 0.00013 ppm in fresh water and 0.0003 ppm in sea water. It is present in marine algae at 0.25 ppm, land plants from 0.06 ppm to 1.4 ppm in accumulator plants growing near silver ore. *Epiogonum ovalifolium* is a silver accumulator and silver indicator plant.

Silver is found at 3.0 to 11.0 ppm in marine animals, 0.05 to 0.7 ppm in terrestrial mammals and at 0.16 to 0.8 ppm in muscle tissue. Even tortoise shell contains silver at 0.05 to 0.7 ppm.

Silver is one of the few metals found in its free state in nature and was known in ancient times and derives its chemical symbol, Ag, from the Latin word *argentums,* which translates to silver.

Silver has been used for money since biblical times and so it is often referred to as a "coinage" metal.

Silver has been employed in human health care and the search for immortality, since the time of the Chinese alchemist 8,000 B.C. Many feel that silver is in fact an essential element, not because it is required by an enzyme system, but rather because it serves as a systemic disinfectant and immune system stimulator.

Sir Malcom Morris reported in the *British Medical Journal* (May 12, 1917) that colloidal silver is free from the drawbacks of other preparations of silver, *viz*. pain caused and discoloration of the skin. Instead of producing irritation, it has a distinctly soothing effect. It rapidly subdues inflammation and promotes healing of the lesions. It can be used with remarkable results in enlarged prostate with irritation of the bladder, in pruritis ani and perineal eczema, and in hemorrhoids.

J. Mark Hovell reported in the *British Medical Journal* (December 15, 1917) that, "colloidal silver has been found to be beneficial for permanently restoring the patentcy of the Eustachian tubes and for reducing nasopharyngeal catarrh. Colloidal silver has also been used successfully in septic conditions of the mouth (including pyorrhea alveolysis - Rigg's disease), throat (including tonsillitis and quincies), ear (including Menier's symptoms and closure to Valsalva's inflation), and generalized septicemia, leucorrhea, cystitis, whooping-cough and shingles."

Taken internally, the particles of colloidal silver are resistant to the action of dilute acids and alkalis of the stomach and intestine. Consequently they continue their catalytic action and pass into the intestine unchanged.

T.H. Anderson Wells reported in *Lancet* (February 16, 1918) that a preparation of colloidal silver was "used intravenously in a case of puerperal septicemia without any irritation of the kidneys and with no pigmentation of the skin."

Silver sulfadiazine (Silvadene, Marion Laboratories) is used in 70% of the burn centers in America. Discovered by D. Charles Fox, Columbia University, silver sulfadiazine has been used successfully to treat syphilis, cholera, and malaria; it also stops the *Herpes simplex* virus responsible for cold sores and fever blisters.

Silver is an anti-bacterial, anti-viral, anti-fungal, anti-metabolite that disables specific enzymes that microorganisms use for respiration. Silver is such an efficient bactericide that our great-grandmothers put silver dollars into fresh milk to keep bacterial counts down and to keep it from spoiling at room temperature.

One of the most common uses of silver in orthodox medicine is in "silver fillings" in dentistry. A typical "filling" is a mix of silver powder and mercury. The silver dissolves in the mercury to form an "amalgam."

The mercury portion of the amalgam has been the subjects of many law suites because of its known toxic effects on the brain (selenium is the specific antidote for mercury poisoning).

Humans can consume 400 mg of silver per day. A silver "deficiency" results in an impaired immune system in *The Body Electric*, Dr. Robert Becker identified a relationship between low levels of tissue and dietary silver and the rate of illness. He stated, "Silver deficiency was responsible for the improper functioning of the immune system" and "silver does more than just kill disease causing organisms; it was also causing major growth stimulation (another criteria for essentiality) of injured tissue."

Human fibroblast (stem) cells were able to multiply at a greater rate, producing large numbers of primitive, embryonic cells in wounds. These stem cells are able to differentiate into whatever cell types that are necessary to heal the wound or replace tissue mass.

Dr. Bjorn Nordstrom of the Carolinska Institute, Sweden has used silver in his alternative cancer therapy programs. According to *Science Digest* (Silver: Our Mightiest Germ Fighter. March, 1978) silver is an antibiotic. Silver kills over 650 disease-causing organisms. Resistant strains fail to develop as they do with prescribed antibiotics. Silver is absolutely non-toxic to humans at standard rates of consumption. CAUTION: chronic overdoses can cause a whole body tattoo that produces a permanent dusky blue discoloration of the skin.

Al-Aluminum is found in igneous rocks at 5,000 ppm, 82,000 ppm in shales, 25,000 ppm in sandstone, 4,200 ppm in limestone, and 71,000 ppm in clay. Aluminum represents 12% of the earth's crust and is the third most abundant element in the earth's crust and the most abundant metal in the earth's crust. Aluminum is nontoxic and is found in high concentrations in all plants grown in the soil, including common organically grown food crops such as beans, tomatoes, squash, apples, bananas, tea, wine, rice, oats, buckwheat and wheat. Aluminum is found in large biological quantities in every plant grown in the soil. You can't eat any grain, vegetable, fruit, or nut or drink any natural water source or juice without taking in large quantities of aluminum.

The aluminum found in plants is organically bound colloidal aluminum and appears not to have any negative or toxic affect and in fact appears to meet all of the requirements to be designated an essential nutrient.

Acid soils yield the highest amounts of soil aluminum to plants. Aluminum is found in marine plants at 60 ppm and is especially high in plankton and red algae. Aluminum is found in terrestrial plants at an average of 500 ppm, with a range of 0.5 to 4,000 ppm. It is found in marine mammals at 19 to 50 ppm. In mammals, the highest levels are found in hair and lungs.

Aluminum is found naturally in significant levels in all healthy plant based foods grown in soil including grains, vegetables, nuts and fruit. The amount of aluminum in infant formulas averages 0.9 mg/kg of body weight per week for milk based formulas and 1.1 mg/kg of body weight per week for soy-based infant formulas. Some soy-based infant formulas contain four times the average levels found in the survey which was conducted and reported July 16, 2008 by European scientists who were rerunning a 2007 report that had been published by WHO.

Aluminum's known biological function is to activate the enzyme succinic dehydrogenase. Deficiencies of aluminum created in laboratory diets results in congenital limb defects (non-genetic birth defects) in laboratory animals and cirrhosis of the liver in mature animals. Aluminum supplementation increases the survival rates of newborns, and according to professor Gerhard Schrauzer, former professor and chairman of the department of chemistry at UCSD, is "probably an essential mineral for human nutrition."

A single faulty study over 35 years ago suggested a link between chronic aluminum exposure and Alzheimer's disease. In a subsequent study that appeared November 5, 1992 in the journal *Nature,* Frank Watt, et al (Oxford University) used a highly accurate technique to quantify the levels of aluminum in the brains of Alzheimer's patients. To their surprise, they found the same levels of aluminum in the brains of the non-Alzheimer's controls as they did in their Alzheimer's patients. The June 1997 issue of the *Berkley Newsletter* reported that there is no link between Alzheimer's disease and aluminum.

In November 2007, the Federal Institute for Risk Assessment issued an updated opinion on the risk of developing Alzheimer's through consuming food with aluminum in it, and they maintained that there is no scientific proof of any risk of developing Alzheimer's disease from the consumption of aluminum found in consumer products.

Am-Americum is a radioactive isotope and has a half life of 7,950 years. Americum is a transition element, one of the elements that follows uranium in the periodic chart. Like all of the transition elements, it is a man made element. Americum was discovered in 1944 by Glenn T. Seaborg at the Metallurgical Laboratory at the University of Chicago, a laboratory that became the Argonne National Laboratory.

Americum-241 emits both alpha particles (helium nuclei) and gamma rays (similar to X rays) and has a half-life of 470 years. It is used in home smoke detectors, in which alpha particles emitted by this isotope ionize the surrounding air by stripping electrons from gas molecules. Ionized air is a relatively good conductor of electricity; smoke particles in the air reduce its electrical conductivity and generate a signal that sets off the alarm.

Americum accumulates in mammalian bone.

Ar-Argon is found in igneous rocks at 3.0 to 5.0 ppm and can be used to date ancient rocks using the potassium/argon dating system. It is found in fresh water and sea water at 0.06 ppm and mammalian blood at 0.75 ppm and constitutes about one percent of the earth's atmosphere making it the third most abundant gas in the air. Argon is a "noble" gas that is chemically inert, is colorless and odorless.

In the year 2000, a group of Finnish researchers demonstrated that in spite of its lack of chemical reactivity it was possible to combine argon with fluorine and hydrogen and form fluorohydride, or HArF.

Argon, discovered in 1894 by the English physicist Lord Rayleigh and the Scottish chemist William Ramsay, was the first noble gas to be identified. Rayleigh was awarded the 1904 Nobel Prize in physics for the discovery. They identified the new element by means of the light it gave off when an electrical discharge was passed through the gas. They called it argon, translated from the Greek word *argos*, meaning "lazy" or "inactive."

Argon gas is used to fill incandescent bulbs to prevent corrosion of the tungsten filament; it is used in the detector probe of Geiger counters to detect radiation; and it is the decay product of an important radioisotope used for dating rock samples. The isotope is potassium-40, a naturally occurring radioactive isotope with an extremely long half-life of 1.25 billion years. Argon is formed as the product of the disintegration of the radioactive potassium - the potassium-argon dating system. Because potassium is present in many rocks, an analysis of the amount of argon present in the rock will effectively reveal the date at which the rock solidified.

As-Arsenic is found in igneous rock at 0.0 to 8.0 ppm, shale at 13.0 ppm, sandstone and limestone at 1.0 ppm, fresh water at 0.0004 ppm, seawater at 0.003 ppm, and soils at 6.0 ppm. Argentina and New Zealand actually have toxic levels of arsenic in some soil regions. Arsenic also accumulates in marine plants at the rate of 30.0 ppm, terrestrial plants at 0.02 ppm, marine animals at 0.005 to 0.3 ppm and terrestrial animals at a rate of less than 0.2 ppm with the arsenic concentrating in the hair and nails.

Arsenic is often thought of as a semimetal or metalloid. Although a small quantity of arsenic does occur in nature in its free form, most arsenic is found in a number of mineral compounds such as realgar and orpiment - both compounds are mixes of arsenic and sulfur. The history of arsenic dates back to ancient China, the Greeks and Romans. Its name is thought to have been derived from the Latin *arsenicum* for orpiment, a common, widely used gold-like yellow pigment.

Arsenic was determined to be an essential nutrient in 1947; the French Academy first identified arsenic in dead human bodies in 1834. Arsenic normally appears in human female blood at 0.64 ppm. Levels rise to 0.93 ppm during menstruation and 2.20 ppm during months five and six of pregnancy. At 90 to 120 ppm, arsenic promotes and enhances the growth rate of chicks. The rate of growth and metamorphosis of tadpoles is enhanced by the presence of arsenic as well.

Compound "606," an arsenic containing compound (arsphenamine) was developed in 1910 by Paul Ehrlich, the German scientist, for the successful treatment and cure of syphilis.

Arsenic in combination with the B-vitamin choline prevents 100% of perosis ("slipped tendon") in poultry. Arsenic deficiency in humans results in a "carpal tunnel syndrome," "TMJ," and other "repetitive motion" type degenerative joint diseases and minute traces stimulate the production of red blood cells.

According to the Memorial Sloan-Kettering Cancer Center in New York, "infusions of arsenic works better than any other drug for the treatment of certain types of leukemia." Their study involved 12 seriously ill patients suffering from acute promyelocytic leukemia (APL).

In the November 5, 1998 issue of The *New England Journal of Medicine*, Dr. Raymond Worrel Jr. stated, "We now know that arsenic can safely bring patients with APL into remission, which may ultimately give them a second chance at life."

Eleven of the 12 patients went into remission within 12 to 39 days after starting the arsenic therapy - eight, of the original APL test group, were still in "remission" ten years after the therapy began. "Based on highly sensitive test results, treatment with arsenic appears to exceed the effectiveness of any single drug to treat APL," said Dr. Steven Soignet, lead author of the study.

Arsenic metabolism is affected by tissue and blood levels of zinc, selenium, arginine, choline, methionine, taurine and quaniacetic acid, all of which affect methyl-group metabolism and polyamine synthesis which is the site of arsenic function in human physiology.

At-Astatine has 20 known radioactive isotopes with an extremely short half-life of 7.2 to 8.0 hours. The isotope with the shortest half-life is astatine-210 with a half-life of 8.3 hours.

Astatine was first made in 1940 by a team of radiochemists from the University of California at Berkeley. They produced astatine by bombarding bismuth with alpha particles. They named the element from the Greek word *astatos,* which translates to "unstable."

Astatine is a member of the halogen family so that it is not surprising that its chemical character is similar to that of iodine; its physical characteristics are more metallic than those of iodine.

Small quantities of astatine are produced naturally as the decay products of isotopes of uranium and thorium. The total amount of astatine estimated to be present in the earth's crust at any one time is estimated to be one ounce.

Astatine is accumulated by the mammalian and human thyroid following ingestion, however, little is retained and it is rapidly excreted.

Au-Gold is found in igneous and sedimentary rocks at 0.004 ppm, fresh water at 0.00006 ppm, sea water at 0.000011 ppm, marine plants at 0.012 ppm, terrestrial plants 0.005 to 0.002 ppm, marine animals at 0.0003 to 0.008 ppm, terrestrial animals at 0.00023 ppm, and in mammalian liver gold forms a colloid.

Gold is considered the most precious of all metals and was used in conjunction with silver and mercury by the ancient Chinese alchemist 8,000 B.C. to provide "immortality". In its pure state, gold is one of the most beautiful of elements. With its bright yellow color and its resistance to corrosion, it has been highly prized since ancient times. Its chemical symbol, Au, comes from the Latin word aurum, which translates to "shining dawn." It has even older origins, coming from the Sanskrit word *jval* and the Anglo-Saxon word *gold,* both meaning "gold."

In nature, gold is usually found as a pure metal, most often in the form of nuggets, flakes or "dust." It also occurs in veins of pure gold or in deposits of a class of minerals called tellurides. It is widely distributed around the world and is always found near deposits of quartz and pyrite.

Gold dissolves in mercury to form an amalgam, or alloy of mercury and gold - this gold-mercury amalgam is used by dentist to fill teeth. A radioactive isotope of gold with a short half-life of 2.7 days is used to treat some forms of cancer. Known as gold-198, it is easily produced by exposing natural gold to a beam of neutrons in a nuclear reactor.

Gold will dissolve very slowly in the solution of hydrochloric and nitric acids that was called "aqua regia" by the alchemists because of its ability to dissolve the king of metals.

Gold concentrates in the horsetail plant (*Equisetum arvense*). Gold compounds (gold sodium thiomalate, gold thioglucose also known as aurothioglucose) are frequently administered by orthodox physicians as an add-on therapy with salicylates (aspirin) for arthritis when added pain relief is required. Gold has been reported only to be effective against active joint inflammation and is not usually helpful for treating advanced destructive rheumatoid arthritis.

B-Boron is found in igneous rocks at 10 ppm, shale at 100 ppm, sandstone at 35 ppm, limestone at 20 ppm, fresh water at 0.013 ppm, seawater at 4.0 to 6.0 ppm, soil from 2.0 to 100 ppm (highest levels are found in saline and alkaline soils), marine plants 120 ppm (highest levels found in brown algae), terrestrial plants at 150 ppm (chenopodiaceae and plumboginaceae are indicator plant families), marine animals at 20 to 50 ppm, and terrestrial animals at 0.5 ppm.

Boron is a scarce element, making up only 0.0003% of the earth's crust. In its pure state, it is a brownish crystal that is almost as hard a diamond. Boron was first isolated in 1808 by the

English chemist Sir Humphry Davy and two French chemists, Joseph Louis Gay-Lussac and Louis-Jacques Thenard.

Boron is never found in its pure form in nature. Boron is commonly found in combination with oxygen, water and sodium in a compound called borax. Boric acid is another important boron compound. It is made by heating borax with either hydrochloric or sulfuric acid. Boric acid is a weak acid that has an antiseptic property and is commonly used as a wound disinfectant and an eye wash.

Boron is essential for bone metabolism including the efficient use of calcium and magnesium and proper function of endocrine glands (i.e. - ovaries, testes and adrenals).

Pure boron is hard and gray and melts at over 4,000 degrees F. Boron is a non-metallic mineral, occurs as a combination in nature (i.e. - borax, boric acid or sassolite, ulexite, colemanite, boracite, and tourmaline).

Prior to 1981, boron was not considered an essential nutrient. Boron was first shown to be an essential mineral for growing chicks. It was not until 1990 that boron was accepted as an essential nutrient for humans.

Boron is required for the maintenance of bone density and normal blood levels of estrogen and testosterone. Within eight days of supplementing boron, women lost 40% less calcium, 33% less magnesium, and less phosphorus through their urine. Women receiving boron supplements had blood levels of estradiol 17B doubled to "levels found in women on estrogen replacement therapy." Levels of testosterone also double in both men and women following boron supplementation.

Industrially, boron is used to make a special heat-resistant type of glass, known as borosilicate glass, which usually carries the commercial name of Pyrex™. The most common use of Pyrex™ is in the kitchen, where Pyrex™ glass baking dishes and measuring cups are used because they can withstand rapid changes in temperature without cracking.

Ba-Barium is found in igneous rocks at 425 ppm, shale at 580 ppm, sandstone at 50 ppm, limestone at 120 ppm, fresh water at 0.054 ppm, sea water at 0.03 ppm, soil at 500 ppm, marine plants at 30 ppm (highest levels in brown algae), terrestrial plants at 14 ppm (the fruit of *Bertholletia excelea* can have up to 4,000 ppm), marine animals 0.2 to 3.0 pm (highest levels in hard tissues such as bone and shell), and terrestrial animals at up to 75 ppm (highest levels found in bone, lung and eyes).

Barium is an abundant element, ranking sixth in abundance of the elements making up the earth's crust. It is found in the minerals witherite, a barium carbonate ($BaCO_3$), and barite, a barium sulfate ($BaSO_4$). Barium was discovered by Sir Humphry Davy, the English chemist in 1808.

Radiologists use barium sulfate to facilitate the examination of a patient's gastrointestinal tract with X-rays. Barium sulfate is a very dense salt that is opaque to X-rays. When a patient drinks a suspension of barium sulfate in water or is given a barium enema, consisting of a similar suspension, the barium sulfate particles temporarily fill all of the hollow organs of the gastrointestinal tract. As the barium sulfate absorbs X-rays and blocks their transmission, the gastrointestinal organs will be clearly outlined in white in an X-ray film.

Barium was considered essential for mammals in 1949.

Be-Beryllium is found in igneous rocks at 2.0 to 8.0 ppm, in shale at 3.0 ppm, sandstone and limestone at < 0.1 ppm, fresh water at 0.001 ppm, sea water at 0.0000006 ppm, soil at 0.001 ppm, marine plants (highest levels in brown algae), terrestrial plants at < 0.1 ppm (highest in plants grown in volcanic soils), and terrestrial animals at 0.0003 to 0.002 ppm in soft tissue.

Beryllium heads the group of elements known as the "alkaline-earth" metals. The most abundant elements in this group are calcium and magnesium, but they all share common chemical and physical properties. Even though several forms of beryllium are found in the earth's crust, it is a relatively rare element, ranking only 32nd in order of the abundance of the elements.

Beryllium in its pure state is a fairly hard, gray-white metal. It is one of the lightest of the metals, however, it is hard enough to scratch glass. As with all the alkaline-earth group, beryllium is much too chemically reactive to be found in its free state. It readily reacts with oxygen and many other elements.

The mineral known as beryl is actually a complex compound of beryllium, silicon, aluminum and oxygen. Its scientific name is beryllium aluminum silicate. Beryllium was discovered in 1798 by the French chemist Louis-Nicolas Vauquelin, while comparing the structures of beryl and emerald

The mineral beryl is the most common source of beryllium. Beryllium was formerly known as "glucinium" because beryllium, like many of its compounds, has a sweet taste.

Crystals of this valuable mineral have been collected and used for jewelry for thousands of years. Both emerald (green) and aquamarine (blue) gemstones are naturally occurring forms of beryl. Gemstones, including emeralds, have been used as sources of exotic minerals in Ayurvedic and Egyptian medicine for thousands of years.

Inhalation of beryllium oxide dust (mining and industrial contaminants) can lead to "berylliosis," a painful and sometimes fatal lung disease.

Bi-Bismuth is found in igneous rocks at 0.17 ppm, shale at 1.0 ppm, sea water at 0.000017 ppm, terrestrial plants at 0.06 ppm, marine animals at 0.09 ppm, and terrestrial animals at 0.004 ppm.

Bismuth is a white, heavy, brittle metal that has a slight yellow cast. Bismuth has been known in the West since the early 15th century; it was often confused with tin or lead.

Claude Geoffroy the Younger, a French Nobleman is credited with its identification in 1753.

Bismuth has been used by the Chinese alchemist to treat gastric ulcers and gastroenteritis for more than 8,000 years; today it is used for over-the-counter GI remedies (Pepto Bismol™) and as a filler, "glitter" and "shimmer" in many cosmetics.

Stress has historically been blamed as the boogy-man as the cause of gastric, peptic, and duodenal ulcers. Animal and human studies have in fact demonstrated that the true cause of ulcers is an infection with a bacterium known as *Helicobacter pylori*.

Australian gastroenterologist Barry Marshall, M.D. and pathologist J. Robin Warren proposed their theory for the bacterial cause of gastric ulcers in 1983. The bacterial cause (*H. pylori*) for gastric ulcers was known in pigs in 1952.

The treatment of choice for gastric ulcers is a course of tetracycline antibiotics, antacids, and bismuth subsalicylate for two to four weeks. You've heard of bismuth used for treating stomach and intestinal disorders if you have ever heard of a pink liquid with the name of Pepto Bismol™.

Br-Bromine is a "halogen" related to iodine. It is found in igneous rocks at 3.0 to 5.0 ppm, shale at 4.0 ppm, sandstone at 1.0 ppm, limestone at 0.2 ppm, fresh water at 0.2 ppm, sea water at 65 ppm, soil at 5.0 ppm, marine plants at 740 ppm (highest levels in brown algae), terrestrial plants at 15 ppm, marine animals at 60 to 1,000 ppm, and terrestrial animals at 6.0 ppm.

Bromine functions in its active form as brominated amino acids. In its pure form, bromine is a diatomic molecule (two bromine atoms) that is a reddish liquid. Bromine and mercury are the only two elements that are liquids at room temperature.

Bromine was discovered by a young French student, Antoine-Jerome Balard, in 1826. He first isolated the element by adding chlorinated water to the brackish water found in the salt marshes near Montpellier, a city in southern France. The addition of the chlorine turned the water brownish. The cause of the color change was found to be a new element that the French Academy named bromine, taken from the Greek word *bromos*, which translates to "stench."

Sodium bromide, a salt of bromine, is a mild sedative that was commonly used in the late 19th and early 20th centuries. People still speak of taking a "bromide" to calm down and ease stress and tension.

There is strong evidence for Bromine's essentiality in mammals and humans.

C-Carbon is found in igneous rocks at 200 ppm, shale at 15,300 ppm, sandstone at 13,800 ppm, limestone at 113,500 ppm, fresh water at 11 ppm, sea water at 28 ppm, soils at 20,000 ppm (up to 90% of the carbon in soil is bound in the humus), marine plants at 345,000 ppm, terrestrial plants at 454,000 ppm, marine animals at 400,000 ppm, and in terrestrial animals at 465,000 (280,000 ppm in bone).

Carbon comprises only 0.09% of the earth's crust by mass, however, it is the element most essential for life on our planet. When we examine the molecules that make up the cells, tissues, organs and bodies of animals and tissues of plants we see that almost all contain carbon. Organic chemistry is the chemistry of organic compounds. Carbon is the center of the "organic" world because of its ability link with other carbon atoms to form long chains that are straight and linear or branched. These carbon chains act as a spine to which other elements are attached, producing an almost endless number of possible carbon-containing molecules.

An example of a well known long-chain carbon molecule is deoxyribonucleic acid, or DNA, found in the genetic material of all living organisms, plant and animal. DNA stores information for the construction of an immense number of proteins manufactured by plant and animal cells, and it can replicate or copy itself. Found in the nuclei of all plant and animal cells, DNA is essential for the reproduction of living organisms.

In addition to its occurrence in organic compounds, carbon also exists in its free state in nature, where it is found in several different physical forms. When an element exists in several different physical forms it is referred to as an allotrope.

In the case of carbon allotropes, it is found as diamond - the hardest of all materials. Carbon is also found as graphite and coal. The atoms of carbon in graphite are arranged in layers, like the pages of a book. Because the bonds between these layers are weak, the layers easily slide over one another, causing graphite to be soft and slippery which makes graphite useful as a lubricant and as a marking material in pencils.

In 1985, a new allotrope form of carbon was created in the laboratory of Harold W. Kroto at the University of Sussex in Brighton, England, and Richard E. Smalley at Rice University in Houston, Texas, using laser beams to vaporize graphite. They named the new allotrope carbon molecule buckminsterfullerene after the American architect Buckminster Fuller, who became famous for designing geodesic dome structures that resembled soccer balls ("buckyballs").

Coal, primarily a mixture of carbon and more than 77 minerals, contains carbon in a noncrystalline form. It is a major source of "solar income" energy for industry and domestic use. Like oil and natural gas, coal is considered a "fossil fuel" because it is the product of the decay of plants and animals over hundreds of millions of years. Hard or anthracite coal is the older form of coal and is thought to be approximately 250 million years old - it contains 80% carbon. Bituminous or soft coal contains only about 40 to 50% carbon, and is the younger form of coal.

The 1991 data from the United States Department of Energy shows that 23.2% of the energy used in the United

States comes from coal, approximately 40% from petroleum, and 24% from natural gas. Fossil fuels provide 90% of the total energy consumed in the U.S.

Industrial, automotive and home use of carbon fuels and respiration of vertebrates and many microorganisms produce large amounts of carbon dioxide (CO_2) as a byproduct.

Carbon dioxide has, since the beginning of time, influenced the temperature of the earth by a process called the "greenhouse effect." Like the glass roof of the green house carbon dioxide allows the "solar income" to pass through the atmosphere and reach the earth's surface - this is essentially a one way event that traps heat in the earth's crust.

While many individuals and organizations, want to blame man's activities and pitifully small biomass for "global warming," we must look to the past for the cycles of Ice Ages and "global warming" that have taken place over and over through the millennia to understand the cyclic nature of these events. The proven method of delaying and/or reducing the "global warming" effects of our times is to simply plant more trees and let the trees convert the CO_2 into oxygen (O_2) and water (H_2O)!

Carbon functions as an essential structural element for all living organisms and organic molecules (i.e.- carbohydrates, fats, amino acids, vitamins, enzymes, etc.).

Carbohydrates & Sugars

In modern times, carbohydrates commonly furnish most of the energy required to move, perform work and for all of the basic biochemical functions of life itself. While carbohydrates and sugars are convenient sources of fuel for energy, they are not essential nutrients as all living organisms can make them by reconfiguring proteins and fats.

The chief sources of dietary carbohydrates include

grains, vegetables, fruits and sugars (i.e. - honey, molasses). Carbohydrates in their simplest form have the formula CH_2O. Hydrogen and oxygen are present in the same ratio that is found in water with one carbon for each molecule of water.

By using the sun's light energy, the carbon dioxide from the air and the chlorophyll dependent process known as photosynthesis, plants are able to manufacture carbohydrates (sugar and starch), vitamins, amino acids, and fatty acids.

To manufacture carbohydrates, plants take CO_2 and H_2O and subject them to a photochemical process known as photosynthesis. In the presence of chlorophyll, a magnesium/carbon ring structure, carbohydrate is produced using the energy from sunlight - O_2 is released to the atmosphere as a by-product of the reaction.

Carbohydrates are classified as monosaccharides (glucose or "grape sugar," fructose, etc.), disaccharides (sucrose = glucose and fructose; maltose = glucose and glucose; lactose = glucose and galactose), oligosaccharides, and polysaccharides (starch, dextrin, fiber, cellulose, and glycogen or "animal starch" are all complexes of glucose units).

Lipids & Fats

Lipids or fats, like carbohydrates, are composed of carbon, hydrogen and oxygen. Fats have the common property of being insoluble in water, soluble in organic solvents such as ether and chloroform, and can be utilized as energy by living organisms.

Fats, as a group of carbon compounds, include ordinary fats, oils, waxes, and unrelated compounds. The primary food sources of lipids are butter, flax seed oil, olive oil, animal fat, nuts, seeds, whole grains, olives, avocados, egg yolks, dairy, etc. Fats serve as a source of immediate or stored energy. A gram of fat contains nine calories per gram compared with 4.5 calories per gram of carbohydrate or protein.

Triglycerides (the primary component of fats and oils) are composed of carbon, hydrogen, and oxygen. Structurally, they are esters of a trihydric alcohol (glycerol) and fatty acids. The fatty acids can have from four to 30 carbon atoms and constitute the bulk of the triglyceride mass. One hundred grams of fat or oil will contain 95 grams of fatty acids.

A fatty acid or hydrocarbon chain is described with regard to three characteristics: chain length, degree of "saturation" with hydrogen, and location of the first "double bond."

The length is a reference to the number of carbon atoms in the chain (i.e. - C:16 has 16 carbons in the chain). The terms "short chain" (less than 6 carbons), "medium chain" (7 to 11 carbons), and "long chain" (12 or more carbons) are used to describe the chains of fatty acids in the structure of triglycerides.

The degree of hydrogen "saturation" in fatty acids is defined by the number of "double bonds" between carbon atoms in the fatty acid chains. A fatty acid chain can contain all the hydrogen it can hold and have no double bonds, in which case, it is referred to as a "saturated" fatty acid. It can contain one double bond (monounsaturated fatty acid) or it may contain several double bonds (polyunsaturated fatty acids).

The location of the first double bond as counted from the "tail" or the methyl end of the fatty acid is referred to as the "omega" number (i.e. - omega-3, omega-6, etc.).

Three polyunsaturated fatty acids (linoleic, linolenic, and arachidonic acids) are essential fatty acids (EFA). Three percent of the total daily calorie intake must be from the EFA - as essential fatty acids, they are required for life but cannot be manufactured. However, only two of the EFA (linoleic and linolenic) are truly regarded as essential because arachidonic acid can be synthesized by humans from linolenic acid when it is present in optimal amounts.

Essential Fatty Acids have essential vitamin-like functions in fat transport and metabolism, and in maintaining the integrity of cell walls (bilipid layer membranes). They are also part of the fatty acids of cholesterol esters and phospholipids in plasma lipoproteins and mitochondrial lipoproteins.

Serum cholesterol can be lowered by the consumption of EFA. EFAs are also the raw material for the human body to manufacture prostaglandins that help regulate blood pressure, heart rate, vascular dilation, blood clotting, bronchial dilation, and central nervous system (brain and spinal cord) function. EFA deficiency in human infants results in a poor growth rate, lowered IQ, seizures, learning disabilities, eczema, asthma, and a lowered resistance to infectious diseases.

Cholesterol is a member of a large group of fats known as sterols. They all have a complex carbon ring structure. Cholesterol is an essential part of the structure of cell walls, brain and spinal cord (myelin), the raw material for the production of vitamin D in the human body, bile acids, adrenal cortical hormones, estrogens (a cholesterol deficiency makes menopause a living hell), progesterone, and testosterone (a cholesterol deficiency will turn hubby into a TV watching steer who is totally disinterested in sex).

Proteins

Proteins, like carbohydrates and fats, contain carbon, hydrogen and oxygen. In addition they also contain 16% nitrogen (the amine group) sometimes in conjunction with other elements such as phosphorus, iron, sulfur and cobalt. The basic structural unit of a protein is the amino acid. Amino acids are united by "peptide bonds" into long chains of various geometric structures to form specific protein. Digestion of proteins breaks the peptide bonds to release individual amino acids.

Classically there are nine essential amino acids that are required in the daily diet as they cannot be manufactured by the human body. Forty-three percent of the dietary protein for human infants must contain the essential amino acids. Growing children require 36% essential amino acids and adults require 19% for maintenance.

To the classic list of essential amino acids, we would add arginine, taurine, and tyrosine. Over the long haul, these three amino acids help prevent certain specific diseases, respectively, these diseases are cancer and PAD, macular degeneration and goiter.

Essential Amino Acids

Amino Acid	Function
Valine	Protein synthesis
Lysine	Protein synthesis
Threonine	Protein synthesis
Leucine	Protein synthesis
Isoleucine	Protein synthesis
Tryptophane	Precursor of niacin and serotonin
Phenylalanine	Precursor of thyroxin and epinephrine
Methionine	Synthesis of choline and creatine phosphate
Histidine	Synthesis of histamine
Arginine	Cancer risk, PAD
Taurine	Macular degeneration
Tyrosine	Synthesis of thyroxin

Use of protein for fuel to provide energy in place of carbohydrate provides 4.5 calories per gram.

An individual consuming protein at even 300 gm per day (almost 3/4 of a pound of meat a day) will have no adverse effects as long as they do not have kidney or liver disease and supplement properly with vitamins and minerals.

Proteins are the fundamental structural components of the living cell (cytoplasm). They are essential parts of the cell nucleus and protoplasm. Proteins are the most abundant of all carbon containing organic compounds in the human body. The greatest mass of body protein is found in the skeletal muscle, the remainder is found in other organs (liver, kidney, hear, stomach, etc.), bones, teeth, blood, and other body fluids (lymph). Enzymes are proteins that do work to facilitate chemical reactions in the body (energy production and utilization, hormone production, nerve impulses, etc.)

Vitamins

Vitamins are a major carbon group of unrelated essential organic carbon compounds needed by the human body in minute quantities each day. They are essential for specific metabolic reactions of the cell and are required for normal growth, development, maintenance, health, longevity and life itself.

Vitamins function as coenzymes or activating side groups for essential subcellular enzyme systems. Vitamins regulate metabolism, facilitate the conversion of carbohydrate, fat and protein to energy, and are required for the formation and repair of tissues in embryos, children, teens, adults, and seniors. Vitamins are essential nutrients in that, they can not be manufactured by humans; they do not supply calories or contribute to body mass.

There are three classifications of vitamins:

1) Fat soluble - A, D, E, and K - Fat soluble vitamins, as the name implies, function in fat (lipid) metabolism in human cells. Fat soluble vitamins can not be absorbed from the intestine when we eat low fat diets. People who have their gall bladders removed should supplement with ox bile to increase the availability of bile salts which are required for the efficient absorption of essential fatty acids, good fats (triglycerides, cholesterol, etc.) and fat soluble vitamins.

2) Water soluble - B-complex, biotin, choline and vitamin C - Water soluble vitamins consists of 10 separate water soluble B vitamins and vitamin C. In general they function as essential nutrients in the metabolic processes of all living cells by acting as cofactors in multiple enzyme systems that drive the oxidation of food and production of energy.

3) Flavanols - Epicatechins and polyphenols - Flavanols and bioflavonoids (polyphenols/epicatechins) are part of a large family of compounds that are generally regarded as a third category of vitamins - fat soluble vitamins, water soluble vitamins and flavanol vitamins.

Flavanols found in dark chocolate, participate in maintaining the strength of capillaries, lower blood pressure, improve blood flow via increased production of nitric acid (a molecule used by the vascular endothelium to signal the surrounding muscle to relax) and have vitamin C-like functions.

Taking optimal levels of essential vitamins goes a long way to preventing birth defects and solving the problems of reduced physical effectiveness and many debilitating degenerative diseases.

Ca-Calcium is found in igneous rocks at 41,500 ppm, shale at 22,100 ppm, sandstone at 39,100, limestone at 302,000 ppm, fresh water at 15 ppm, sea water at 400 ppm, soils at 7,000 to 500,000 ppm (lowest in acid soils and highest in limestone or alkaline soils), marine plants at 10,000 to 300,000 ppm (highest in calcarious tissue, - red, blue-green and green algae and diatoms), terrestrial plants at 18,000 ppm, marine animals at 1,500 to 20,000 ppm (350,000 ppm in calcarious tissue - sponges, coral, mollusks and echinoderms), terrestrial animals at 200 to 85,000 ppm (260,000 ppm in mammalian bone, 200 to 500 ppm in soft tissue and 5 ppm or less in red blood cells). The metal, calcium, was isolated in 1808 by Sir Humphry Davy.

Calcium is an extremely active element and is not found in a pure form in nature. It reacts with water to form calcium hydroxide ($Ca(OH)_2$) and with the atmospheric oxygen to form calcium oxide (CaO). Pure calcium metal is hard and has the characteristic silvery-white color of all the alkaline-earth metals.

In the 1st century, the Romans used a compound of calcium they called calx (lime) in Latin.

Calcium is essential for all living organisms and is found in the cell walls of plants, in all calcareous tissues, and mammalian bones and teeth. Calcium also helps to regulate electrochemical functions in cells and is a required cofactor necessary to activate several enzymes.

Calcium is the fifth most abundant mineral element in the earth's crust and biosphere. There is evidence that clearly shows humans are designed to consume and use high calcium diets. The late Paleolithic period of 35,000 to 10,000 years ago was the most recent time that our human forebears lived in the environment for which they had been biochemically designed.

The agricultural revolution occurred 10,000 years ago and it reduced the wide variety of wild foods in the human food chain while increasing food energy (calories). These dietary changes universally and forever decreased man's dietary intake of minerals, trace minerals and rare earths. The uncultivated food plants and wild game commonly available to Stone Age humans would supply 1600 mg of calcium at basal energy intakes and between 2,000 and 3,000 mg of calcium at the energy levels required to support hunting and work.

During the 20th century, American adults had a calcium intake of only one-fifth to one-third as much as did Stone Age humans. The National Health & Nutrition Examination Survey II reported a median calcium intake for American women of between 300 and 508 mg per day and only 680 mg for men.

Common Calcium Deficiency Diseases

Osteoporosis (osteopenia)
Peripheral neuropathies
Kyphosis
Dowager's hump
Lordosis
Legg-Perthe's disease
Compression fractures
Spontaneous fractures
Receding gums
Periodontal disease
Osteomalacia
Osteoarthritis
Degenerative arthritis
Ankylosing spondylitis
Hypertension (glaucoma)
Insomnia
Kidney stones

Bone spurs (heel spurs)
Calcium deposits
Cramps and twitches
PMS
Sciatica
Low back pain
Bell's palsy
Tinnitis
Wallach's vertigo (Meneire's disease)
Trigeminal neuralgia
Spinal stenosis
Nutritional secondary hyperparathyroidism (elevated blood calcium)
Osteofibrosis
Myelofibrosis (myelosclerosis)
Tetany
Panic attacks
Elevated blood calcium (hypercalcemia / hyperparathyroidism)
Anemia
Prolonged clotting time
Restless leg syndrome

Other nutrients that are commonly found in the American diet can aggravate the national calcium deficiency crisis. Diets rich with an overabundance of fiber, salt and phosphates (soft drinks) result in an increased calcium "cost." In effect, these foods increase the dietary requirements for calcium. Urinary calcium loss increased from 96 mg per day to 148 mg per day when food was excessively salted. As phosphate intake is doubled, the output of urinary calcium increases by 50%.

There are no less than 147 deficiency diseases that can be attributed to calcium deficiencies or imbalances. The most recent clinical research clearly points out that the entire scope of American diets are critically deficient in calcium. The only practical way to obtain enough sufficient amounts of calcium is through supplementation. Interestingly, the allopathic physicians who did the study failed in their duty. Instead of simply recommending effective calcium supplementation, they recommended eating five cups of broccoli per day as a valuable source of calcium. Try and get a kid to eat five cups of broccoli each day.

The most common calcium deficiency diseases are easy to recognize and range from poor clotting time of the blood when you nick yourself shaving (calcium is a cofactor in the clotting mechanism), arthritis (which physicians treat with pain killers, anti-inflammatory drugs and surgery), to the dozens of variations of osteoporosis.

Famous people who have suffered from an advanced degree of calcium deficiency include Pope John Paul II (fractured hip/osteoporosis), Elizabeth Taylor (osteoporosis/multiple hip replacement surgeries), "Bo" Jackson (fractured hip/osteoporosis), Bill Walton, a vegan of professional basketball fame (osteoporosis, arthritis, fractures), etc.

Calcium is the most abundant mineral in the human body. The average male has 1,200 grams and the average female has 1,000 grams. Calcium makes up two percent of the adult body weight (water makes up 65 to 75%). Calcium also composes up to 39% of the total mineral reserves (ash after cremation). Ninety-nine percent of body calcium is found in bones and teeth. The other one percent is found in the blood, extracellular fluids, and within cells where it is a cofactor and activator for numerous enzyme systems.

Calcium, in bones, is found in the form of hydroxyapatite salts composed of calcium phosphate and calcium carbonate in a classic crystal structure bound to a protein framework called "bone matrix."

To extract the calcium from a bone and reveal the protein matrix, put a chicken "drumstick" bone in a quart of vinegar for two weeks and the calcium will be leached out of the bone leaving the protein matrix.

Hydroxyapatite crystals are found in the enamel and dentine of teeth; however, little calcium is readily available from teeth to contribute to rapidly available Ca to maintain blood levels.

In addition to being a major structural mineral, Ca is also required as a cofactor for the release of energy from ATP for muscular contraction, and blood clotting. In the blood clotting process, ionized Ca stimulates the release of thromboplastin from platelets and converts prothrombin to thrombin. Thrombin helps to convert fibrinogen to fibrin, and fibrin is the protein web that traps red blood cells to create blood clots.

Calcium mediates the transport function of cell and organelle membranes. Calcium affects the release of neurotransmitters at synaptic junctions. It also mediates the synthesis, secretion, and metabolic effects of hormones and enzymes. Calcium helps to regulate the rate and strength of the heart rate, muscle tone and muscle receptivity to nerve stimulation.

Calcium is primarily absorbed in the duodenum, where the environment is still acid. Once the food in the intestine converts to an alkaline pH, the absorption rate of calcium will decline. Calcium is absorbed from the small intestine by active cellular transport and by simple diffusion. Metallic calcium absorption may be limited to one to three percent or less and can be affected by many substances in the gut. Under ideal circumstances calcium is highly absorbable, up to 98% in the organically bound plant derived colloidal mineral and water soluble chelated form.

Causes of a calcium deficiency can include, a deficiency or lack of vitamin D; the lack of stomach acid or hypochlorhydria can result from a restricted NaCl (salt) intake; lactose intolerance; celiac disease; high fat diet; low protein diet; and a high fiber and phytate consumption.

Phytic acid is a phosphorus containing acid compound found in the bran of grains, seeds, as well as the stems and roots of many plants. Oatmeal and whole wheat especially contain phytic acid. When phytic acid combines with calcium it forms an insoluble product called calcium phytate which cannot be absorbed by the body.

Oxalic acid in rhubarb, spinach, chard, and mustard greens combines with calcium to form an insoluble calcium oxalate, which is not absorbed. Fiber itself, besides the phytate content, prevents calcium absorption. Alkaline intestinal environment, gut hypermobility (too rapid transit time brought on by too much fiber, fruit, etc.), and pharmaceuticals (anti-seizure drugs, diuretics, etc.) result in decreased absorption and retention. Excesses of sugar, carbonation and caffeine from coffee, tea, colas, etc. will reduce the efficiency of absorption and will leach stored calcium from the bones.

Under optimal conditions, parathormone secreted by the parathyroid gland and calcitonin secreted by the thyroid gland, maintain a serum calcium of 8.5 to 10.5 mg% by drawing on calcium reserves from the bones. The parathormone can also affect the kidney so that it retains more calcium. The same hormone can cause the gut to be more efficient in absorption. When blood calcium begins to rise above 10.5 mg% from too much parathyroid activity, the calcitonin produced by the thyroid gland reduces the availability of calcium from the bones.

In 1980, McCarron et al theorized that chronic calcium deficiency probably led to hypertension. More than 30 subsequent studies supported the original theory of calcium deficiency as the cause of hypertension. In addition, recent studies have shown that serum ionized calcium is consistently lower in humans with untreated hypertension. In a recent review article, Sower and others noted that the association of calcium intake and high blood pressure is most clear in people with daily calcium intakes of less than 500 mg per day.

The phenomenon of salt sensitive hypertension consists of a rise in blood pressure and a sustained increase in urinary loss of calcium in response to excess salt consumption and a coexisting calcium deficiency. Among black and elderly whites with essential hypertension, restricted intakes and deficiencies of calcium and potassium, rather than elevated salt consumption is responsible for "salt sensitivity." In a four-year study of 58,218 nurses, hypertension was more likely to develop in females who took in less than 800 mg of calcium per day.

Up to 75% of ingested elemental calcium is lost in the feces. Two percent is lost in the urine and sweat (15 mg per day is lost in normal sweating - this can double or triple in active athletes or individuals engaged in physical labor). In cases of excess urine loss of calcium (osteoporosis, hyperactive parathyroid glands, excess dietary phosphorus and phytates, etc.), kidney stones, bone spurs and calcium deposits will develop.

Bone and heel spurs and calcium deposits always develop at the sites of insertions of tendons and ligaments during a raging and progressive osteoporosis. Bone spurs, heel spurs, calcium deposits and the elevated blood calcium of hyperparathyroidism can be reversed and eliminated by supplementing with significant amounts of chelated and colloidal chelates of calcium.

Nutritional secondary hyperparathyroidism, resulting from a raging calcium deficiency, produces a significant elevation in blood calcium levels. The parathyroid glands will attempt to compensate and will enlarge in an attempt to absorb more calcium from the gut. This scenario will almost always result in the surgeon calling the enlarged or hypertrophied parathyroid glands a "tumor" and they will recommend surgery. Supplementation with the appropriate amounts of usable calcium will result in a rapid and complete resolution of the problem - DO NOT GET SURGERY!

Not only are most of our soils and foods deficient in calcium, additionally the diet of the industrialized world is rich in phosphorous, which is found in just about everything we eat. Ideally, the calcium to phosphorous (Ca:P) ratio in our daily diet should be 2:1. The ideal ratio is not possible by simply eating food. You would have to eat 25 pounds of broccoli every time you ate a 16 oz. T-bone steak! The only possible way to approach the 2:1 ideal is to avoid as much as possible the food items containing high levels of phosphorous (i.e. - raw vegetables (phytates), colas, etc.) and supplement with plant derived colloidal and chelated calcium.

Cd-Cadmium is found in igneous rocks at 0.2 ppm, shale at 0.3 ppm, sandstone at 0.05 ppm, limestone at 0.035 ppm, fresh water at 0.08 ppm, sea water at 0.00011 ppm, soils at 0.06 ppm, marine plants at 0.4 ppm, terrestrial plants at 0.6 ppm, marine animals at 0.15 to 3.0 ppm and in land animals at 0.5 ppm (accumulates in kidney tissue).

Cadmium is a silver-colored metal that is soft enough to cut with a knife. Its chemical properties are similar to those of zinc. It is a rare metal with an abundance level of only one-thousandth of that of zinc in the earth's crust. It is generally collected as a byproduct of zinc refining.

Cadmium was isolated and recognized as a separate element in 1817 by Friedrich Strohmeyer, a pharmaceutical chemist who was investigating the compound zinc oxide, known as calamine.

A cadmium alloy, Wood's metal, consists of bismuth with 12.5% cadmium. It has an extremely low boiling point of 70 degrees C and is used to seal overhead sprinkler systems. A fire will melt the Wood's metal seal before it becomes too hot, releasing water to snuff out the fire.

Cadmium is used to make nickel-cadmium, or "nicad," batteries. The "nicad" battery can be recharged an infinite number of times.

Tobacco accumulates cadmium, as a result, both

smokers and victims of second hand smoke inhale dangerous cadmium ashes.

Cadmium functions in nature by stimulating the hatching of nematode (round worm) cysts. Cadmium-bound proteins have been isolated from molluscs and horse kidneys - cadmium is known for its ability to replace zinc in zinc dependent enzyme reactions.

Ce-Cerium, a rare earth, is found in igneous rock at 60 ppm, shale at 59 ppm, sandstone at 92 ppm, limestone at 12 ppm, sea water at 0.0004 ppm, soil at 50 ppm, terrestrial plants accumulates cerium at 320 ppm, and terrestrial animals at 0.003 ppm (accumulates in bone).

Cerium is the most abundant of the rare earth minerals. It was simultaneously isolated and identified as a new element in 1803 by the Swedish chemist Jons Jakob Berzelius and the German chemists Wilhelm Hisinger and Martin Klaproth, as an impurity in the mineral bastnasite. It was named for the asteroid Ceres, which was discovered in 1801.

Cerium is found in the mineral ores called monazite and bastnasite. Monazite sand contains all of the rare earth elements and is found in Florida beach sand, and in river sand from India and Brazil. Large deposits of bastnasite are found in Southern California.

Cerium nitrate is used as a topical disinfectant for severe 4th degree burn patients.

Cl-Chlorine is found in igneous rocks at 130 ppm, shale at 180 ppm, sandstone at 10 ppm, limestone at 150 ppm, fresh water at 7-8 ppm, sea water at 19,000 ppm, soil at 100 ppm (higher in alkaline soils, near the sea and in deserts - a major exchangeable anion in many soils), marine plants at 4,700 ppm, terrestrial plants at 2,000 ppm, marine animals at 5,000 to 90,000 ppm (highest in soft coelenterates), and in land animals at 2,800 ppm. In land animals, Cl's highest concentration is found in mammalian hair and skin. Chlorine is essential for all living species' electrochemical and catalytic functions, activates numerous enzymes, and is the basic raw material for our stomachs to make stomach acid (HCl) required to activate protein digestion by the enzyme pepsin, B_{12} absorption (intrinsic factor activation) , and for absorption of minerals. Salt (NaCl) is the universal source of chloride ions for all living things.

Cm-Curium is found in igneous rocks at 0.0001 ppm. All isotopes are radioactive with a 2.5 x 108 years half-life. Curium is a man-made element.

It was isolated in 1944 by Glenn T. Seaborg, Ralph A. James and Albert Ghiorso, when they bombarded plutonium-239 with alpha particles. They named the new element after Pierre and Marie Curie, who themselves discovered radium and polonium. Curium exists in some molybdenites.

The radiation these isotopes emit are easily converted into electricity with compact units that are useful for powering pacemakers, remote navigational buoys, and instruments employed in space missions.

The element curium accumulates in mammalian bone.

Co-Cobalt is found in igneous rock at 25 ppm, shale at 19 ppm, sandstone at 0.3 ppm, limestone at 0.1 ppm, fresh water at 0.0009 ppm, sea water at 0.00027 ppm, soils at 8 ppm (higher in soils derived from basalt or serpentine; vast areas of the earth are known to be totally devoid of cobalt), marine mammals at 0.5 ppm and terrestrial animals at 0.03 (greatest concentrations in bone and liver).

Cobalt is a rare element, making up only 0.003 percent of the earth's crust. Cobalite is one of its common ores, a compound made up of cobalt, arsenic and sulfur. The pure metal, which has a characteristic bright bluish-white color, is obtained by roasting this ore in air. Cobalt metal was first isolated by the Swedish chemist Georg Brandt in 1739.

Many thousands of years ago the ancient Egyptians

manufactured a form of blue glass that was made with traces of cobalt. The name cobalt was derived in the 18th century from the German word "kobald" that refers to an evil gnome or spirit. Cobalt miners commonly blamed mining accidents on the evil "kobald" or cobalt.

Cobalt is well known for its ability to be magnetized. It is easily magnetized and retains its magnetism at temperatures far higher than those that demagnetize iron. Twenty five percent of all of the cobalt produced in the world is used to make a super magnetic substance called "alnico." Alnico is an alloy of aluminum, nickel and cobalt and is used for making industrial magnets.

Cobalt is essential for all forms of life including blue-green algae, some bacteria and fungi, some plants, insects, birds, reptiles, amphibians and mammals including man. Cobalt functions as a cofactor and an activator for enzymes, "fixes" nitrogen during amino acid production, and a single cobalt atom is the central metal component of vitamin B_{12}, which itself is a cofactor and activator (cobamide coenzymes) for several essential enzymes.

B_{12} cobalt is chelated in a large tetrapyrrole ring similar to the porphyrin ring found in hemoglobin (iron) and chlorophyll (magnesium). The original B_{12} molecule isolated in the laboratory contained a cyanide group, thus the name cyanocobalamine. There are several different cobalamine compounds that have B_{12} activity, with cyanocobalamine and hydroxycobalamine being the most active.

Vitamin B_{12} is a red crystalline substance that is water soluble. The red color is due to the cobalt atom in the molecule. Vitamin B_{12} is slowly deactivated by exposure to acid, alkali, light, and oxidizing or reducing substances. About 30% of B_{12} activity is lost during cooking (electric, gas, microwave, wood, charcoal, etc.).

In 1948 B_{12} was isolated from liver extracts and demonstrated anti-pernicious anemia activity. The essentiality of cobalt is unusual in that the requirement is for a cobalt complex known as cyanocobalamine or vitamin B_{12}. A pure cobalt requirement is only found in some bacteria and algae and the need for B_{12} cobalt is thought by some to represent a symbiotic relationship between microbes which generate and manufacture B_{12} from elemental cobalt and vertebrates that require B_{12}.

Ruminants (i.e. cows, sheep, goats, deer, antelope, buffalo, giraffe, etc.) can use elemental cobalt because the microbes fermenting and digesting plant material in their first stomach (rumen) convert elemental cobalt into vitamin B_{12}, which the animal then uses.

Carnivores can get their B_{12} from their ruminant prey by consuming stomach contents, liver, bone, and muscle from their kills.

Poultry, lagomorphs (rabbits and hares), and rodents actively eat feces during the night (coprophagy) and in the process obtain vitamin B_{12} that has been manufactured by intestinal microorganisms.

Metallic cobalt itself is absorbed at the rate of 20 to 26.2% by mice and in humans if intrinsic factor is present in the stomach and the stomach pH is 2.0 or less. Intrinsic factor is a mucoprotein enzyme known as Castle's intrinsic factor and is part of normal stomach secretions. If a person has hypochlorhydria (low stomach acid- usually a NaCl deficiency) the intrinsic factor will not work and B_{12} cobalt is not absorbed - this is why doctors frequently give B_{12} shots to older people on salt restricted diets. Sublingual (under the tongue) and oral spray B_{12} is available. Plant derived cobalt is very bioavailable; however, because of low salt diets and cobalt depleted soils, vegetarians frequently have B_{12} deficiencies.

The B_{12} intrinsic factor complex is primarily absorbed in the terminal small intestine or ileum. Calcium is required for the B_{12} to cross from the intestine into the blood stream as well as an active participation (active transport) by intestinal cells. Simple diffusion can account for only one to three percent of the vitamin's absorption. There is an enterohepatic (intestine direct to the liver) circulation of vitamin B_{12} that recycles B_{12} from bile and other intestinal secretions which explains why B_{12} deficiency in vegans may not appear for five to ten years after giving up meat.

The maximum storage level of B_{12} is 2 mg which is slowly released to the bone marrow as needed. Excess intake of B_{12} above the body's storage capacity is shed in the urine (expensive urine). Vitamin B_{12}/cobalt joins with folic acid, choline, and the amino acid methionine to transfer single carbon groups (methyl groups) in the synthesis of the raw material to make RNA and the synthesis of DNA from RNA. DNA and RNA are directly involved in gene function; remember the concept of preconception nutrition to prevent birth defects. Growth, myelin formation (converts cholesterol into the insulating material myelin found around nerves in the brain, spinal cord, and large nerve trunks), and red blood cell synthesis are dependent on B_{12}. Cobalt is also required as a necessary cofactor for the production of the thyroid hormone thyroxin.

The discovery of the essentiality of cobalt came from observing a fatal disease ("bush sickness") in cattle and sheep from Australia and New Zealand. It was observed that "bush sickness" could be successfully treated and prevented by cobalt supplements. Bush sickness was characterized by emaciation (unsupplemented vegans), dull stare, listless and starved look, pale mucus membranes, anorexia, and pernicious anemia (macrocytic/hypochromic).

In humans, a failure to absorb B_{12}/cobalt results in a deficiency disease. This can result from a surgical removal of parts of the stomach (eliminates zones of intrinsic factor production), or surgical removal of the ileum portion of the small bowel, small intestinal diverticulae, parasites (tapeworm), celiac disease (allergies to wheat gluten, barley, rye, oats and cows milk albumen), and other malabsorption diseases. Pernicious anemia and demyelination of the spinal cord and large nerve trunks are classic diseases that are the result of B_{12}/cobalt deficiency.

Less than 0.07 ppm Co in the soil results in cobalt deficiency in animals and people who eat crops grown from those soils; 0.11 ppm Co in the soil prevents and cures Co deficiency.

The human RDA for B_{12}/cobalt is 3 to 4 mcg per day, however 250 to 400 mcg gives a respectable safety margin. Pregnant and nursing mothers should especially take care to supplement with the optimum levels of B_{12}. A baby being nursed by a deficient mother has their congenital deficiency extended over a longer period of time, which can result in a serious and permanent form of nerve damage.

Cobalt excess in man (20 to 30 mg/day) may create an accelerated erythropoiesis (RBC -red blood cell- production) by stimulating an increased production of the kidney hormone erythropoiten.

Cr-Chromium is found in igneous rocks at 100 ppm, shale at 90 ppm, sandstone at 35 ppm, limestone at 11 ppm, fresh water at 0.00018 ppm, sea water at 0.00005 ppm, soils at 5 to 3,000 ppm (highest in soils derived from basalt and serpentine), marine plants at 1 ppm, terrestrial plants at 0.23 ppm, marine animals at 0.2 to 1.0 ppm and in terrestrial animals at 0.075 ppm, where it accumulates in RNA and insulin.

Chromium was discovered by French chemist Louis-Nicolas Vauquelin in 1797 and named from the Greek word *chroma*, which translates to "color."

This word chromium was chosen because all of the chromium compounds display a color; however, the pure metal is a silver-white color. Although brittle, chromium is quite hard.

Chromium metal is commonly extracted from chromite, an oxide of chromium. Chromium oxide (Cr_2O_3) is among the 10 most abundant compounds in the crust of the earth. When exposed to air, chromium forms an almost invisible oxide that makes it extremely resistant to corrosion and very useful for decorative and protective coatings over other metals including brass (bathroom fixtures), bronze (jewelry) and steel (car bumpers). Chromium added to steel at the rate of 18% produces "stainless steel."

The beautiful and radiant colors, of many precious gems, are also due to the presence of trace amounts of chromium. The red color of rubies is produced by small amounts of chromium in the form of corundum. The characteristic green color of emeralds is produced by the presence of the chromium bearing mineral beryl.

One of the more exotic precious stones that contain chromium is alexandrite, which contains a small amount of chromium in the base mineral chrysoberyl. Alexandrite changes color depending on the light source - when seen in firelight it is a bright red, when seen in daylight it is a brilliant blue.

Chromium activates phosphoglucosonetase and other enzymes and is closely associated with glucose tolerance factor (GTF). Glucose tolerance factor is a combination of chromium III, dinicotinic acid and glutathione. The reported plasma levels of chromium in humans over the past 20 years has ranged from 0.075 to 13 ng/ml. Concentrations of chromium in human hair are ten times greater than in blood, making hair analysis a much more accurate view of chromium tissue stores and function in the human. There is an average of 1.5 mg of chromium in the human body.

Very little inorganic chromium is stored in the body. Once inorganic chromium is absorbed, it is almost entirely excreted in the urine (therefore urine chromium levels can be used to estimate dietary chromium status). Dietary sugar loads (i.e. colas, apple juice, grape juice, honey, candy, table sugar, fructose, etc.) increase the natural rate of urinary Cr loss by 300% for 12 hours. The average intake of 50 to 100 ug of inorganic chromium from food and water supplies only 0.25 to 5 ug of usable and retainable chromium. By contrast, 25% of chelated chromium is absorbed and up to 98% of colloidal chromium is absorbed. The chromium RDA for humans is a range of 50 to 200 ug of usable chromium per day for adults.

The concentration of chromium found in newborn animals and humans is higher per pound of body weight than it is in older individuals. In fact, the chromium levels of unsupplemented human tissue, steadily decreases throughout life. Of greater concern has been the steady decline in the average American serum chromium since 1948.

Mean Chromium Blood Levels (ug/l)	**Year**
28 (city) 1000 (rural)	1948
13	1971
10	1972
4.7 - 5.1	1973
0.73 - 1.6	1974
0.16	1978
0.43	1980
0.13	1985

The fasting level of plasma chromium is lower in pregnant women than in non-pregnant women. Increasing impairment of glucose tolerance in "normal" pregnancy is well documented and reflects a chromium deficiency that oftentimes results in pregnancy onset diabetes. One study demonstrated abnormal glucose tolerance in 77% of clinically "normal" adults over the age of 70. According to Richard Anderson of the USDA, "Ninety percent of all Americans are deficient in chromium."

Gary Evans, Bemidji State University, Minnesota, very clearly showed an increased lifespan in laboratory animals by 33.3%, when they were supplemented, with chromium. Prior to this study, gerontologist, led by Dr. Roy Walford, felt a Calorie Restricted diet was the only way to extend life past the expected average age. Deficiencies of chromium in humans are characterized by a wide variety of clinical diseases as well as a shortened life expectancy. The clinical diseases of chromium deficiency are aggravated by concurrent vanadium deficiencies and increased sugar or alcohol intakes.

Diseases and Symptoms of Chromium Deficiency

Hypoglycemia (low blood sugar)
Prediabetes (Metabolic Syndrome)
Diabetes (adult onset, type II)
Hyperinsulinemia (narcolepsy)
Hyperactivity
Learning disabilities
ADD/ADHD
Autism
Hyperirritability
Depression
Manic depression
Bi-polar disease
Anxiety attacks
Panic attacks
Dr. Jekyll/Mr. Hyde rages ("Bad Seeds")
Impaired growth
Peripheral neuropathy

Negative nitrogen balance - protein loss
Elevated blood triglycerides (Metabolic Syndrome)
Elevated cholesterol (Metabolic Syndrome)
Coronary blood vessel disease
Aortic cholesterol plaque
Infertility
Decreased sperm count
Shortened life span
Obesity

Cs-Cesium is found in igneous rocks at 1 ppm, shale at 5 ppm, sandstone and limestone at 0.5 ppm, fresh water at 0.0002 ppm, sea water at 0.00005 ppm, soils at 0.3 to 25 ppm, marine plants at 0.07 ppm, terrestrial plants at 0.2 ppm, terrestrial animals at 0.064 ppm (highest concentrations in muscle).

As an alkaline mineral, cesium behaves chemically in a similar manner as sodium, potassium and rubidium. Cesium and potassium enter into a solute complex, which participates in ion antagonism, osmosis, permeability regulation, and maintenance of the colloidal state in the living cell. The increase in supplemental potassium increases the rate of excretion or loss of cesium.

Cesium was discovered in 1860 by the German chemists Robert Bunsen and Gustav Kirchhoff. They isolated cesium by observing colors or spectral emission lines, that cesium emits when it is heated. The color lines were bright blue, which prompted them to name the element cesium after the Latin *coesius* ("sky blue").

Cesium chloride is used as part of alternative cancer therapy programs. Cesium provides "high pH therapy" for cancer by entering the cancer cell and producing an alkaline environment. It has been recommended for all cancers including sarcomas, bronchiogenic carcinoma and colon cancer.

Cu-Copper is found in igneous rocks at 55 ppm, shale at 45 ppm, sandstone at 5 ppm, limestone at 4 ppm, fresh water at 0.01 ppm, sea water at 0.003 ppm, soils at 2 to 100 ppm (copper is strongly bound and retained by humus, but there are known areas in the world with extreme copper deficiency), marine plants at 11 ppm, terrestrial plants at 14 ppm, marine animals at 4 to 50 ppm (accumulates in the blood of annelid worms, crustaceans and mollusks, especially cephalopods), and in terrestrial animals at 2 to 4 ppm with highest levels being found in the liver.

Despite the common use of copper, it makes up only 0.007% of the earth's crust. Copper gets its name from the Latin word, *cuprum,* which translates to "from Cyprus," a reference to the fact that the Romans mined their copper from the island of Cyprus.

Copper is easily refined from many different ores and was known and employed by many ancient civilizations, copper jewelry dating back to 9000 B.C. was discovered in Iraq. Copper is soft and had to be mixed with tin (bronze), zinc (brass) or nickel (monel) to make harder alloys for tools and weapons.

Copper is an essential nutrient for all living organisms and is a universally important cofactor for many hundreds of metalloenzymes. Copper deficiency is widespread and common and copper deficiency diseases have an important impact on human populations.

Copper deficiency Symptoms and Diseases

White, grey and "silver" hair

Vitiligo (loss of skin pigment)

Dry brittle hair ("steely wool" in sheep)

Ptosis (sagging tissue - eye lids, "crows feet," skin, arm

flappers, breasts, belly)
Hernias (congenital and acquired)
Varicose veins (including hemorrhoids)
Spider veins
Aneurysms (cerebral artery, coronary artery, aorta and large artery "blowouts")
Kawasaki disease (congenital aneurysms with streptococcal infections)
Anemia (especially common in high milk and vegan diets)
Hypo and hyperthyroid dysfunction
Arthritis (especially where immature bone growth plates are involved)
Disc disease (ruptured, bulging, degenerative)
Liver cirrhosis
Violent behavior, blind rage, explosive outbursts and "criminal" behavior
Learning disabilities (ADD, ADHD, some forms of autism)
Cerebral palsy, aplasia and hypoplasia of the cerebellum
Enzootic ataxia in sheep
Mad Cow Disease in cattle (same disease as enzootic antoxia-sheep)
Krotzfeld-Jakob Disease (Humans-madcow disease)
Elevated blood cholesterol (above 350)
Iron storage disease (hemosiderosis)
Reduced carbohydrate tolerance
Neutropenia (low neutrophil count)

Copper is required for many subcellular and physiological functions: RNA, DNA, Lysyl oxidase (elastic fiber cofactor), melanin production (skin and hair), electron transport for subcellular respiration, tensile strength of elastic fibers in skin, hair, wool ("steely wool"), cartilage, tendons, ligaments, vertebral discs, blood vessels, etc.

Neonatal "enzootic ataxia" (sway back, lamkruis) was recognized as a clinical and disease entity in 1937 as a copper deficiency in pregnant sheep. Copper supplements prevented the syndrome, which was characterized by demyelination of the cerebellum and spinal cord.

"Mad Cow Disease" and Krotzfeld-Jakob Disease in humans, while thought by many, to be an infectious disease of cattle and humans that is transmitted by "prions," a needle-like protein crystalloid that is neither a bacteria, fungus or virus, has not been experimentally transmitted to any laboratory animal, livestock or humans.

Efforts to transmit Mad Cow Disease have been a failure. The brain lesions of Bovine Spongioform Encephalopathy (BSE) appear to be similar to those of Enzootic Ataxia in sheep - a copper deficiency.

Cavitation or gelatinous lesions of the cerebral white matter, chromatolysis, nerve cell death and myelin aplasia (failure to form during embryonic development) were also identified as a copper deficiency disease in sheep - these congenital lesions are identical to those of the classical changes of human cerebral palsy.

Famous people affected or dying of an obvious copper deficiency include: Albert Einstein (ruptured aortic aneurysm), Franklin D. Roosevelt (ruptured cerebral aneurysm), Paavo Airola (ruptured cerebral aneurysum), Conway Twitty (ruptured abdominal aortic aneurysm), John Ritter (ruptured abdominal aortic aneurysm), George and Barbara Bush (thyroid disease and white hair). Four to six out of every 100 Americans autopsied have died of a ruptured aneurysm; an additional 40% of Americans autopsied have aneurysms that have not ruptured.

The average well-nourished adult human body contains between 80 to 120 mg of copper. Concentrations are higher in the brain, liver, heart and kidneys. Bone and muscle have lower percentages of copper but contain 50% of the body's total copper reserves because of their mass. It is of interest that the greatest concentrations of copper are found in the newborn.

The daily copper requirement for the newborn is 0.08 mg/kg; toddlers require 0.04 mg/kg; and adults only 0.03 mg/kg.

The average plasma copper levels of women ranges from 87 to 153 mg/dl; for men the range is 89 to 137 mg/dl. About 90% of the plasma copper is bound in a protein called ceruloplasmin.

Copper functions as a cofactor and activator of numerous cupro-enzymes that are involved with the development and maintenance of the cardiovascular system. Deficiency of copper in the pregnant female results in congenital defects of the heart and vascular system (Kawasaki disease) and brain (cerebral palsy, atrisia and hypoplasia of the cerebellum)). Deficiency of copper also results in reduced lysyl oxidase activity causing a reduction in conversation of proelastin to elastin causing a decrease in the tensile strength of venous and arterial walls (spider veins, varicose veins, hemorrhoids and aneurysms).

Deficiency of copper also results in a reduced skeletal, connective tissue and muscular integrity which can produce a specific type of arthritis in children that forms bone spurs in the bone growth plates.

Lack of copper can result in myelin defects, anemia, poor hair keratization and loss of hair color. Neutropenia (reduced numbers of neutrophillic WBCs or white blood cells) and leucopenia (reduced total WBC count) are the earliest indications of a copper deficiency in an infant. Infants whose diets are primarily cow's milk frequently develop copper deficiency anemia and/or iron storage disease.

Menkes' Kinky Hair Syndrome is thought to be a sex-linked recessive genetic defect of copper absorption. The affected infants exhibit retarded growth, defective keratin formation of the hair, loss of hair pigment, low body temperature (low thyroid function, anemia), degeneration and fractures of aortic elastin (aneurysms), arthritis in the growth plates of long bones, and a progressive mental deterioration. Mental deterioration results from brain tissue being totally devoid of the essential copper dependent enzyme cytochrome oxidase.

Because of the absorption problems of elemental copper, injections of copper and liver extracts and the employment of a diet program designed for celiac patients will be useful for children with the Menkes' Kinky Hair Syndrome.

Serum and plasma copper increases 100% in pregnant women and women using oral contraceptives. Serum copper levels are also elevated during acute infections, liver disease, and pellagra (niacin deficiency).

Accumulations of copper in the cornea form Kayser-Fleischer Rings.

Dy-Dysprosium, a rare earth, is found in igneous rocks at 3.0 ppm, in shale at 4 to 6 ppm, sandstone at 7.2 ppm and limestone at 0.9 ppm. and in terrestrial animals at 0.01 ppm (accumulates in the bones).

Of the rare earths, dysprosium is a metal that ranks ninth in abundance. It was discovered in 1886 by the French chemist Paul-Emile Lecoq de Boisbaudran who was working with a sample of erbium oxide. It was named for the Greek word *dysprositos*, which translates to "hard to get at."

Dysprosium is a metal that is soft enough to be cut with a knife; it is a shiny, silvery element that is fairly stable in air. Dysprosium forms alloys whose magnetic features are employed to help compact discs function efficiently.

Er-Erbium, a rare earth, is found in igneous rock at 2.8 ppm, shale at 1.9 ppm, sandstone at 1 ppm, limestone at 0.36

ppm, terrestrial plants accumulate erbium (up to 46 ppm in *Carya spp.*), marine animals at 0.02 to 0.04 ppm and terrestrial animals primarily in bone.

Erbium is a scarce rare earth metal that was discovered in 1843 by Carl Gustaf Mosander. The main sources of erbium are the minerals xenotime and euxerite. Erbium, along with other rare earths is considered an impurity in these ores.

Erbium is employed in special alloys with metals such as vanadium to improve their workability characteristics. Erbium is frequently added to glass and enamel to tint them pink, this glass is commonly used for sunglasses and costume jewelry.

Eu-Europium is a "light" rare earth found in igneous rocks at 1 to 2 ppm, shale at 1.1 ppm, sandstone at 0.55 ppm, limestone at 0.2 ppm, terrestrial plants at 0.021 ppm (accumulates up to 16 ppm in *Carya spp.*), marine animals at 0.01 to 0.06 ppm, and terrestrial animals at 0.00012 ppm in soft tissue and 0.2 ppm in bone.

Europium is one of the most-rare of the rare earth elements. It was isolated in 1901 by the French chemist Eugene-Anatole Demarcay, who named the new element for the continent of Europe.

Europium is found mixed in ores containing monazite and bastnasite. Monazite contains all of the rare earths along with thorium and calcium. Monazite is found in river sands from India and Brazil and in beach sand in Florida. Large deposits of bastnasite are located in Southern California.

Europium is the most soft of all of the rare earths and will ignite spontaneously in air at temperatures above 150 degrees C.

Europium supplementation has extended the life expectancy of laboratory species over their expected lifespan by 100%. Europium is found in higher concentrations in breast milk from women in third world countries than in American women.

F-Fluorine is found in igneous rocks at 625 ppm, in shale at 740 ppm, sandstone at 270 ppm, limestone at 330 ppm, fresh water at 0.09 ppm, sea water at 1.3 ppm, and soils at 200 ppm (fluoride can be "fixed" or tightly bonded in several types of clay).

Fluorine is a member of the halogen family or "salt formers." The other members are chlorine, bromine, iodine and astatine. All halogen atoms react chemically by accepting electrons from other atoms and easily combine with metals to form compounds known as salts. Fluorine is the smallest, lightest and most reactive member of the halogen family.

Fluorine is a pale yellow gas whose molecules contain two atoms. Fluorine is far too reactive to be found in nature in its diatomic form. Fairly large quantities of fluorine occur in the minerals fluorite or calcium fluoride (oftentimes called fluorspar).

The French chemist Henri Moissan won the Nobel Prize in 1906 for being the first to produce fluorine in its pure elemental form. The name fluorine is derived from the Latin word *fluere*, which translates to "to flow." It took 75 years of continuous effort on the part of many chemists before fluorine was finally isolated by Moissan in 1886.

Certain types of fluorine rich soils in Madras, Spain South America are toxic to grazing livestock. Fluorine is found in marine plants at 4.5 ppm, terrestrial plants at 0.5 to 40.0 ppm (accumulates in *Dichapetolum cymosum*), marine animals at 2.0 ppm (accumulates in fish bones), and terrestrial animals at 150 to 500 ppm in mammalian soft tissue and 1,500 ppm in teeth and bones.

Teeth are protected by a hard "enamel" that is composed of a mineral called hydroxyapatite. This mineral is not soluble under normal circumstances, however, in the presence of weak acids that oral bacteria produce from high sugar foods and drinks, some dissolving of the hydroxyapatite structure occurs.

The resulting loss of the hydroxyapatite enamel

promotes the initiation of tooth decay or "caries." One of the body's defenses against the breakdown of hydroxyapatite is to generate new enamel continuously (remineralization).

In the presence of sodium fluoride, the remineralization process manufactures a form of enamel referred to as fluorapatite. Fluorapatite is considerably more resistant to damage from acid than the natural enamel. It is this process that has motivated the producers of toothpaste to add sodium fluoride to their products.

Prior to 1972, fluoride was considered essential in animals because of its apparent benefit for tooth enamel in warding off dental caries ("cavities"). In 1972, Schwarz proved that fluoride was in fact an essential mineral for animals and humans.

The skeletal reserves of fluoride in an adult man can reach 2.6 gm (2,600 mg); the average daily intake by Americans is 4.4 mg from combined sources of food, water, toothpaste and nutritional supplements.

The universal fluoridation of drinking water is still highly controversial. Some studies show that fluoridated water helps reduce fractures from osteoporosis, while other studies showed an increase in hip fractures. Clinical toxicity is observed as dental fluorosis at fluoride concentrations of 2 to 7 ppm and osteosclerosis at 8 to 20 ppm. Chronic systemic toxicity appears when the daily fluoride intake levels are above 20 to 80 ppm over several years.

Approximately 10,000 American towns and cities serving a total of 100 million people have added fluoride to their municipal drinking water at the rate of 1 mg/L, which has reportedly reduced dental caries by 60 to 70%. In certain western states in the U.S., there is an excess of fluoride, reaching levels of 10 to 45 ppm with a resultant mottling of teeth in children.

As a result of epidemiological studies by Yiamouyiannis and Burk in 1977, full scale congressional hearings were held to examine the charge that 10,000 excess cancer deaths were caused by fluoridation of certain public water systems. As a result of those hearings, the committee mandated that the U.S. Public Health Service conduct animal studies to confirm or refute the theory that fluoridated water increased the rate of cancer deaths. The studies were carried out by the National Toxicology Program under the supervision of the U.S. National Public Health Service with a special focus on oral, liver and skeletal cancers.

In 1990, the results of the fluoride study showed an increase in rat precancerous lesions in mucus membrane cells. There was an increase in cancers of the oral mucus membranes (squamous cell carcinoma). A rare form of osteosarcoma appeared at double the rate in males as females, and there was an increase in thyroid follicular cell tumors and liver cancer (hepatocholangio carcinoma).

Fe-Iron is found in igneous rocks at 56,000 ppm, shale at 47,200 ppm, sandstone at 9,800 ppm, limestone at 3,800 ppm, fresh water at 0.67 ppm, sea water at 0.01 ppm, and soils at 38,000 ppm (iron content is responsible for most soil color). Iron is most available in acid soil and availability is greatly determined by bacterial activity in the soil. It's found in marine plants at 700 ppm (very high in plankton), terrestrial plants at 140 ppm, marine animals at 400 ppm (high in the blood of annelid worms, echinoderms, fish, and in the eggs of cephalad molluscs).

Iron is the fourth most abundant element in the earth's crust and is second only to aluminum as the most abundant metal. The "core" or interior of the earth is theorized to be made up of magnetized, molten iron.

Iron is rarely found in its pure form in nature, most iron ores are iron mixed with oxygen; two of the most important iron-containing minerals are hematite and magnetite.

Iron was identified, as a useful metal, thousands of years ago. The ability to extract iron from the red-brown ores was a milestone in human development - known as the Iron Age

(1100 B.C.). The discovery of iron and man's understanding of it allowed the production of tools and weapons that were harder and more durable than those of the Stone Age and the Bronze Age (3000 B.C.). Today, iron makes up 90% of all metals that are extracted from ore.

Today, iron is one of the most commonly used metals in all human cultures. Iron and its alloys (steel) play a universal role in every aspect of daily life. Whenever we use a tool or appliance, vehicle (car, truck, train, boat, airplane, etc.) or build something (frame, nails, screws, bolts, pipe, etc.), the importance and utility of iron as a structural material is obvious.

Iron is an essential nutrient for all terrestrial species of animals. It is the four iron atoms in each hemoglobin molecule that are central to its structure and physiological function. Oxygen actually bonds to the iron atoms in the lung capillaries, and then are transported via the circulation to distant cells.

Carbon monoxide, a byproduct of imperfect combustion, is bound to the hemoglobin iron 200 times more tightly than oxygen - this phenomenon can lead to "carbon monoxide poisoning!"

In the 1860's, Boussingault, was the first to regard iron as an essential nutrient for animals. During the 1920s, feeding rats on an exclusive milk diet created an animal model for iron deficiency research.

In a healthy adult human there is three to five grams of iron, the newborn infant has nearly double the amount of iron per kg than adults. Sixty to 70% of tissue iron is used as essential or functional iron, and 30 to 40% as storage iron.

Essential iron is found as an integral part of hemoglobin, myoglobin (muscle oxygen storing pigments - particularly rich in deep diving animals such as whales, dolphins, walrus, seals, etc.), and subcellular respiratory enzymes involved with oxidation and electron transfer processes.

Functions of iron include cofactor and activator of enzymes and metallo enzymes, respiratory pigments (iron is to hemoglobin what magnesium is to chlorophyll), and electron transfer for the subcellular utilization of oxygen.

Iron is stored in bone marrow and liver (i.e. hemosiderin and ferritin). Heme iron from meat is 10% available for absorption, while iron from fresh plant sources are only one percent available because of the endogenous phytates in the plant. Iron absorption takes place primarily in the duodenum where the intestinal environment is still acid.

Experimental evidence shows very clearly that "pica" is a specific sign of iron deficiency. The pica behavior can drive children and adults to eat ice (pagophagia), dirt (geophagia), lead paint, excess food ("munchies," obesity), alcohol (alcoholism) and sugar (sweet tooth).

Iron deficiency can be the result of unsupplemented pregnancy, dysmenorrhea, chronic infections, hypochlorhydria (low stomach acid from a salt-restricted diet), chronic diarrhea, chronic bleeding (i.e. cancer, ulcers, parasites, blood thinners, nutritional deficiencies, etc.) and impaired absorption (i.e. high fat diets, high fiber diets, celiac disease, etc.).

Symptoms of iron deficiency include listlessness, fatigue, heart palpitations on exertion, reduced cognition, memory deficits, sore tongue, angular stomatitis, dysphagia (poor appetite, pica, etc.), obesity and hypochromic microcytic anemia.

Stomach hydrochloric acid is required for optimal absorption of iron. Ascorbic acid increases the absorption of iron; clays and dietary fiber (phytates) decrease the absorption of iron. The RDA of 18 mg per day as metallic iron is too low for those individuals consuming high fiber, high phytate diets (vegans, vegetarians, etc.).

"Excesses of iron can result in cirrhosis of the liver, fibrosis of the pancreas, diabetes and heart failure. These diseases are not the direct result of toxic affects of iron, but rather, the increased iron consumption produces an increased need for selenium, chromium, vanadium, copper, zinc, etc.

Fr-Francium is found only as radioactive isotopes. The longest lived of its isotopes has a half life of 22 minutes. Of its 30 known isotopes, only francium-223 exists in nature. It is estimated that the earth's crust contains less than one ounce of francium.

The element was discovered in 1939 by Marguerite Perey, when she worked at the Curie Institute in Paris. Francium was named for France where it was discovered.

Ga-Gallium is found in igneous rocks at 15 ppm, shale at 19 ppm, sandstone at 12 ppm, limestone at 4.0 ppm, fresh water at 0.001 ppm, sea water at 0.00003 ppm, soils at 0.4 to 30.0 ppm, marine plants at 0.5 ppm, terrestrial plants at 0.06 ppm, marine animals at 0.5 ppm, and in terrestrial animals at 0.006 ppm.

Gallium belongs to the same family of elements as aluminum and shares many of the same chemical properties. It is an extremely soft metal that can easily be cut with a knife. It also has an extremely low melting point of 29.8 degrees C, allowing gallium to liquefy when it is held in the hand. Gallium has an extremely high boiling point of 2,403 degrees C, allowing gallium to be in its liquid form in a range greater than that of any known metal.

The history of gallium is unique as it is one of the elements that was predicted to exist by Mendeleyev (creator of the periodic chart) in 1871. Paul-Emile Lecoq de Boisbaudran identified gallium in 1875 and named it for *Gallia,* the Latin word for France.

Gallium was claimed to be an essential element in 1938 and again in 1958. Gallium has specific areas of metalloenzyme activity in the human brain and has been reported to specifically reduce the rate of brain cancer in laboratory animals. British research has shown that diets, of pregnant women that are supplemented with gallium, significantly reduces the rate of brain cancer in children.

Gallium-67 was one of the first artificially produced

radioactive isotopes to be used in medicine. Because of its short half-life (78 hours), it rapidly loses its radioactivity and its destructive properties. This isotope has the property of accumulating in certain cancers (melanoma) and is used to treat these cancers without damage to surrounding tissues.

Gd-Gadolium, a rare earth, is found in igneous rocks at 5.4 ppm, shale at 4.3 ppm, sandstone at 2.6 ppm, limestone at 0.7 ppm, terrestrial plants (*Carya spp.*) can concentrate gadolium up to 70 ppm, and in marine animals at 0.06 ppm. Terrestrial animals accumulate gadolium in bone and liver almost immediately after absorption.

Ge-Germanium is found in igneous rocks at 5.4 ppm, shale at 1.6 ppm, sandstone at 0.8 ppm, limestone at 0.2 ppm, sea water at 0.00007 ppm, soil at 1.0 ppm in humus in alkaline soils and in marine animals at 0.3 ppm.

The existence of the "metalloid" element germanium or eka-silicon, had been predicted by Mendeleyev in his periodic table in 1871, however, it was not until 1886 that Clemens Winkler, a German scientist, isolated the silicon-like element germanium. Germanium is a poor conductor of electricity and therefore is relegated to a semi-conductor status.

The addition of small amounts of other elements such as arsenic, gallium, or antimony is called "doping" - this process greatly increases its ability to conduct electricity. Doped germanium is used to manufacture transistors, which essentially become micro-computers.

Symptoms of a typical germanium deficiency include reduced immune status, arthritis, osteoporosis, low energy, fatigue and cancer.

Twenty to 30 mg per day is the recommended maintenance dose for germanium. Fifty to 100 mg per day doses are commonly used when an individual has a serious germanium deficiency.

Radio-do-it-yourself kits from the 40s and 50s utilized

the germanium diode crystal to attract the radio signal to the radio. The germanium atom is structured so it accepts and transmits electrons effectively acting as a semiconductor. It is not too surprising that germanium is closely related to silica and carbon. Biologically, germanium is a highly effective electrical impulse initiator intracellularly and acts as a metallic cofactor for oxygen utilization.

In 1950, Dr. Kazuhiko Asai, a Japanese chemist, found traces of germanium in fossilized plant life. Russian researchers quickly attributed anti-cancer activity to germanium.

Dr. Asai was able to connect the healing properties of certain herbs to relatively high levels of germanium. Many of these herbs are germanium accumulator plants. Germanium is known to enhance the effectiveness of the immune system by stimulating the production of natural killer cells, lymphokines, such as IFN(y) interferon, macrophages, and T-suppresser cells.

Asai synthesized Ge-132, carboxyethyl germanium sesquioxide, in 1967 by a hydrolysis reaction. This organic germanium structure forms a cubic structure with three negative oxygen ions at the base of a cubic triangle. As an organic or chelated form of germanium, GE-132 is absorbed at the rate of 30% efficiency and the total intake is completely excreted in one week.

Food plants and animals contain small amounts of germanium (i.e. beans - 4.67 ppm; tuna - 2.3 ppm). Healing herbs such as garlic, aloe, comfrey, chlorella, ginseng, watercress, Shiitake mushroom, pearl barley, sanzukon, sushi, waternut, boxthorn seed and wisteria knob contain germanium in amounts ranging from 100 to 2,000 ppm.

The "Holy Waters" at Lourdes, France, known world wide for their healing properties, contains large amounts of germanium and lithium.

H-Hydrogen is found in igneous rocks at 1,000 ppm, shale at 5,600 ppm, sandstone at 1,800 ppm, limestone at 860 ppm, fresh water at 111,000 ppm, sea water at 108,000 ppm, soil at 600 to 24,000 ppm (in very acid soils it can become the major exchangeable cation), marine plants at 41,000 ppm, terrestrial plants at 55,000 ppm, marine animals at 52,000 ppm, and in terrestrial animals at 70,000 ppm.

Hydrogen is the most simple of all atoms, consisting of a single proton, its nucleus, which is circled by a single electron. Its simple and basic structure partially explains why hydrogen is the most abundant element in the universe. Enormous quantities of hydrogen gas is found in interstellar space, and is by far the most dominant element found in the stars. Hydrogen atoms make up a whopping 93% of all the atoms in the universe.

It is surprising, with the great and diverse role played by hydrogen in the universe, that there is only a small quantity of hydrogen gas in the earth's atmosphere. Out of 100 million liters of atmospheric air, hydrogen would only make up 5 liters!

Hydrogen gas is typically a diatomic molecule, meaning that a hydrogen molecule is made up of two hydrogen atoms (H_2). Hydrogen gas is colorless, odorless and tasteless; however, hydrogen is extremely flammable.

When hydrogen burns in air, it reacts violently with oxygen to form large amounts of heat and water. It is this reaction with oxygen that gave hydrogen its name, which is translated from the Greek words *hydro* (water) and *genes* (creator).

The identification of hydrogen as an element is credited to the English chemist Henry Cavendish (1731-1810) after whom the Cambridge University's Cavendish Laboratory was named.

Cavendish, a frugal, shy, stuttering and eccentric scientist, was the son of an extremely wealthy English aristocrat. Cavendish never spoke directly to women; he gave instructions to his female servants by handwritten letters, and would summarily fire them if they came into his line of sight as he walked through his laboratory or house. He spent little of his great fortune and spent his entire life buried in his laboratory "in the pursuit of knowledge."

In 1766, Cavendish was the first to produce hydrogen gas in the laboratory by placing a piece of zinc in hydrochloric acid. He deduced that the "inflammable air," was a distinct and separate substance and in fact a separate element.

Cavendish accurately calculated the mathematical value for the gravitational force (G) and the mass of the earth.

Hydrogen in its free form is a very light gas, weighing so little, that the gravitational pull of the earth, was not strong enough to keep the hydrogen gas from escaping into outer space. Most of the hydrogen gas found on earth is bound in the water of oceans and lakes.

By contrast, larger planets such as Saturn and Jupiter have a greater gravitational force and their atmosphere has a much higher percentage of hydrogen gas.

Hydrogen is widely known for being a gas that is lighter than atmospheric "air." A balloon of any size that is filled with hydrogen gas will quickly rise, float and drift away. The low density of hydrogen gives it its enormous lifting power. Hydrogen was once the main lifting power for manned balloons and "blimps." A discharge spark from a grounded docking line set the hydrogen containing German blimp, Hindenburg, on fire in 1937, causing the "lighter than air" airship industry to abandon the gas and switch to the non-flammable helium.

Hydrogen makes up a small portion of the gaseous atmosphere; hydrogen functions as a major constituent of water and all organic molecules. Seventy percent of the human body is water. The regulation of the acid-base balance in the human body is in fact the regulation of the hydrogen ion (H+) levels of cellular and extracellular fluids.

The acidity of the body is critically regulated within a narrow range by numerous and complex homeostatic mechanisms. The pH of healthy blood ranges from 7.36 to 7.44.

When the pH falls below 7.30, the patient has acidosis; when the blood pH rises above 7.44, the individual has alkalosis.

Blood pH below 6.8 and above 7.8 is rapidly fatal. Intracellular pH ranges between 6.0 and 7.4. Rapid metabolism (hyperthyroid, Grave's disease) or decreased blood flow (heart attack) increases the carbon dioxide levels and therefore decreases pH or acidifies the blood. In contrast to the internal body, the pH of secretions and excretions can be more variable and range from 1.0 (stomach acid) to 8.2 (pancreatic juice) and alkaline urine in vegans.

Hydrogen ions circulate in the body in two forms, volatile and non-volatile (metabolic hydrogen ions). Volatile hydrogen ions are found as a weak acid (carbonic acid), which must continuously be excreted from the lungs as carbon dioxide and water.

Non-volatile (metabolic) hydrogen ions are produced by the normal metabolic processes of the body or are taken in as food. The largest amounts of hydrogen ions are produced by normal and abnormal metabolism. Large amounts of hydrogen ions may be generated and/or retained as part of a disease activity (i.e. emphysema, diabetes, anxiety or loss of chloride ions, NaCl [salt] deficiency, cystic fibrosis, Addison's Disease, etc.).

Hydrogen ion concentration (pH) is controlled by the body by means of dilution, buffering respiratory control of volatile hydrogen ion concentrations and kidney-control of non-volatile hydrogen ions. Buffer systems react to hydrogen ion concentrations in fractions of seconds, respiratory controls react in minutes, and the kidneys may require as much as an hour to several days to respond.

Metabolic hydrogen ions must be excreted by the kidney in one of three forms: 60% as ammonium ions, 40% as weak acids, or trace amounts as free hydrogen ions. It is the amount of free hydrogen ions in the urine that determines the urine's pH.

Acidifying the urine with unsweetened cranberry juice

can often times control bladder infections (cystitis). Acidifying the urine and saliva can also be accomplished by consuming meat. Alkalinizing the urine and saliva can be accomplished by consuming vegetables.

Hydrogen is found in an innumerable number of organic or carbon-containing compounds, and biological compounds found in living organisms. It is commonly combined directly with carbon in organic molecules (hydrocarbons).

Hydrocarbons are long chain-like molecules that make up natural gas and oil which are burned to produce the energy that is used to drive industry, vehicles and provide raw materials for the production of many commercial products (i.e. plastics, pesticides, fertilizer, clothing, dyes, perfumes, etc.).

Hydrogen is also a significant part of the molecules that make up living organisms such as carbohydrate, sugar, fats, proteins, enzymes, DNA, RNA, etc. In the commercial preparation of "food," enormous quantities of hydrogen are used in the "hydrogenation" process and in the production of "trans fatty acids." This process is accomplished by adding hydrogen gas to liquid vegetable oils (i.e. soy, corn, cotton seed, rape seed, sunflower, sesame seed, olive, etc.) in order to convert it to the solid "margarine."

Hydrogenated and partially hydrogenated vegetable oils, once touted by the medical trade as a safe substitute for butter in the prevention of arteriosclerosis, atherosclerosis and stroke, are now known to be the direct cause of these diseases. The consumption of fried foods, super-heated carbohydrates (breads, French fries, croutons, etc.), margarines, cooking oils and trans fatty acids are now known to produce the "inflammation" that damages the intima or arterial lining that produces clogged and blocked arteries, blood clots, thrombosis and stroke.

He-Helium is found in igneous rocks at 0.008 ppm and sea water at 0.0000069 ppm. One only has to add a second proton and two neutrons to the hydrogen nucleus to produce the helium molecule. Helium is found in the periodic table at the head of the "noble gas" column - these "noble gases" are inert and gave the "impression that they were keeping aloof from the other elements."

Helium was discovered on the sun before it was discovered on earth. In 1868, the French astronomer Pierre Janssen (1824-1907) observed an unusual and unexpected spectral line during his analysis of the spectral emission of the sun. Janssen reasoned quite correctly that the new spectral line was the emission of an unknown element. He named the new element helium, translated from the Greek word *helios*, meaning sun. In 1895 the Scottish chemist William Ramsay discovered helium gas in a sample of uranium ore.

Spectral emissions refer to the wavelengths of light given off by each element when it is heated. Each element gives off colors that are unique to its self. Scientists use these color emissions to identify unknown elements much in the same manner that finger prints are used to identify people.

Helium is colorless, odorless and is so inert that it will not even react or combine with itself. It is so inert that it is one of those few elements that are found in nature in its pure elemental form. No stable compound of helium has ever been manufactured.

Helium is second only to hydrogen as the most abundant element in the universe. Helium makes up seven percent of all the existing atoms. Together, helium and hydrogen make up 99.9% of elements in the universe. Helium ranks sixth amongst the gasses found in the earth's atmosphere.

Almost all of the helium gas on earth is found in "natural gas," produced by the decay of uranium and radon radioactive isotopes. The more common name for these helium nuclei is "alpha particles," named by their discoverer, Sir Ernest Rutherford, a professor of physics at the Cavendish Laboratory at Cambridge University.

Divers use helium/oxygen "air" when working at great depths; helium being less soluble than nitrogen dissolves at a low percentage in blood, therefore reducing the risk of "bends."

The "bends" is a condition that is produced by a diver coming to the surface too quickly, the lower pressure at the water's surface results in the dissolved gasses to bubble out of solution. The effect is like fizzing of an opened bottle or can of carbonated soft drinks. In the human body these gas bubbles become trapped in the joints, causing severe pain and causing the diver to "bend" in a fetal position.

Inhaling pure helium produces a dramatic change in the pitch and speed of vocalizations, producing a "Donald Duck" speech.

A mixture of helium and neon gases was used to produce the first gas "laser." The term laser is an acronym for "Light Amplification by Stimulated Emission of Radiation." A common application of the helium-neon laser is found in retail outlets, where it is used to read bar codes on price tags at the checkout line.

Hf-Hafnium is found in igneous rocks at 3 ppm, shale at 2.8 ppm, sandstone at 3.4 ppm, limestone at 0.3 ppm, sea water at 0.000008 ppm, soil at 3.0 ppm, marine plants at 0.4 ppm, terrestrial plants at 0.01 ppm and terrestrial animals at 0.04 ppm.

Hafnium is a common and abundant metal, however, it was not discovered until 1923. Numerous investigators, including the creator of the periodic table Mendeleyev, predicted the existence of "element 72," however, the ever present diamond-like twin zirconium overshadowed the existence of hafnium. Ultimately, Dirk Coster, a Dutch physicist and George Karl von Hevesy, a Hungarian physicist found the element. To honor Bohr, Coster and de Hevesy named their new element for his native city, Copenhagen, using the Latin translation, *Hafnia.*

Hafnium is a bright, silvery-white metal, its elemental properties and history are joined with the element zirconium.

Hafnium, is more dense than zirconium, however, the two metals are chemically similar and it is almost impossible to work with one without working with the other.

Hg-Mercury is found in igneous rocks at 0.08 ppm, shale at 0.4 ppm, sandstone at 0.03 ppm, limestone at 0.04 ppm, fresh water at 0.00008 ppm, sea water at 0.00003 ppm, soil at 0.03 to 0.8 ppm (lowest in the surface layers of the soil because it leaches to the subsoil and it also volatilizes), marine plants at 0.03 ppm, terrestrial plants at 0.015 ppm (*Arenaria setacia* is an accumulator plant), terrestrial animals at 0.046 ppm (accumulates in the brain, kidney, liver and bone) and marine animals at 0.0009 to 0.09 ppm. Mercury is the only metal that is liquid at room temperatures. It is an extremely dense metal, and therefore a heavy metal with a silvery-white color that has resulted in the common name of "quicksilver."

Mercury is rarely found as a pure metal in nature, rather it is found bound in a bright red ore called cinnabar or vermillion. Cinnabar is primarily mercury sulfide and is found in large deposits in Spain and Italy. Spain has mercury mines that have been operating continuously for more than 2,000 years. Metallic mercury is produced from cinnabar by heating the ore and condensing the mercury vapor.

Like many heavy metals, mercury is an accumulative poison that binds with enzymes in the body, producing a reduction or loss of function as a catalyst of biological functions. It is easily absorbed into the body through the gastrointestinal tract and can enter the body via trans-dermal routes. The vapor is considerably more dangerous than the elemental metal. It has been estimated that the vapors from the volume of mercury as small as a teaspoon can saturate a large room within a week and make it unsafe to work in.

Mercury occurs universally in the bios and has long been known as a potentially toxic element, even though the early Chinese alchemists insisted that the regular consumption of mercury or "potable gold" was the path to immortality.

Mercury was well known to the ancient Chinese and Egyptians, samples of the metal have been found in tombs dating back to 1500 B.C. Mercury takes its name from the planet Mercury and chemical symbol, Hg, from the Latin word *hydragyrum*, which translates to "liquid silver."

The first Chinese Emperor (210 B.C.), Jing Shi Huang, in a failed attempt to attain immortality, inadvertently killed himself by drinking several doses of a mercury spiked elixir over an extended period of time.

Prior to his death, Jing became paranoid ("mad as a hatter"), had many of his loyal inner circle, advisors, scholars and academics executed and had hundreds of life sized terra cotta likenesses of his loyal palace guard constructed, painted and dressed to be with him throughout a thousand year reign (he knew that the average man only lived to be 45 to 60).

Mercury is concentrated in the environment by industry, mining operations, agriculture, dental repairs (amalgams), and microorganisms that methylate mercury in the sediments at the bottoms of fresh water or salt water rivers, lakes, oceans and seas. Mercury has been detected in all tissues of accident victims, with no known mercury exposure except dental mercury amalgam fillings.

Historically, the property of being able to dissolve other metals and form alloys (amalgams) was used by dentists to create silver-mercury and gold-mercury amalgams to fill caries (cavities in teeth).

Mercury in fish is present as methyl mercury. People who rarely eat fish have low levels of mercury (2-5ug/kg); moderate fish consumers have 10 ug/kg; high fish consumers (especially if they eat shark, tuna, or swordfish) have higher values ranging up to 400 ug/kg.

Mercury mineworkers accumulate mercury, which can reach tissue levels that produce clinical disease. The biological half life of methyl mercury in humans is 70 days and only four days for inorganic mercury. The placenta acts as a barrier against the passage of inorganic mercury but not for methyl mercury. Methyl mercury transfers very easily to the fetus ("congenital" Minamata Disease in Japanese infants).

The main industrial source of mercury is the chloralkali industry. Additional sources of mercury that are associated with human activity include the manufacture of electrical appliances, paint, dental amalgams, pharmaceuticals, vaccines, slimicides and algaecides (paper and pulp industries), seed treatments as agricultural fungicides - especially dangerous as methyl mercury, and burning of fossil fuels.

The metabolic antagonism between mercury and selenium, results in the protection from selenium poisoning by mercury and protection against mercury poisoning by selenium supplements. Because a mutual antagonism between Hg and Se exists, Se protects the human kidney from necrosis (tissue death) by mercury poisoning and the placental transfer of mercury. Mercury vapor off-gassing from dental amalgam has been shown to increase the percent of antibiotic resistant bacteria in the gut from nine percent to 70% in monkeys given dental mercury fillings. The drug resistant bacterial population dropped to 12% when the fillings were removed.

Mercury poisoning from inhalation of mercury vapors was reported during the Victorian Age in "hatters" who used mercuric nitrate paste to prevent molds from growing on felt hats and as a result, commonly developed serious problems, including hair loss, loss of teeth, loss of memory, bizarre behavior and various forms of insanity, hence the expression "mad as a hatter" from *Alice in Wonderland*. Goldsmiths and mirror workers could also suffer from inhalation poisoning.

In modern times dentists and dental patients have developed high rates of several diseases thought to be related to mercury exposure including multiple sclerosis, ALS (Lou Gehrig's Disease) and Parkinson's Disease depending on what part of the brain was most severely affected. Annette Funicello contracted multiple sclerosis, which is believed to be caused by vapors from dental mercury amalgams.

The manifestations of direct mercury poisoning are

primarily neurological (i.e. tremors, vertigo, irritability, moodiness (suicidal, depression, etc.), salivation, inflammation of the mouth, stomatitis and diarrhea.

Poisoning with inorganic mercury targets the liver and kidneys. Poisoning with the more toxic alkyl mercury results in progressive lack of coordination, loss of vision, heart palpitations, loss of hearing, and mental deterioration caused by a toxic neuroencephalopathy in which the neuronal cells of the cerebral and cerebellar cortex are selectively affected.

In 1962, in the small fishing village of Minamata, Japan, mercury contaminated factory effluent (waste water) was dumped directly into the bay, which in turn contaminated aquatic plants (kelp and algae) and bacteria, which were then eaten by fish. Subsequently it was learned that certain species of bacteria and plants can metabolize mercury safely.

The contaminated fish were eaten by the bay residents with disastrous results. The Minamata disaster was characterized by a high incidence of "congenital" (damage to the fetus) mental retardation, cerebral palsy, neural tube defects and high rates of infant mortality.

The Minamata disaster was the eco-disaster event that resulted in the creation of The Center for the Biology of Natural Systems.

The cause of autism is thought by some to have a relationship to the mercury preservatives in some vaccines. It is of interest to note that none of the other countries (Third World or Industrialized) using the same vaccines and vaccine manufacturers have registered the same complaints, level of diagnosis or law suites regarding a relationship between autism and vaccinations.

The rate of autism in America in 1980 was 1/150,000 and 2008 it is claimed to be 1/150. A few autistic babies (10%) are born with the disease, 90% are born normal and then develop it somewhere between the ages of two and six years of age.

Since 2006 much of the mercury preservatives have been removed from childhood vaccines because of universal concerns and class action law suites.

In Iraq, a large scale methyl mercury poisoning was reported when large numbers of people were fed bread made with mercurial fungicide treated seed grain and meat (liver and kidneys) from animals fed the treated grain. The result of consuming the mercury contaminated grains was thousands of babies born retarded and having a high incidence of congenital brain defects including neural tube defects and cerebral palsy.

Ho-Holmium, a rare earth, is found in igneous rocks at 1.2 ppm, shale at 0.6 ppm, sandstone at 0.51 ppm, limestone at 0.17 ppm, terrestrial plants at 16 ppm (*Carya spp.*), marine animals at 0.005 to 0.01 ppm and terrestrial animals at 0.5 ppm in bone.

In 1878, two Swiss chemists noticed holmium's characteristic spectral lines, but could not identify them, so they referred to the unknown element as "element X." In 1979, a Swedish chemist, Per Teodor Cleve isolated and identified the element and called it *Holmia,* Latin for his home town of Stockholm.

I-Iodine is found in igneous rocks at 0.5 ppm, shale at 2.3 ppm, sandstone at 1.7 ppm, limestone at 1.2 ppm, fresh water at 0.002 ppm,sea water at 0.06 ppm, soil at 5 ppm, (strongly bound in humus- large areas of earth are known to be devoid of iodine), marine plants at 30 to 1,500 ppm; terrestrial plants at 0.42 ppm, marine animals at 1.0 to 150 ppm, and in terrestrial animals at 0.43 ppm (concentrates in the thyroid gland and hair).

Iodine is a violet-black solid that vaporizes to give a violet gas. It is found in sea weed and brine wells, in the sea, in the form of inorganic salts and organic iodides. It is the heaviest element in the halogen family and is highly reactive. Iodine was discovered in 1811 by Bernard Courtois, who noticed a purple vapor emanating from a sample of kelp to which he had added sulfuric acid. The color of the gas determined its name, translated from the Greek word *iodes*, meaning "violet-colored." A drop of iodine will turn starch a deep blue (potato, flour, etc.).

Commercial quantities of iodine are extracted from sodium iodate, which is found in "saltpeter" or potassium nitrate, mined in Chile. At one time Chile was one of the largest producers of iodine. Historically iodine was extracted from the ashes of burnt seaweed. The ocean contains large quantities of iodine which concentrates in various kinds of seaweed, including the giant kelp that grows of the coast of California. Iodine can also be recovered from the natural brines found in underground wells in Arkansas and Oklahoma.

Historically, one of the most common uses of iodine was in the form of an alcohol tincture, which was used as a wound antiseptic for treating minor lacerations and scrapes of the skin.

Because iodine kills bacteria, the military, campers and scouts use iodine tablets to "purify" water.

Iodine-131 is used by the medical trade to treat thyroid cancer and hyperthyroidism and iodine-125 along with an isotope of palladium is used to treat prostate cancer.

Iodine is known to be essential to red and brown algae and all vertebrates. In combination with the amino acid tyrosine, iodine is manufactured into the thyroid hormone thyroxin. Iodine intake is typically low to begin with, but since Americans have been restricting their salt intake at the advice of their doctors, hypothyroidism and goiter have become epidemic diseases.

The average American takes in 170-250 mcg/day of elemental iodine. Humans lose considerable amounts of iodine in their sweat - a loss, of as much as 146 mcg/day, with only moderate exercise. Metallic iodine is not toxic with long term intakes of up to 2,000 mcg/day.

Goiter develops in Japanese living along the sea coast despite high daily iodine consumption. Japanese subjects being fed Chinese cabbage (bok choi), turnips, buckwheat, noodles, 2.0 mcg iodine, soybean or sea weed developed goiter in all groups except the sea weed fed group.

Northern parts of the Adictis Islands had more clinical goiter than the southern areas while the southwest was goiter-free. Forty-six percent of the population of Pisila, 40% of the population of Polje, and only three percent of the population of Milahnici were affected. There is an identical iodine content of the soil in all three locations. A severe copper deficiency in the soils of the north and south cause the deficiency state because copper is a cofactor required for the efficient utilization of iodine.

Some one million Americans have either a hypothyroid (low, under active) or a hyperthyroid (overactive) condition. Thyroid hormones control and regulate digestion, heart rate, metabolism, body temperature, sweat gland activity, nervous and reproductive systems and body weight.

Symptoms of Hypothyroidism

Hashimoto's disease
Fatigue
Cold intolerance
Muscle aches and pains
Heavy or more frequent periods (dysmenorrhea)
Loss of libido (low sex drive)
Brittle nails
Weight gain
Hair loss
Muscle cramps
Depression
Constipation

Elevated blood cholesterol
Puffy face
Dry skin and hair
Inability to concentrate
Poor memory
Goiter
Wilson's syndrome

Symptoms of Hyperthyroidism

Grave's disease
Insomnia
Heat intolerance
Excessive sweating
Lighter/less frequent periods (dysmenorrhea)
Hand tremors
Rapid pulse
Exophthalmos ("bug eyes," Rodney Dangerfield eyes, etc.)
Weight loss
Increased appetite
Muscle weakness
Frequent bowel movements
Irritability
Nervousness
Goiter

Many foods and food additives are known as "goitrogens" because they interfere with the normal thyroid metabolism and produce thyroid disease. These substances include nitrates and nitrites (i.e. ham, bacon, sausage, bologna, salami, pastrami, pepperoni, jerky, deli-meats, etc.) and cruciferous vegetables (i.e. broccoli, Brussel sprouts, cabbage, cauliflower, etc.).

In-Indium is found in igneous rocks at 0.05 to 1.0 ppm, terrestrial plants at 0.62 ppm, and terrestrial animals at 0.016 ppm. Indium is a rare, soft, bluish-white metal that is corrosion resistant. When it is vigorously rubbed against other metals it will leave small residues of itself; when bent rapidly, indium emits a bizarre "shrieking" noise. Commercial sources of indium are produced as a byproduct of refining zinc.

Indium was discovered in 1863 by the German chemist Ferdinand Reich while studying zinc ore. It was identified by the bright violet light that it gave off during spectroscopic analysis. Its name is taken from the Latin word *indicum,* which translates to "violet" or "indigo."

Ir-Iridium is found in igneous rocks at 0.001 ppm, terrestrial plants at 0.62 ppm and terrestrial animals at 0.00002 ppm. Iridium is one of the hardest and most corrosion resistant metals known. It is considered a precious metal similar to platinum.

The English chemist Smithson Tennant discovered iridium in 1803, using the same process that led him to the discovery of osmium; he isolated iridium from the residues of platinum ores he treated with aqua regia (a mixture of nitric and hydrochloric acids).

Tennant named the new metal iridium after the Latin word, *iris,* which translates to "rainbow" because of the highly colored salts.

K-Potassium is found in igneous rocks at 20,000 ppm, shale at 26,000 ppm, sandstone at 10,700 ppm, limestone at 2,700 ppm, fresh water at 2.3 ppm, sea water at 380 ppm, soil at 14,000 ppm (a major exchangeable cation in all soils, but in highest amounts in alkaline soils), marine plants at 52,000 ppm, terrestrial plants at 14,000 ppm, marine animals at 5,000 to 30,000 ppm, and terrestrial animals at 7,400 ppm (highest levels are found in soft tissue).

Potassium is a silver-white metal with a characteristic putty or wax-like nature that is so soft that it can easily be cut with a knife. It is a member of the family of alkali metals along with the elements lithium and sodium, and like them is never found as a pure metal in nature.

A naturally occurring radioactive isotope of potassium is potassium-40, which has a half-life of 1.25 billion years. Potassium-40 is used to date rocks. When potassium-40 decays, it becomes the noble gas argon. To determine the age of a rock, it is necessary to know how much argon is present in the rock. The oldest rocks on earth have been dated by this method as being 3.8 billion years old.

The human body contains approximately 140 grams of potassium and since the natural level of potassium-40 is 0.012 percent, we all contain small amounts of this isotope - it is a natural and life-long contributor to our background radiation load.

Potassium was first isolated by Sir Humphrey Davy in 1807 using electrolysis as a means of separating elemental potassium from its compounds.

Sodium and potassium are chemically similar and are found in equal abundance in the crust of the earth. Although both metals occur in silicate minerals and sea water, however, the large bodies of salt water (oceans, seas and lakes) contain considerably more sodium than potassium. Potassium is essential for plant growth, while sodium is not - plants therefore preferentially take up potassium allowing dissolved sodium to flow to the oceans.

Almost all of the potassium chloride that is mined is used as plant fertilizer. In fact, plants (crops and trees) were the early source of essential minerals including potassium for humans. Wood and other plants were burned in pots or under pots to produce a potassium-rich ash ("potash").

The original "chemical fertilizer," first produced in the 1700s by the German chemist Liebig, was made up of NPK (nitrogen, phosphorus and potassium) which he formulated after the ash he produced by burning bread and then analyzing the mineral content of the ash.

The name, potassium, has its origin from the term potash, from the early source of the element - wood ashes, the byproduct of daily living, that was produced by heating and cooking with wood.

Potassium nitrate, KNO_2, is an important compound that has been used by many cultures for centuries. It is commonly called "saltpeter" or "rocksalt." The name is taken from the Greek word *petra,* which translates to rock. It looks like table salt and when dissolved in water, it tastes like salt.

Saltpeter is commonly used as a preservative and fertilizer. Gunpowder is a mixture of saltpeter, charcoal and sulfur.

Potassium is essential to all organisms and is the major cation in cell cytoplasm with a wide variety of electrochemical and catalytic functions for enzyme systems. Potassium constitutes five percent of the total mineral content of the body. It is the major cation of the intracellular fluid and there is a small amount in the extracellular fluid. With sodium, the other "electrolyte," potassium participates in the maintenance of normal water balance, osmotic equilibrium and acid-base balance. Potassium participates with calcium in the regulation of neuromuscular activity.

Potassium is easily absorbed. Ninety percent of ingested potassium is excreted through the urine. Essentially there is no storage of potassium in the human body, thus requiring a significant daily intake of 5,000 mg.

Muscular weakness and mental apathy are features of a potassium deficiency. Hypokalemic cardiac failure is the most serious potassium deficiency event. Diuretics (both natural and prescribed), water toxicity (over drinking water), sweating, colds and flu, vomiting and diarrhea increase the rate of loss of all minerals, including potassium, when compared to the normal expected excretion rate.

Kr-Krypton is found in igneous rock at 0.0001 ppm and sea water at 0.0025 ppm. Krypton is legendary as the home planet of "Superman" and the source of the mineral "kryptonite" which had a crippling effect on "Superman." In fact krypton in its natural elemental form is a noble gas, totally harmless to humans and may in fact be an essential element for all vertebrates.

As none of the Noble gases had been discovered when Mendeleyev first constructed the periodic table in 1869, he made no provision for them in the original table. It was only the discovery of argon in 1894 that produced the need for a new column in the table. In 1898, the English chemist Sir William Ramsay isolated and identified krypton as a new element. He named it for the Greek word *kryptos,* which translates to "hidden."

The chemical inertness of krypton was challenged by the celebrated American chemist and two time Nobel Prize winner, Linus Pauling, who in 1933 used quantum mechanics to demonstrate that a molecule containing krypton and fluorine should be stable enough to exist. In 1966, Neil Bartlett of the University of British Columbia produced krypton fluoride (KrF_4) as Pauling had predicted.

La-Lanthanum is a "light" rare earth and is found in igneous rocks at 30 ppm, shale at 20 ppm, sandstone at 7.5 ppm, limestone at 6.2 ppm, sea water at 0.000012 ppm, soil at 30 ppm, marine plants at 10 ppm, terrestrial plants at 0.085 ppm, marine mammals at 0.1 ppm, and in terrestrial animals at 0.0001 ppm in soft tissue and 0.27 in bone.

Notably the yeast *Candida albicans* accumulates lanthanum at the rate of 370 ppm/day. It is theorized that this is how *C. albicans* produces a debilitating, energy sapping "chronic fatigue" disease, by "stealing" lanthanum from the victim.

The growth of the protozoa *Blepherisma* and *Tetrahymena pyriformis* is stimulated and their life span doubled by the presence of the rare earth lanthanum at concentrations of 0.32 ppm.

Li-Lithium is found in igneous rocks at 20 ppm, shale at 66 ppm, sandstone at 15 ppm, limestone at 5 ppm, fresh water at 0.0011 ppm, sea water at 0.18 ppm, soil at 30 ppm (lithium is freely mobile in the soil), marine plants at 5 ppm, terrestrial plants at 0.1 ppm, marine animals at 1.0 ppm, and terrestrial animals at 0.02 ppm. Lithium's density is so low that a small piece can actually float on water.

Lithium was discovered in 1817 by the Swedish chemist Johan August Arfvedson during a routine chemical assay of ore from a mine in Sweden. It was named for the Greek word *lithos*, which translates to "stone."

Lithium is an extremely reactive metal. It reacts vigorously with water, to produce hydrogen gas, and with oxygen to form lithium oxide (Li_2O). To prevent these reactions from occurring, free lithium is usually stored in oil or kerosene.

Since 1915, the risk of clinical depression nearly doubles with each succeeding generation. Myrna M. Weissman, a psychiatrist at Columbia University, New York City, says that, "Depression is a world wide phenomenon happening at younger and younger ages."

In 1935, the age of the early onset of depression was in the early 20s, by 1955, the age of early onset of clinical depression dropped to between 15 and 20 years of age.

One in four women and one in ten men will develop depression. Prozac™, America's leading antidepressant pharmaceutical, was introduced to the public in 1987. Sales soared to $350 million in 1989, more than was spent on all antidepressants just two years earlier. Prosac™ sales topped $1 billion in 1995 as a result of 650,000 prescriptions per month!

While the professional psychiatrist says that depression and manic depression are due to feelings that "we are out of control of our lives," negative thinking, and self recrimination ("I'm a loser"), they treat depression successfully with the trace mineral lithium. Depression and manic depression with all that implies, are simply a lithium deficiency aggravated by a high consumption of sugar.

Lithium carbonate is regularly used to treat patients with the severe form of bipolar disorder. More than 3 million prescriptions for this trace mineral are filled yearly. The role of lithium is thought to be related to the role the brain cells play and respond to certain hormones and neurotransmitters.

Animal studies show that a deficiency of lithium results in reproductive failure, infertility, reduced growth rate, shortened life expectancy, and behavioral problems.

In humans, manic depression, depression, "bi-polar" disease, rage, road rage, "going postal," Dr. Jekyll/Mr. Hyde behavior, hyperactivity, ADD, ADHD, certain forms of autism and "bad seeds" are all hallmarks of a lithium deficiency aggravated by a high sugar or alcohol intake.

Chelated lithium supplemented at 1,000 to 2,000 ug/day causes a dose related increase in hair lithium levels. Hair lithium levels increased after four weeks of supplementation and leveled off and became stationary after three months. When the lithium supplementation was stopped, hair lithium levels dropped to presupplement values in two months. This scenario is not seen with the supplementation of metallic lithium carbonate. A comparison of 2,648 subjects showed that 65% had hair lithium values ranging between 0.04 and 0.14 ug/G; 16% had hair lithium values of more than 0.14 ug/G; and 18.4% had less than 0.04 ug/G. The highest levels of lithium were found in university students from Tijuana,

Mexico. The lowest levels found in hair analysis were found in Munich, Germany.

Normal controls showed almost 400 times more hair lithium than do the violent criminals from California, Florida, Texas and Oregon. The EPA estimated daily intake of lithium ranges from 650 to 3,100 ug/day, however,, much of the ingested lithium is metallic and not necessarily biologically available.

Lu-Lutetium, a rare earth, is found in igneous rocks at 0.5 ppm, shale at 0.33 ppm, sandstone at 0.096 ppm, limestone at 0.067 ppm, terrestrial plants at up to 4.5 ppm (*Carya spp.*), marine animals at 0.003 ppm, terrestrial animals at 0.003 ppm, and terrestrial animals at 0.00012 ppm in soft tissue and 0.08 in bone. As with most of the other rare earth metals, lutetium is silvery-white and corrosion-resistant. As the last lanthanide in the periodic table, it is the hardest and heaviest rare earth element.

Lutetium is one of the least abundant of the rare earth elements. It was discovered in 1907 by the Austrian mineralogist Baron Carl Auer von Welsbach and the French scientist Georges Urbain as an impurity in a mineral sample thought to contain ytterbium.

Urbain created the name for the new element from *Lutetia,* the ancient name for the city of Paris. Welsbach had chosen the name *cassiopium,* a name derived from the constellation Cassiopia. Many German scientists still refer to lutetium by the name *cassiopium.*

Though he never published his findings, the American chemist Charles James, known to his colleagues and students as "King James," is now believed to have independently identified lutetium in 1907.

Mg-Magnesium is found in igneous rocks at 23,300 ppm, in shale at 15,000 ppm, sandstone at 10,700 ppm, limestone at 2,700 ppm, fresh water at 4.1 ppm, seawater at

1,350 ppm, and soil at 5,000 ppm (highest in soil derived from basalt, serpentine, or dolomite). Magnesium is the second most common exchangeable cation in most soils. Magnesium is found in marine plants at 5,200 ppm, land plants at 3,200 ppm, marine animals at 5,000 ppm, and in land animals at 1,000 ppm where it accumulates in mammalian bone.

Magnesium is a white silvery metal that is very light weight, its name is derived from the ore magnesite (dolomite) which is primarily magnesium carbonate. Magnesite is believed to have been originally mined in Magnesia, a district in ancient Greece.

Magnesium was identified as a separate element by the British chemist Sir Humphry Davy in 1808, using electrolysis to extract it from magnesium oxide.

Magnesium is the seventh most abundant element in the earth's crust; it is present in such large quantities in sea water that the earth's oceans constitute an unlimited supply of the dissolved metal.

Milk of magnesia is a suspension of magnesium hydroxide, $Mg(OH)_2$, in water, it is used as an everyday OTC laxative. Another OTC remedy containing magnesium is Epsom salts. These salts are a hydrated form of magnesium sulfate; it was first discovered in well water from Epsom, England in the mid 17th century. Epsom salts are still used today as a wound disinfectant and for reducing the swelling and inflammation of bruises, strains and sprains.

Magnesium oxide is an important commercial compound of magnesium and is extracted directly from magnesite. It is used as a source of metallic magnesium for animal and human dietary supplements. It is also the metallic atom found in chlorophyll of all green plants, which plays an essential role in photosynthesis, the photochemical process that converts the sun's solar energy into a stored "solar currency" for a source of chemical energy for all plants and all animals and humans. Magnesium, the source of the deep green color of plants, is the ultimate source of all biological energy!

Magnesium, as a mineral is essential to all living organisms and has cofactor, electro-chemical, catalytic, and structural functions. It activates numerous enzymes and is a constituent of all chlorophylls.

The adult human contains 20 to 28 grams of total body Mg. Approximately 60% is found in bone. Twenty-six percent is associated with skeletal muscle and the balance is distributed between various organs and body fluids. Serum levels of Mg range from 1.5 to 2.1 mEq/L (a measure of electrolytes) and is second to potassium as an intracellular cation. Half of the Mg, including most that is bound in bone, is not exchangeable.

Magnesium is required for the production and transfer of energy for protein synthesis, for contractility of muscle and excitability of nerves, and as a cofactor in a myriad of enzyme systems. AN EXCESS OF MAGNESIUM WILL CAUSE DIARRHEA AND INHIBIT BONE CALCIFICATION.

Calcium and magnesium have antagonistic roles in normal muscle contraction, calcium acting as the stimulator and magnesium as the "relaxer." An excessive amount of calcium can induce signs of magnesium deficiency.

Perhaps the most important manifestation of magnesium deficiency in modern times is "malignant calcification." Malignant calcification appears as calcium deposits in soft tissue, especially the media or middle layer of arterial walls. Magnesium deficiency appears to be the basic root cause of arteriosclerotic calcium deposits, not elevated blood cholesterol or triglycerides!

Magnesium Deficiency Diseases

Asthma

Anorexia

Menstrual migraines

Growth failure

ECG changes

Neuromuscular problems

Tetany (convulsions with muscle cramping)

Depression

Muscular weakness

Muscle "ties"

Tremors

Vertigo

Calcification of arterial media

"Malignant calcification" of soft tissue

The rate of absorption of magnesium ranges from 24 to 85%. The lesser absorption rate is for metallic sources of Mg, the higher rates of absorption are associated with plant derived colloidal mineral sources. Vitamin D has no effect on Mg absorption. The presence of dietary fat, phytates, and calcium reduces the efficiency of absorption. High performance athletes lose a considerable amount of Mg in sweat.

The RDA for Mg is 350 mg/day for adult males, 300 mg/day for adult females, and 450 mg/day for pregnant and lactating females. If the kidneys are healthy, there is no evidence of toxicity at supplemental doses of up to 6,000 mg/day.

Mn-Manganese is found in igneous rocks at 950 ppm, shale at 850 ppm, sandstone at 50 ppm, limestone at 1,100 ppm, fresh water at 0.012 ppm, sea water at 0.002 ppm, soil at 850 ppm (can be a major exchangeable cation in very acid soil), marine animals at 1.0 to 6.0 ppm (lowest in fish), and in terrestrial animals at 0.2 ppm with the highest concentration in mammalian liver and kidney.

Manganese is a hard, gray-white metal that has chemical

and physical properties that are similar to iron. Manganese does not occur as a pure mineral in nature, it is usually found combined with oxygen in pyrolusite, a mineral that is made up chiefly of manganese dioxide (MnO_2).

Manganese was identified in 1774 by Carl Wilhelm Scheele who named it from the Latin word *magnes*, which translates to "magnet," referring to the magnetic properties of pyrolusite.

The United States has no deposits of manganese of any commercial quantities. Rich ores containing up to 40% manganese are found in South Africa and India. A unique source of almost pure manganese is found on the floor of the world's seas as "manganese nodules." These nodules, spherical in shape, are made up primarily of manganese and iron oxides, and are thought to be the byproduct of microorganisms that have the ability to extract manganese from sea water.

One of the most common compounds of manganese found in chemical laboratories is potassium permanganate ($KMnO_4$), which is employed as an indicator for acid solutions. When dissolved in water, it produces a deep purple color. If an acid is added to the solution, its color instantly turns to a pale pink. It is also used to purify community water supplies and to absorb toxic gases.

The total body content of manganese in humans is only 10 to 20 mg. Manganese is known to be essential for all living organisms. Manganese activates numerous enzyme systems including those involved with glucose metabolism, energy production and antioxidant properties of superoxide dismutase (SOD). It is a major constituent of several metalloenzymes, hormones, and proteins essential to all vertebrates and humans.

Manganese is an essential part of the developmental process and the physical structure of the three fragile ear bones and joint cartilage.

Excessive levels of manganese found in certain

community water supplies and in some industrial processes can produce a Parkinsonian syndrome or a psychiatric disorder (locura manganica) resembling schizophrenia.

Deficiency diseases of manganese are very striking, ranging from severe birth defects (congenital ataxia, cerebral palsy, deafness, chondrodystrophy), asthma, convulsions, retarded growth, skeletal defects, disruption of fat and carbohydrate metabolism to joint problems in children and adults (i.e. TMJ, Repetitive Motion Syndrome, Carpal Tunnel Syndrome, etc.).

Deficiency Diseases of Manganese

Congenital ataxia
Cerebral palsy
Deafness (congenital malformations of otolithes)
Asthma
Chondromalacia
Chondrodystrophy
"Slipped tendon"
Defects of cartilage formation and maintenance
Defects of chondroitin sulfate metabolism
TMJ
Repetitive Motion Syndrome
Carpal Tunnel Syndrome
Convulsions
Infertility (failure to ovulate, testicular atrophy)
Still births/ spontaneous abortions (miscarriages)
Loss of libido in both males and females
Retarded growth
Shortened long bones

Repetitive stress injury or repetitive motion syndrome now costs America $20 billion per year and accounts for 56% of the 331,600 gradual onset work related illnesses and disabilities.

In 1991, orthopedic surgeons performed 100,000 carpal tunnel operations (at $4,000 per surgery) with lost work, wages and medical costs of over $29,000 per case.

At risk for the repetitive motion syndrome are those working in the world of computers: journalism, airline reservations, directory assistance, law research, data entry, graphic design and securities brokerage. Chief among blue collar victims are the auto assembly workers, chicken pluckers, meat cutters, postal employees, dock workers, etc.

Repetitive motion syndrome was observed three centuries ago in monks who were scribes and was described in 1717 by Bernardo Ramazzini, an Italian physician (considered the father of occupational medicine).

Repetitive motion syndrome victims have reached such numbers that federal legislation has been passed in the form of OSHA and Americans with Disabilities Act (ADA) to ensure work place safety. Large numbers of ergonomically correct keyboards and furniture have been developed. We now see literally millions of people in the work place with Velcro wrist, neck, elbow, finger, knee, back and hip supports - all for simple manganese deficiencies!!

Mo-Molybdenum is found in igneous rocks at 1.5 ppm, shale at 2.6 ppm, sandstone at 0.02 ppm, limestone at 0.4 ppm, fresh water at 0.00035 ppm, sea water at 0.01 ppm, soil at 2.0 ppm (strongly concentrated by humus, especially in alkaline soils; a few soils worldwide are rich enough in molybdenum to cause molybdenum poisoning in animals consuming the plants). Numerous soils are known to be molybdenum deficient. Molybdenum is found in marine plants at 0.45 ppm, terrestrial plants at 0.9 ppm, marine animals at 0.6 to 2.5 ppm, and terrestrial animals at 0.2 ppm with the highest levels being found in the liver and kidneys.

Molybdenum is a hard, silvery metal that is extracted from an ore called molybdenite (MoS_2). There are large deposits of "Moly" molybdenite in Colorado.

In 1778, molybdenum was originally extracted from molybdenite and identified as a new element by the Swedish chemist Carl Eilhelm Scheele who identified it as a new element.

Molybdenum is essential for all organisms as a constituent of numerous metalloenzymes. Molybdenum is known to be an integral part of no less than three essential enzymes: Xanthine oxidase, Aldehyde oxidase and Sulfite oxidase.

The average American daily intake of Mo in food ranges from 76 to 1,109 mcg per day. The RDA for Mo is 250 mcg per day. Toxicity occurs at 10 mg per day; clinical signs of toxicity appear as a gout-like disease and interference with copper metabolism.

N-Nitrogen is found in igneous rock at 20 ppm, fresh water at 0.23 ppm, sea water at 0.5 ppm, soils at 1,000 ppm (99% present as non-basic N bound in humus), marine plants at 15,000 ppm, terrestrial plants at 30,000 ppm, marine animals at 75,000 ppm, and in terrestrial animals at 100,000 ppm.

Nitrogen in its free state is a gas, and as a gas nitrogen is relatively inert and is colorless, tasteless and odorless. Nitrogen makes up 78% of the earth's atmosphere by volume. Although a relatively non-reactive gas, nitrogen is part of hundreds of thousands of compounds that are essential for life, agriculture and industry. Even though nitrogen is relatively stable, some of its compounds are extremely unstable and explosive.

Nitrogen was discovered in 1772 by David Rutherford (1749-1819), an English chemist and physician. Rutherford used a bell jar to limit a sample of atmospheric air, he then removed all of the oxygen from the trapped air by consuming it by burning a substance in it; he then placed a mouse in the oxygen free jar, which rapidly asphyxiated; he then demonstrated that "nitrogen" could not sustain life.

Many compounds found in nature and contain nitrogen are crucial for plant and animal life. Included in the plethera of biological molecules that have nitrogen as a significant functional component are proteins and nucleic acids. Despite the lack of reactivity of nitrogen, there are several natural mechanisms for converting nitrogen from the atmosphere into usable nitrogen compounds called nitrogen "fixing."

During electrical storms, the extremely high temperatures of the lightening supply enough energy to break apart the diatomic nitrogen molecule (N_2). The free nitrogen atoms that are formed can then combine with oxygen to form nitrogen oxide (NO), and nitrogen dioxide (NO_2).

Most of the nitrogen dioxide dissolves in rainwater and then falls to the earth's surface, where nitrogen-fixing bacteria in the soil called cyanobacteria use the nitrogen dioxide to build nutrients such as proteins and amino acids. These nutrients are then taken up by the roots of plants, which are in turn eaten by animals, in whose tissues the nitrogen is used to create animal proteins. Bacteria in the soil then convert the inevitable waste products of nitrogen metabolism, such as urea, into amino acids and ammonia. These same denitrifying bacteria also breakdown these compounds to form gaseous nitrogen, which is then returned into the atmosphere.

Nitric acid (HNO_3), is of major commercial value in the United States, where it is used to manufacture fertilizer (ammonium nitrate), as well as for the manufacture of explosives and plastics (nylon, polyurethane, etc.). Nitric acid was known to early chemists as *aqua fortis*, which in Latin translates to "strong water."

More than 15 billion pounds of nitric acid were produced in the US alone in 1992, chiefly by the Ostwald process. This process was discovered in 1902 by the German chemist Wilhelm Ostwald (1853-1932), who received the

Nobel Prize in 1909 for his research into the importance and value of catalysts in chemical reactions.

In the Ostwald process, high temperatures and platinum catalysts convert ammonia into nitric acid which can then be used to make explosives.

When nitric acid combines with glycerol, a syrup-like alcohol, it produces nitroglycerine, which is extremely dangerous to handle, because it can explode with the smallest of shocks.

Dynamite, a useful and much safer derivative of nitroglycerine was invented in 1867 by Alfred Nobel (1833 - 1896). He showed that when nitroglycerine is mixed with clay, it forms a relatively safe, shock-resistant explosive - TNT. Nobel eventually established the Nobel Prize with an investment of $900,000 with some of the fortune he accumulated from the sale and royalties from TNT.

When nitric acid is neutralized with bases including sodium and potassium hydroxide, it forms compounds called nitrates. Nitrates and nitrites are added to canned foods and preserved meats to help prevent the growth of bacteria and to color meat red.

Nitrates and nitrites are converted to nitrosamines in the acid environment of the stomach; these compounds can be converted to cancer causing chemicals (carcinogens) and can suppress thyroid function.

Nitrogen functions as a structural atom in protein, nucleic acids (RNA, DNA), and in a wide variety of organic molecules. Dietary nitrogen (as protein) furnishes the amino acids for the synthesis of tissue protein and other special metabolic functions:

1. Proteins are used to repair worn out body tissue

2. Proteins are used to build new tissue (muscle, infant growth, childhood development, teenager puberty, pregnancy (embryonic growth), maintenance and repair).

3. Proteins can be an emergency source of heat and energy (albeit more "expensive" in biological terms than energy derived from fat or carbohydrate).

4. Proteins make up a major percentage of essential body secretions and fluids (i. e. enzymes, hormones, mucus, milk, semen, etc.).

5. Blood plasma proteins maintain osmotic fluid balance (hypoproteinemia results in edema and acites).

6. Proteins help to maintain acid-base balance of blood and tissue.

7. Proteins aid in the blood transport of other essential substances (i.e. minerals, fats, vitamins, etc.).

8. Proteins make up basic immunoglobulins (antibodies).

9. Proteins provide a nitrogen pool for the synthesis of amino acids and new proteins.

Classic protein deficiency results in infertility, poor growth, lowered immune status, edema, and Kwashiorkor (potbellied, thin children of Third World countries). The availability and usability of nitrogen from various foods are quite different and must be considered when choosing N sources.

Nitrogen/Protein Utilization Values of Common Foods

Nitrogen Source (Protein)	Chemical Score	% Utilization
Whole egg	100	94
Human milk	100	87

Cow's milk	95	82
Soy bean	74	65
Sesame	50	54
Peanut	65	47
Cotton seed	81	59
Maize (corn)	49	52
Millet	63	44
Rice	67	59
Wheat	53	48

Mixing protein sources such as beans and rice, wheat and legumes, or vegetable and animal tends to improve the utilization of the vegetable protein source and make up for missing amino acids.

Na-Sodium is found in igneous rocks at 23,600 ppm, shale at 9,600 ppm, sandstone at 3,300 ppm, limestone at 400 ppm, fresh water at 6.3 ppm, sea water at 10,500 ppm, soil at 6,300 ppm (it is a major exchangeable cation in soils, especially alkaline soil), marine plants at 33,000 ppm, terrestrial plants at 1,200 ppm, marine animals at 4,000 ppm, and in terrestrial animals at 4,000 ppm.

Sodium is a highly reactive, bright, silvery metal, light enough to float on water and soft enough to cut with a knife. It is the sixth most abundant element in the crust of the earth.

The English chemist, Sir Humphry Davy first isolated and identified sodium as a new element in 1807 by separating it from molten sodium hydroxide. The name, sodium is taken from the English word soda, which itself is derived from the Latin word *sodanum*, a common headache remedy of ancient Rome.

Sodium chloride, the chemical name for common table salt, is mined in large quantities from ancient salt mines on every continent on earth. Sea water is another common source of salt, every gallon of sea water contains a quarter pound of salt.

Salt has been used and traded as a nutrient, preservative and flavoring condiment since before Roman times. The word salary, is derived from the Latin word *sal*, which translates to "salt." Roman soldiers were paid a "salary" or allowance in the form of salt.

"Salt hunger" dates back to the beginning of time and is one of the basic cravings of vertebrates. Carnivores (man or beast) do not always show obsessive cravings for salt because meat contains relatively large amounts of NaCl. By contrast herbivorous animals and human vegetarians demand large quantities of NaCl in grains, vegetables, nuts and fruit. The average dietary intake of sodium per day in western cultures is five to 12 grams per day, while the Japanese, who outlive Americans by an average of four years, consume an average of 28 grams of sodium per day!

Sodium, chlorine and potassium are three indispensable "electrolytes" so intimately associated in the human body that they can be presented together. Sodium makes up two percent, potassium five percent and chlorine three percent of the total mineral content of the human body. All three are widely distributed throughout the body tissues and body fluids, however, Na and Cl are primarily extracellular (outside the cell), while K is an intracellular (inside the cell) mineral. Sodium, potassium and chlorine are involved in at least four important physiological functions in the body:

1. Maintenance of normal water balance and distribution.

2. Maintenance of normal osmotic equilibrium.

3. Maintenance of normal acid-base balance.

4. Maintenance of normal muscular irritability.

Hormonal control of Na, K and Cl balance is regulated by the adrenal cortex hormones as well as by the anterior pituitary gland. Addison's Disease, a loss of function of the adrenal cortex, results in the loss of Na and K retention with clinical signs of general weakness, muscle cramps, weight loss, and a marked "salt hunger." The symptoms can be relieved with the supplementation of NaCl or by administering adrenal cortical hormones (steroids).

Deficiencies of NaCl occur primarily in hot weather (i.e. the American heat wave of 1993), heavy work in a hot climate, or exercise when large volumes of sweat are produced for body cooling. "Water intoxication" occurs in infants fed low sodium formulas (because of doctor's insane paranoia with sodium) and death occurs as a result of the resultant brain swelling. The treatment for sodium deficiency is water and salt, either orally (salt food to taste) or IV (saline administered at 0.9%).

Nb-Niobium is found in igneous rocks at 20 ppm, shale at 11 ppm, sandstone at 0.05 ppm, limestone 0.3 ppm, sea water at 0.00001 ppm, terrestrial plants at 0.3 ppm, and marine animals at 0.001 ppm.

Niobium is a soft, steel-gray metal that is primarily found in the mineral columbite, an ore that also contains iron and manganese. Niobium was discovered by the Englishman Charles Hatchett in 1801, while he was analyzing a sample of columbite that was owned by the British Museum in London. The new element was named *niobium* for the mythological goddess Niobe.

Nd-Neodymium, a rare earth, is found in igneous rock at 28 ppm, shale at 16 ppm, sandstone at 11 ppm, limestone at 4.3 ppm, marine plants at 5 ppm, terrestrial plants accumulates up to 460 ppm (*Carya spp.*), marine animals at 0.5 ppm, and accumulates in the liver and bone of terrestrial animals.

Neodymium is a "light rare earth" proven to enhance normal cell growth and double the lifespan of laboratory species.

Neodymium was discovered in 1885 by an Austrian amateur mineralogist, Baron Carl Auer von Welsbach. He divided a mineral called didymium into two new and distinct elemental salts, one of which contained neodymium. Welsbach created the name for this new element from two Greek words, *neos,* which translates to "new" and *didymos,* which translates to "twin."

Neodymium and its oxides, which tend to be rose colored, are used to make colored glass for welder's goggles and the synthetic "ruby" for powerful lasers.

Neodymium is a magnetic substance and is used to create the most powerful magnets on earth. Disc magnets made from neodymium are powerful enough to recognize the magnetic materials in the printing ink used to print paper money and are used to detect counterfeit paper money.

Ne-Neon is found in igneous rocks at 0.005 ppm and sea water at 0.00014 ppm. Neon is a "noble" gas, inert and unreactive, it does not form any compound with any other element. It is a colorless and odorless gas and is the fifth most common element in the earth's atmosphere. Its concentration in air is 0.002%, or about one-tenth that of carbon dioxide.

Neon was discovered in 1898 by the English chemist Sir William Ramsy during his experiments with the fractional distillation of liquid air, he named it neon after the Greek word *neos,* which translates to "new."

The "neon signs" we see in store and restaurant windows are glass tubes that contain neon gas that glows when it is energized by electricity. The term "neon sign" is now used generically for all such glowing tubes, many of which contain gases other than neon. Different gasses produce signs of different colors; every gas, when electrically excited, radiates its own characteristic color, argon produces a purple light, xenon produces a blue-green light.

Ni-Nickel is found in igneous rocks at 75 ppm, shale at 68 ppm, sandstone at 2.0 ppm, limestone at 20 ppm, fresh water at 0.01 ppm, sea water at 0.0054 ppm, soils at 40.0 ppm (higher in soils derived from serpentine), marine plants at 3 ppm, terrestrial plants at 3.0 ppm (accumulated by *Alyssum bertalonii*), marine animals at 0.4 to 25 ppm, and terrestrial animals at 0.8 ppm (primarily in RNA).

Nickel is a silvery metal found in an ore called millerite, which is a compound of nickel and sulfur. Nickel is considered a rare element because only one one-hundredth of one percent of the earth's crust is nickel. The molten core of the earth is thought to be primarily iron and nickel. Nickel is a common element found in meteorites.

While nickel compounds were known since ancient times, the pure metal was only identified in 1751 by a Swedish chemist named Axel Fredrik Cronstedt. Nickel is a German word for Satan, and the element is thought to be named for the German Kupfernickel, or "Satan's copper." Like cobalt, nickel was known in the ancient world as a method for coloring glass - nickel turns glass green.

The "nickel" or the five cent U.S. coin is made of copper and nickel, with nickel being 25% of the alloy.

Like iron, nickel can be made magnetic; the alloy named alnico, formed from aluminum, nickel and cobalt, is used to produce some of the most powerful magnets.

An important use of nickel is the nickel-cadmium (Ni-Cad) battery.

Symptoms of Nickel Deficiency

Poor growth

Anemia

Depressed oxidative ability of the liver

Increased newborn mortality

Rough dry hair

Dermatitis

Delayed puberty

Poor zinc absorption

Less than 10% of ingested metallic nickel is absorbed. Nickel deficiency was first reported in 1970. Nickel functions as a cofactor for metalloenzymes and facilitates gastrointestinal absorption of iron and zinc.

Optimal tissue levels of vitamin B_{12} are necessary for the optimal biological function of nickel. Vitamin B_{12} deficiency results in an increased need for nickel in animals and humans.

Np-Neptunium is a highly reactive silvery metal, known only as radioactive isotopes. The half-life of neptunium is 2.2 x $10^{(6)}$. Neptunium accumulates in mammalian bone after ingestion. Neptunium has been found in fresh water organisms in the Hanford River (USA).

Neptunium was the first manmade transuranium element. Neptunium derives its name from the planet Neptune, because that is the planet beyond Uranus (the planet from which the name uranium was derived from).

Currently there are 18 known isotopes of neptunium, the most important of which is neptunium-237, with a half-life of 2.1 million years.

O-Oxygen is found in igneous rocks at 464,000 ppm, shale at 483,000 ppm, sandstone at 492,000 ppm, limestone at 497,000 ppm, fresh water at 889,000 ppm, sea water at 857,000 ppm, soils at 490,000 ppm, marine plants at 470,000 ppm, terrestrial plants at 410,000 ppm (except for anaerobic organisms), marine animals at 400,000 ppm, and terrestrial animals at 186,000 ppm. Terrestrial oxygen consists of 99.76% $O^{(16)}$ with a half-life of less than two minutes.

The English chemist, Joseph Priestly (1733 - 1804) is credited with the discovery of oxygen. In his most famous experiment, Priestly heated an oxide of mercury, and noted that the gas it gave off "caused a candle to burn with a remarkably brilliant flame."

Credit for naming oxygen is given to the French chemist Antoine Laurent Lavoisier (1743 - 1794) who was beheaded during the French Revolution. The word oxygen is derived from the Greek *oxys*, which translates to acid and *gens*, which translates to creator or former.

Oxygen is one of the most important and abundant elements on earth. It exists in the atmosphere as a gas, in water as part of the water molecule, and in rocks and minerals in the earth's crust. In its most common elemental form, oxygen is found in the atmosphere as diatomic oxygen - O_2. Oxygen is colorless and odorless; many natural chemical reactions consume oxygen, including combustion and decay of organic matter.

Oxygen is constantly being "produced" through the solar-chemical process unique to green plants - photosynthesis. Photosynthesis is a chlorophyll dependant process. The green plant will use the suns solar light energy to cut CO_2 into carbon atoms and O_2. The oxygen is pumped into the environment, thus replenishing the oxygen supply.

The carbon atoms that are a byproduct of photosynthesis are used to construct carbon chains which are then in turn used to produce, wood (cellulose), complex carbohydrates, sugars, amino acids, fatty acids, oils and vitamins.

The solar energy stored in wood, carbonaceous plant materials, carbohydrates and sugars is referred to as "solar income."

Almost 46% of the earth's crust is oxygen, and it is by far the most abundant element in the earth's crust. Oxygen is essential to life and is part of almost every biological molecule in our body. The combustion of various fuels depends upon oxygen and provides most of the energy for industry and for heating.

Oxygen is a structural atom of water (in and out of living systems) and all organic compounds of biological interest, O_2 is required for respiration by all aerobic organisms. We can live for 30 days without food, three to seven days without water, under ideal circumstances, however, we can only survive for four minutes without gaseous oxygen.

This critical requirement for oxygen makes it the most important of all elements from the standpoint of immediate survival and maintenance of human life.

Oxygen is transported across the alveolar (microscopic air sacs) membranes in the lungs into capillaries and is transported to the bodies trillions of cell attached to a large complex protein molecule - hemoglobin. This molecule is very large, consisting of 574 amino acids. Found only in the red blood cell, hemoglobin chemically binds oxygen to itself and then releases it to our cells. When loaded with oxygen, hemoglobin is bright red and gives oxygenated blood its characteristic color. When the oxygen is released, hemoglobin turns color to a dark bluish red.

According to the 1980s U.S. Geological Survey, our earth's atmosphere had 50% oxygen at the time when dinosaurs flourished. These oxygen levels were arrived at by inserting microneedles into trapped air bubbles in polar ice and determining the oxygen levels in the dated prehistoric ice.

Some paleontologists claim that the simultaneous and universal demise of the dinosaurs followed the widespread quieting of the earth's volcanoes, which reduced the atmospheric levels of CO_2, which in turn reduced the oxygen levels to 38%. It is theorized that the 12% drop in the earth's oxygen levels was sufficient to cause the apocalyptic end of the dinosaurs.

The Geological survey also reported that the earth's atmosphere still contained 38% oxygen as late as 100 years ago. During the 1950s the percentage of oxygen in our atmosphere dropped to 21% and today oxygen is only 19% of our gaseous atmosphere. The continued drop in oxygen levels reflects an increase in oxygen consuming species and fossil fuel combustion (i.e. vehicles, electric and power generating plants). Combined with increased consumption is lower oxygen production (i.e. decreasing acreage of the rain forests and aquatic algae). The net result of this continued drop in atmospheric oxygen levels is a relative "anaerobic state" compared with the 38% of just 100 years ago and a very dramatic shift to the "anaerobic state" compared with the 50% oxygen levels of 75 million years ago.

Most pathogenic organisms (disease producing germs) are by themselves anaerobic. They are "happier," and flourish and reproduce with more vigor in the absence of oxygen. You know them as gangrene organisms, type A "flesh eating" Streptococcus, MRSA, etc. They are able to survive and grow in and around living cells weakened by low oxygen environments, which are also conducive for the growth of viruses, yeast, fungi, cancer, etc.

The question is, why have anaerobic diseases "suddenly" appeared in the 80s and 90s, diseases that we have little or no human history or experience?

Regardless of the name, tuberculosis, consumption, or scrofula can be found in five thousand-year-old mummies from Egypt and China, one thousand-year-old corpses from

Peru, and in ancient writings from the Greeks and Romans. The "new" modern day anaerobic diseases have little or no history with humans, nor will you find anything in biblical or ancient writings describing HIV, EBV, CMV, Herpes II, Hanta virus, SARS, H5N1 Avian Flu, *Candida albicans*, yeast, Toxic Shock Syndrome, *E. coli*, MRSA, or type A "flesh eating" *Streptococcus Sp.*

The most plausible theory is that the anaerobic disease causing organisms laid around in a dormant state as long as the atmospheric oxygen remained high (i.e. 50, 38, or even 21%) and inhibited their activity and growth. With the precipitous dip in atmospheric oxygen we are having an "oxygen counter revolution" with a return to the anaerobic bios.

Anaerobic Diseases of Humans

Disease	Year of Appearance
Viral	
Mycoplasma (rheumatoid arthritis And "Desert Storm Syndrome")	1958
Herpes II (sexually transmitted herpes)	1978
HIV (AIDS virus)	1982
EBV, CMV (Chronic Fatigue Syndrome)	1982
Hanta Virus (Four Corners Disease)	1993
Ebola virus	1996
SARS	2000
H5N1 Avian Flu	2004

Bacteria

Staphylococcus (Toxic Shock Syndrome)	1982
E. coli (Toxic Shock Syndrome)	1993
Type A Streptococcus ("Flesh-eating" Strep)	1994
MRSA (Methacillin Resistant *Staphlococcus aureus*)	2000

Yeast/Fungus

Candida albicans ("Candida")	1982
Coccidioidomycosis ("Valley Fever")	1900 - 35/year 1992 - 1,450/year

Cancer

Cancer (all types)	1900 - 1/10 1994 - 2/3

Dr. Otto Warburg of the Max Plank Institute, Germany, was the recipient of two unshared Nobel Prizes. Linus Pauling was the only other individual to be awarded two unshared Nobel Prizes. One of Warburg's Nobel Prizes was awarded for his discovery of the amino acid and for describing the basic chemical composition of proteins and the second for discovering that the metabolism of the cancer cell is fermentative and anaerobic while the metabolism of the normal noncancerous cell is aerobic. During the 1950s, Warburg was able to demonstrate clearly that cancer cells ferment sugar under anaerobic conditions and die in the presence of oxygen.

Neutrophils, a type of white blood cell that help

defend us by identifying, engulfing, and destroying invading micro-organisms (i.e. viruses, bacteria, yeast, fungus, malaria, etc.), parasites, and cancer cells, use hydrogen peroxide as their "lethal weapon." Neutrophils tend to be very sloppy, dribbling their over-production of hydrogen peroxide freely into the blood stream.

The potential danger of hydrogen peroxide free in the blood stream could be a loose cannon, but fortunately, we humans are blessed with a protective ubiquitous enzyme called catalase. Catalase literally covers our red blood cells and coats the inside walls of our blood vessels. The function of catalase is to rapidly facilitate the decomposition of hydrogen peroxide down to water (H_2O) and a singlet oxygen atom (O).

There are concerns by the uninitiated regarding the "free radical" status of singlet oxygen which has a free electron. When singlet or atomic oxygen comes into direct contact with tissue cells outside of the circulatory system (i.e. cell culture, test tube, wounds, etc.) the cells will die. In the whole animal or human, other factors come into play to prevent "free radical" damage.

When ingested in proper dilution on an empty stomach or administered intravenously under proper conditions, food grade hydrogen peroxide is readily absorbed through the stomach and duodenal walls directly into the blood stream where it is immediately broken down into water and singlet oxygen. The free electron of the singlet oxygen either combines with a free electron of a carcinogenic free electron or with the free electron of a second singlet oxygen, becoming O_2.

Carcinogenic free electrons frequently remain free electrons under many circumstances. They are actually quite happy with their free electron status. On the other hand, the free electron of the singlet oxygen does not like to be a singlet electron and if it doesn't locate another free electron to attach to, it will grab onto another singlet oxygen in nanoseconds becoming atmospheric oxygen (O_2) - the required stuff of respiration.

$$\text{Ozone } O_3 \longrightarrow H_2O_2 + O- \xrightarrow{\text{catalase}} H_20 + O_2$$

Oxygen in the form of hydrogen peroxide has been used topically, intravenously and orally since the Civil War. It has been used widely in Europe for over 50 years for alternative cancer therapies, circulatory disease, arteriosclerosis, emphysema, asthma, gangrene and more recently as a therapy for stroke patients.

Stroke patients have inactive but living cells surrounding the stroke site known as "sleeping beauty" cells that can be reactivated or jump started when they are exposed to several atmospheres of oxygen in hyperbaric chambers. Athletic injuries can also be treated by putting the injured athlete into a hyperbaric oxygen chamber. The healing time is shortened significantly so the athlete can return to play in weeks instead of months.

Os-Osmium is found in igneous rocks at 0.0015 ppm. It oxidizes organic matter as OsO_4 and is reduced to Os.

Osmium is a hard, brittle, bluish-white metal with an extremely high melting point (3,054 C). Osmium was discovered in 1803 by the English chemist Smithson Tennant, who found the new element while examining the residue formed by treating platinum ores with aqua regia, a mixture of nitric and hydrochloric acids. Tennant named his newly discovered element for its odor, using the Greek word *osme*, which translates to "smell."

P-Phosphorus is found in igneous rocks at 1,050 ppm, shale at 700 ppm, sandstone at 170 ppm, limestone at 400 ppm, fresh water at 0.005 ppm, sea water at 0.07 ppm, and soil at 650 ppm, where it has been "fixed" by hydrous oxides of Al and Fe in acid soil. Phosphorous is found in marine plants at 3,500 ppm, terrestrial plants at 2,300 ppm, marine animals at 4,000 to

18,000 ppm, and terrestrial animals at 17,000 to 44,000 ppm.

Phosphorus is a nonmetal element that was discovered by the German physician Hennig Brand in 1669. Brand carried out experiments in the fashion of the ancient alchemists. He distilled the residue from boiled-down urine and obtained a new element that glowed in the dark and burst into flames when exposed to warm air. He had discovered white phosphorus, a waxy, white solid that melts at 44 C. The name given to the new element was taken from the Greek word *phosphorous* which translates to "bearer of light."

In many ways, the chemistry of phosphorus is similar to that of nitrogen. Phosphorus occurs in nature as phosphate rocks, which consists mainly of calcium phosphate and fluorapatite, a mineral containing calcium, fluorine, and phosphate. Almost all of the elemental phosphorus produced commercially is in the form of phosphoric acid. Phosphoric acid is a solid that is most often sold as an 85% solution in water. Its primary use is for the production of triple-phosphate fertilizers - soil that is devoid of phosphorus is barren.

The original use of NPK (nitrogen, phosphorus, potassium) as a fertilizer began in the 1700s was a creation of the German chemist Liebig, who burned bread, grain and vegetables, analyzed the ash and then produced a cheap chemical fertilizer from these three elements.

Phosphorous is an extremely important essential mineral, however, it gets little or no attention from nutritionists because it is widely available in all foods. Phosphorous is a major structural mineral for bones and teeth. It has more functions in the human body than any other mineral, including its role as a vital constituent of nucleic acids, activating enzymes, and for several steps of the ATP energy cycle, and for RBC metabolism.

A complete discussion of phosphorous would require a discussion of every metabolic function in the human body. Second in abundance only to calcium in the human body, it comprises 22% of the body's total mineral content. The human body contains about 800 grams of phosphorous, just short of two pounds, of which 700 grams are found in bones and teeth as insoluble calcium phosphate.

The balance of phosphorous in the human body is found as biologically active intra and extracellular colloidal P in combination with carbohydrates, lipids, protein and a wide variety of other biologically active organic compounds including the blood's major buffer system. B-complex vitamins function as coenzymes to intracellular metabolic functions only when combined with phosphorus.

Phosphorus is part of most proteins and as such becomes problematic because elevated P intake increases Ca requirements when "high protein diets" are consumed. Under those circumstances P can aggravate osteoporosis, arthritis, high blood pressure, loosen teeth, periodontal disease, etc. Phosphorus is present as phytates in cereals and whole grain flours, therefore, if bread is made from unleavened flours, the phytic acid will complex with Ca, Fe, Zn, and other minerals further lowering their absorption rate.

The average adult human dietary intake of P is 1,000 to 1,500 mg/day. In adults and older children, the absorption of metallic P is limited to about three to five per cent and as high as eight to 12% in infants. Mixed dietary sources of chelated P may be absorbed at the rate of 40 to 50%. Optimal absorption of metallic and chelated P occurs when the dietary Ca:P ratio is 1:1. Organically bound colloidal P is absorbed up to 98%.

Deficiencies of P have long been recognized in livestock. Symptoms of P deficiency include the behavior of pica and cribbing and fractures. Phosphorus deficiency has only recently been recognized in humans. The widespread, universal, and ultimately fatal results of P deficiency are the result of its widespread biological functions, significantly as the result of a decrease in ATP synthesis (complete metabolic energy failure) with associated neuromuscular, skeletal, blood and kidney disease.

Clinical P depletion and resultant low blood P

(hypophosphatemia) without P supplements, excessive use of antacids, hyperparathyroidism (low calcium/high phosphate diets are the cause of this disease).

Improper treatment of diabetic acidosis, use of diuretics, sweating during exercise, and work and alcoholism with and without liver disease can create a P deficiency.

Vegetarians and vegans who do supplement with minerals rarely have P deficiency, however, because of their high phytic acid intake, they tend to always have other mineral deficiencies including Ca, Cu, Cr, V, Li, Fe, Co and zn.

Pa-Protactinium is found in igneous rocks at 1.4 x $10^{(-6)}$ ppm and sea water at 2.4 x $10^{(-31)}$ ppm. All isotopes of protactinium are radioactive with a half-life of 32,000 years. Protactinium accumulates in mammalian bone after ingestion.

Protactinium is one of the most rare and most expensive of the naturally occurring elements. It is found in pitchblende, where it is produced as one of the decay products of uranium.

Protactinium was discovered by the German physicists Kasimir Fajans and O. H. Gohring in 1913 during a study of the elements produced by the decay of uranium ore.

The two Germans originally named their new element "brevum," however, the name was later changed to protactinium in 1949. Its name is derived from the Greek word *protos*, which translates to "first," and actinium, because the decay product of protactinium is actinium. There are 22 known isotopes of protactinium. The pure metal was eventually purified in 1934.

Pb-Lead is found in igneous rocks at 12.5 ppm, shale at 20 ppm, sandstone at 7 ppm, limestone at 9 ppm, soil at 10 ppm (higher in limestone soils and humus), fresh water at 0.005 ppm, sea water at 0.00008 pm, marine plants at 8.4 ppm, terrestrial plants at 2.7 ppm (many plant species are adapted to grow in lead-rich soils and accumulate lead including

Amorpha canescens), marine animals at 0.5 ppm (highest in fish bones), and in terrestrial animals at 2.0 ppm. The highest lead levels are found in bone, liver and kidney. Lead is known to be part of and required for the RNA/DNA duplicating system.

Lead has an ancient history, lead coins and lead sculpture have been found in Egyptian tombs dating back to 5,000 years B.C. The alchemists associated lead with the planet Saturn and not only believed lead to be the oldest metal but also believed that all other metals eventually transmutated into lead.

The metal, lead, takes its name from the Anglo-Saxon word *lead*, and its chemical symbol from the Latin word for the element, *plumbum*. Lead is rarely found in nature as the pure metal, the most common lead ore is galena, which is made up of lead sulfide.

Mineral deficient animals and children with the symptoms of pica and cribbing, a craving for non-food items (i.e. paint, sand, dirt, etc.), are very susceptible to lead poisoning ("plumbism"). Infants and children with pica will will chew on their toys, cribs, windowsills, caulking, furniture, and paint. A chip of lead paint the size of a penny can contain as much as 50 to 100 ug of lead. Consuming this much lead daily over a three month period will result in lead poisoning. Like many heavy metals, lead disables enzymes that are catalysts for subcellular biochemical reactions.

The "normal" background blood lead level is below 40 ug/dl. Children with blood lead levels above 60 to 80 ug/dl have symptoms of vomitting, irritability, weight loss, muscular weakness, headaches, abdominal pain, insomnia and anorexia.

Children with blood lead levels above 80 ug/dl show anemia, kidney disease, peripheral neuritis, ataxia and muscular incoordination, joint pain, and encephalopathy (brain damage, learning disabilities, etc.) with eventual death.

The best approach to treating lead poisoning is to supplement with all 90 essential nutrients to eliminate pica and cribbing and further ingestion of lead, restoring fluid and electrolyte balance. In addition, the use of IV or IM chelation therapy using EDTA (ethylenediaminetetraacetic acid) and BAL (British Anti-lewisite) for a minimum of five days. It is not unusual for as many as 25% of Pb poisoned individuals to have residual loss of IQ, loss of coordination, hyperactivity, learning disabilities and impulsiveness.

Pd-Palladium is found in igneous rocks at 0.01 ppm and terrestrial animals at 0.002 ppm. Palladium accumulates in mammalian liver and kidney. Palladium is relatively rare and, like rhodium and ruthenium, is frequently found mixed with platinum; it was discovered in 1803 by William Hyde Wollaston, who named it after the asteroid *Pallas*.

Palladium is commonly used for the treatment of malignant tumors. These Palladium compounds inhibit cell division of the cancer, yet are free of negative side effects. Radioactive palladium pellets, the size of a grain of rice, are commonly used as a treatment for prostate cancer. With a half-life of only 17 days, the palladium-103 isotope delivers doses of radiation and then disappears.

Oral compounds of thiamine, lipoic acid and palladium began to be used as a non-prescription OTC (home remedy) cancer treatment after the year 2000.

Pm-Promethium is a synthetic rare earth element created in nuclear accelerators and nuclear reactors; its isotopes are radioactive with a half-life of 2.6 years. Promethium is an important fission product that has now entered the biosphere. Prior to man-made nuclear explosions, promethium did not exist in nature.

Very little is known about the chemical or physical properties of pure promethium although pure salts have been produced; the radiation produced by pure promethium salts causes the surrounding air to glow in the dark with a brilliant blue light.

Promethium is named after the Greek god Prometheus

who stole fire from the heavens; promethium has been identified in the spectrum of several stars in the Andromeda Galaxy.

The existence of promethium was predicted in the early 20th century, however, it was only in 1947 that it was isolated by J. A. Mirinsky, L. E. Glendenin and C. D. Coryell, a team of scientists working at the National Laboratory at Oak Ridge, Tennessee. They found promethium among the plethora of different nuclei of intermediate size, known as fission fragments. When neodymium is bombarded with intense neutron radiation it is transmutted to promethium.

Twenty-eight isotopes of promethium have so far been synthesized, all of which are radioactive. Promethium-145 is the longest-lived isotope with a half-life of 17.7 years. The electrons given off by promethium-147 nucleus disintegration, are used to produce light from phosphors to produce heat in nuclear-powered batteries, to produce X-rays in portable X-ray units and to measure the thickness of thin sheets and film such as paper and metal sheets and foil.

Promethium accumulates in mammalian bone and liver after ingestion.

Po-Polonium is found in igneous rocks at $2 \times 10^{(-10)}$ ppm. The discovery of polonium by Marie and Pierre Curie in 1898 was one of the "great moments in the history of science." Their discovery of this radioactive element (originally called "radium") eventually produced the modern concept of the atomic nucleus and a basic understanding of its structure.

The Curies were looking for the source of the radioactivity in the uranium-bearing mineral pitchblende. Their curiosity was aroused when they removed the uranium from pitchblende, radioactivity was still present. Their investigations eventually led to the isolation of two new elements, polonium and radium.

Polonium was named for Poland, the native country of Marie Curie. It is a rare element in nature, being formed by the decay of radioactive uranium and thorium. Polonium is found in uranium mines in concentrations as little as 100 millionths of a gram per ton of ore.

Polonium has 27 known isotopes, more than any other element, and all are radioactive. The most common isotope is polonium-210. It has a half-life of only 138 days, making it 5,000 times more radioactive than radium.

Polonium-210 is a silvery metalloid that is extremely volatile; it will almost completely vaporize at temperatures as low as 60 C. As it decays, polonium emits alpha particles, each of which is a nucleus of a helium atom. When polonium-210 ejects an alpha particle, it is transmutted into lead-206, a very stable isotope of lead.

The Nuclear Regulatory Commission has established a quantity of 0.8 million millionths of a gram as the maximum allowable amount of polonium-210 that can be ingested; this makes polonium-210 approximately 100,000 million times more toxic than cyanide.

Pr-Praseodymium is a "light" rare earth found in igneous rock at 8.2 ppm, shale at 6 ppm, sandstone at 2.8 ppm, limestone at 1.4 ppm, marine plants at 5 ppm, terrestrial plants accumulate Pr at 46 ppm (*Carya spp.*), marine animals at 0.5 ppm,and terrestrial animals at 1.5 ppm (accumulating in liver and bone after ingestion).

Praseodymium was isolated in 1885 by Carl Auer von Welsbach, an Austrian baron who had a passion for mineralogy. He separated a mineral called didymium into two new and distinct elements, one of which contained praseodymium; it was named from two Greek words, *prasios*, which translates to "green," and *didymos*, which translates to "twin." The name refers to the green color of the element's oxide; the second element was neodymium. Praseodymium was not produced in its pure elemental state until 1931. It is a soft, silvery-white metal that tarnishes to form a green oxide.

Praseodymium is found primarily in monazite and bastnasite ores. Monazite sands contain all of the "rare earth" elements, often in concentrations greater than 50%. Monazite is found in river sand in India and Brazil and in Florida beach sand. Large deposits of bastnasite are found in Southern California

Pt-Platinum is found in igneous rocks at 0.005 ppm and land animals at 0.002 ppm. Platinum is a precious metal, like gold, is highly prized for jewelry and is used as a medium of exchange world wide.

Platinum is a durable, heavy, silver-white metal that is resistant to corrosion, does not react with oxygen and is found in nature as the pure element. Most of the world's supply of platinum comes from South Africa.

Platinum was discovered in 1741 by an Englishman, Charles Wood, however, there is considerable evidence that points to the wide spread use of platinum by the pre-Columbian Indians. Platinum is derived from the Spanish word *platina,* which translates to "silver." A bar of platinum-iridium alloy is stored in a vault in Paris where it serves as the world's standard for the kilogram.

Platinum is used in the medical treatment of ovarian cancer and testicular cancer (cis-platinum) as it specifically inhibits the growth of ovarian and testicular cancer cells.

Platinum is commonly used in the mechanism of cardiac pacemakers.

Pu-Plutonium isotopes are all radioactive with a half-life of 24,000 years. Plutonium was released into the earth's atmosphere by nuclear explosions. Marine plants show 4,000 times the background level of sea water, terrestrial plants record 0.4 to 2.2 disintegrations/sec/kg, and terrestrial animals show 0.07 to 6.8 disintegrations/sec/kg. Plutonium accumulates in mammalian bone after contact or ingestion.

Plutonium is the most important of all of the transuranium elements, all of which are synthetically created. Plutonium was the second transuranium element, following neptunium. In 1941, the American chemist, Glenn T. Seaborg, at the University of California at Berkeley discovered plutonium, however, because of security reasons, the announcement of the discovery was not made until 1946. Plutonium was named for Pluto, the planet that is found outside the orbit of Neptune in our solar system.

Plutonium has 15 known isotopes, all of which are radioactive. Plutonium-239 has a half-life of 24,000 years, is the most important because it readily fissions when bombarded by thermal neutrons.

Ra-Radium is found in igneous rocks at $9 \times 10^{(-7)}$ ppm, shale at $11 \times 10^{(-7)}$ ppm, sandstone at $7 \times 10^{(-7)}$ ppm, limestone at $4 \times 10^{(-7)}$ ppm, fresh water at $3.9 \times 10^{(-110)}$, sea water at $6 \times 10^{(-11)}$ ppm, soils at $8 \times 10^{(-7)}$ ppm, marine plants at $9 \times 10^{(-4)}$ ppm, terrestrial plants at $10^{(-9)}$ ppm, marine animals at $0.7^{(-15)} \times 10^{(-9)}$ ppm, and in terrestrial animals at $7 \times 10^{(-9)}$ ppm. The highest concentrations are found in mammalian bone; all isotopes of radium are radioactive.

Radium was discovered in 1898 by the Polish-born French chemist Marie Sklodowska Curie and her husband, Pierre Curie. It is generally agreed that the discoveries of radium, the electron and Einstein's theory of relativity "ushered in the beginning of the modern era in science."

During their analysis of the radioactive properties of a uranium-containing mineral (pitchblende), the Curies realized when they extracted all of the uranium from the pitchblende, the remainder was still radioactive. Sifting through tons of ore, they were able to isolate a radioactive mix that was mostly barium.

The barium was employed as a precipitating reagent for polonium and other elements in the ore. When they heated the precipitate in a flame to create spectral lines, the Curies observed an unexpected red color - a new element. The Curies named their new element (radium) from the Latin word *radius*, which translates to "ray." They also discovered polonium in the same ore. It takes seven tons of pitchblende to produce one gram of radium.

It took four more years for the Curies to produce a pure sample of radium, which they isolated from a solution of radium chloride by electrolysis. In 1911, Marie Curie was awarded the Nobel Prize in chemistry for her discovery of these new elements. It was her second Nobel Prize, as she had shared her first with her husband and the French scientist, Henri Becquerel in 1903 for the accidental discovery of radioactivity.

Radium has 25 known isotopes, the most common and the one discovered by the Curies, is radium-226, which has a half-life of 1,630 years.

The international standard for the measurement of radiation is called the Curie in honor of the Curies.

Rb-Rubidium is found in igneous rocks at 90 ppm, shale at 140 ppm, sandstone at 60 ppm, limestone at 3.0 ppm, fresh water at 0.0015 ppm, sea water at 0.12 ppm, soil at 100 ppm ("fixed" by clay bearing soils), marine plants at 7.4 ppm, terrestrial plants at 20 ppm, marine animals at 20 ppm, and terrestrial animals at 17 ppm (the highest levels are found concentrated in the liver and muscle, the lowest levels are found in bone.

In 1861, the German chemists Robert Bunsen and Gustav Kirchhoff discovered rubidium. They identified it as an impurity mixed with the alkali metals they were investigating; they identified rubidium as a new element from the spectral lines it emitted, one of which is a deep red color. The name rubidium is taken from the Latin word *rubidus*, which translates to "deep red."

It is documented that rubidium can replace the electrolyte function of potassium in many species, including bacteria, algae, fungi, and certain invertebrates (echinoderms - starfish).

Re-Rhenium is found in igneous rocks at 0.005 ppm, marine plants at 0.014 ppm, and marine animals at 0.0005 to 0.006 ppm, Terrestrial animals accumulate rhenium in the thyroid.

Rhenium is one of the most-rare of all earthly elements. It takes one million pounds of molybdenite ore to produce one gram of rhenium, resulting in a price of $10,000 per gram in 1928.

In 1925, the existence of rhenium was predicted by and then discovered by the German chemists Ida Tacke, Walter Nodack, and Otto Carl Berg. They named rhenium from the Latin word *Rhenus*, which translates to the Rhine River.

Rh-Rhodium is found in igneous rock at 0.001 ppm. Rhodium is very rare and is usually found mixed in platinum ores. It was discovered by the Englishman William Hyde Wollaston in 1803. He named it after the Greek word *rhodon*, which translates to "rose" for its characteristic rose color.

The catalytic converter of carbon fuel vehicles are filled with small catalytic beads that are made of platinum, palladium and rhodium, that act to convert hot exhaust gases that flow through them into harmless byproducts.

The carbon monoxide and unburned hydrocarbons are converted into carbon dioxide and water and the nitrogen dioxide is converted to nitrogen and oxygen.

Rn-Radon gas is found in igneous rocks at $4 \times 10^{(-13)}$ ppm, fresh water at $1.7 \times 10^{(-15)}$ ppm and sea water at $6 \times 10^{(-16)}$ ppm. All 20 known isotopes of radon are radioactive with a half-life ranging from 54 seconds to 3.8 days. Radon is carcinogenic and highly toxic when inhaled. Radon is a common household pollutant and hazard; it is colorless and odorless. Detection requires the use of OTC detection kits which are generally available.

Radon is produced as one of the radioactive decay products of uranium and thorium. This noble gas is the heaviest known gas, being eight times heavier than air and is chemically non-reactive..

Radon was originally discovered by the German physicist Friedrich Ernst Dorn in 1900 while analyzing the decay products of radium; he named the new gaseous element "radium emanation." William Ramsay and R. W. Whytlaw, two early radon investigators, renamed the gas "niton," from the Latin word *nitens*, which translates to "shining." In 1923 the name of this gas was changed again to radon.

Radon-222 is the longest-lived isotope of radon, with a half-life of 3.82 days. Radon-222 is found naturally in the soil in large concentrations as the result of trace levels of uranium that are found throughout the earth's crust. The gas diffuses through the soil and into the air. Radon can diffuse into family dwellings and businesses through basement floors and walls. This dangerous pollution risk is particularly high during the winter months when doors and windows are kept closed.

As early as the 16th century, it was well known that uranium miners in Bohemia often died from strange diseases of the lungs. When radon-222 is inhaled, it decays and emits alpha particles, which are the nuclei of helium atoms. This decay product, lead-210 is also radioactive and settles into the lower reaches of the lung.

Lead-210 has a radioactive half-life of 20.4 years; it is this extended exposure of the lungs to radiation of lead-210 that causes cancer. Experts believe that 10% of all lung cancers are caused by radon and it's decay byproducts.

Smoking cigarettes poses a radiation risk as well as the well known chemical risk. While it is growing, tobacco is a victim of contamination by radon in the soil, and the phosphate fertilizers commonly used by farmers are rich in uranium. When the tobacco leaf is burned, the inhaled smoke subjects the smoker to levels of radiation that are 1,000 times higher those suffered by nuclear power plant employees.

Ru-Ruthenium is found in igneous rocks at 0.001 ppm, terrestrial plants at 0.005 ppm, and in terrestrial animals at at 0.002 ppm. RuO_4 is very toxic.

Ruthenium is a rare element that is a byproduct of refining platinum ores. Its discovery was noted by the Estonian chemist Karl Karlovitch Klaus, who named it from the Latin word *Ruthenia*, which translates to "Russia."

A current use of ruthenium is as a catalyst for a reaction that splits water into hydrogen gas and oxygen. This catalytic method of splitting water to obtain hydrogen and oxygen depends upon the ruthenium being "excited" or energized by exposing it to solar radiation. This alternative source of fuel does not require electricity to generate energy and therefore ruthenium has an obvious importance in the 21st century as part of a method that can produce cheap fuel at a low cost of man generated energy and it is environmentally green.

S-Sulfur is found in igneous rocks at 260 ppm, shale at 2,400 ppm, sandstone at 240 ppm, limestone at 1,200 ppm, freshwater at 3.7 ppm, sea water at 885 ppm, soils at 700 ppm, marine animals at 5,000 to 19,000 ppm (highest in coelenterates and molluscs) and in terrestrial animals at 5,000 ppm (highest levels in cartilage, tendons, keratin, skin, intervertebral discs, hair and nails). Its lowest concentrations are in bones. In soils, 90% of sulfur is bound tightly in humus, SO_4 is a major exchange anion in many soils, and occurs in soils near to volcanoes. In terrestrial plants sulfur occurs at a rate of 3,400 ppm with the lowest concentrations found in bryophytes and gymnosperms.

Sulfur is an important structural atom in most proteins as sulfur amino acids (cystine, cysteine and methionine) and small organic molecules. Glutathione, a tripeptide containing cysteine, is essential to normal cellular reactions involving sulfur amino acids in proteins. Sulfur is found in a reduced form (-SH) in cysteine and in an oxidized form (-S-S-) as the double molecule cystine. This "sulhydryl group" is important for the specific configuration of some structural proteins and for the biological activities of some enzymes (proteins that do work).

Sulfur-containing proteins work in indirect ways to maintain life:

Hemoglobin

Hormones (insulin, adrenal cortical hormones)

Enzymes

Antibodies

Sulfur also occurs in carbohydrates such as heparin, an anticoagulant that concentrates in the liver and to lesser degrees other tissues, chondroitin sulfate (cartilage, ligaments, tendon, discs, connective tissue, etc.), the vitamins thiamine (B_1) and biotin have sulfur bound in their molecule.

The toxic characteristics of arsenic are the result of its ability to combine with sulfhydryl groups.

A deficiency of sulfur results in osteoarthritis, osteoporosis and a degeneration of cartilage, weakened tendons, weakened ligaments, erythematosis, sickle cell anemia, lupus and other "collagen diseases."

Sb-Antimony is found in igneous arocks at 0.2 ppm, shale at 1.5 ppm, soil at 2.0 to 10 ppm, terrestrial plants at 0.06 ppm, and in terrestrial animals at 0.0006 ppm, where it concentrates in mammalian heart tissue. Antimony potassium tartrate (tarter emetic) is still used today as the preferred treatment for blood flukes (schistosomiasis or bilharziasis).

In its pure state, the metal antimony, is a hard, brittle, grayish crystalline metal. The ore that produces the most antimony element is stibnite (antimony sulfide), which has been known for thousands of years. A black compound, stibnite was used in the ancient days to darken women's eyebrows (mineral makeup).

The ancient alchemists often mistook lead bearing ore for stibnite. The chemical symbol for antimony (Sb) was taken from its original Greek word, *stilbium*, named after the mineral stibnite. In 1855, the safety match was created by the Swedish chemist Jerry Eugene Lundstom. The head of the match consisted of a mixture of antimony trisulfide and an oxidizing molecule such as potassium chlorate. The tip of the match, above the head, contains red phosphus that, when struck against a rough surface, ignites and generates enough heat to set fire to the head of the match (bursts into a bright flame).

Sc-Scandium is found in igneous rock at 22 ppm, shale at 13 ppm, sandstone and limestone at 1.0 ppm, and in terrestrial animals at 0.00006 ppm, where it concentrates in mammalian heart and bone.

Scandium is a rare element that is found in the crust of the earth at 0.0025%, it is found in a higher rate in the sun and a few other stars. Scandium, using the periodic chart in 1871, was one of the elements that Mendeleyev predicted would exist. In 1879, scandium was discovered by Lars Fredrik Nilson, who named the element after his homeland. Scandinavia.

Se-Selenium is found in igneous rock at 0.05 ppm, shale at 0.6 ppm, sandstone at 0.055 ppm, limestone at 0.08 ppm, fresh water at 0.02 ppm, sea water at 0.00009, soils at 0.2 ppm, marine plants at 0.8 ppm, terrestrial plants at 0.2ppm, and terrestrial animals at 1.7 ppm where the highest concentrations are found in liver, kidneys, heart and skeletal muscle. Keep in mind that selenium is not universally distributed.

Selenium is a metalloid that can exist in two different forms, red and gray, called allotrops. Red selenium is an amorphous, glasslike solid, while the gray form of selenium is a soft, bluish-gray metal.

Selenium was discovered by the Swedish chemist Jons

Jakob Berzelius in 1817. Selenium was named for the Greek word *selene,* which translates to moon.

Vast areas earth are deficient or totally devoid of selenium; where it occurs selenium is found in the humus of alkaline soils.

Selenium is found in the humus of alkaline soils. Selenium is the most efficient antioxidant; it is used at the subcellular level in the glutathione peroxidase enzyme system and metalloamino acids (selenomethionine, etc.).

Selenium prevents cellular and subcellular lipids and fats from being peroxidized, which literally means it prevents body fats from going rancid. "Rancid" body fats are seen externally as "age spots" or "liver spots." These golden brown pigments of aging are technically known as ceroid lipofuscin.

Lipofuscin gradually fills cells as the individual ages. The medical theory is that these pigments eventually fill the cell and render them helpless and this "aging" process eventually kills the organism.

In fact the accumulation of ceroid lipofuscin is preventable and can be reversed.

Selenium also functions to protect cellular and organelle bi-lipid layer membranes from oxidative damage. High intakes of vegetable oils, including salad dressing and cooking oils, concurrent with a selenium deficiency is the quickest route to a cardiomyopathy heart attack, arteriosclerosis (build up of plaque in the arteries resulting from free radical damage to the "intima" or lining of the artery), cataracts, macular degeneration, dementias, multiple sclerosis, cancer, etc.

The polyunsaturated configuration of oils when heated or treated with hydrogen ("trans fatty acids") literally causes the rancidity ("free radical" damage) of cellular fat.

The clinical diseases associated with a selenium deficiency are diverse and to the uninformed shrouded in mystery. Selenium deficiency is one of the more costly mineral deficiency complexes affecting embryos, the newborn, toddlers, teens, young adults, and seniors alike.

Selenium Deficiency Diseases

<u>Direct Result</u>

Anemia

"Age spots" & "Liver spots"

Fatigue

Muscular weakness

Myalgia (muscle pain and soreness)

Fibromyalgia

Scoliosis

Muscular dystrophy (MD, White Muscle Disease, Stiff Lamb Disease)

Cardiomyopathy (Keshan Disease, "Mulberry Heart" Disease)

Heart palpitations

Atrial fibrillation

Liver necrosis and cirrhosis

Pancreatitis

Pancreatic Atrophy

Infertility

Low birth weight

High infant mortality

SIDS (Sudden Infant Death Syndrome)

Cystic Fibrosis (congenital and immediately post natal)

Wilson's Syndrome (hypothyroidism with normal TSH, T3 and T4)

Indirect Deficiency Results

HIV (increases rate of conversion to AIDS)

ALS (Lou Gehrig's disease)

MS (Multiple sclerosis)

Alzheimer's Disease

Cancer (deficiency increases risk significantly)

Selenium deficiency can result in infertility in both men and women. Congenital selenium deficiency (during pregnancy) can result in a wide variety of problems ranging from failure to conceive, miscarriages, low birth weight, high infant mortality, SIDS, muscular dystrophy, Cystic Fibrosis, cardiomyopathy heart disease and liver cirrhosis. Selenium deficiency in growing children can result in "crib death" or SIDS (Sudden Infant Death Syndrome).

Sixty-five percent of SIDS death occurs in children being fed commercial infant formulas low or devoid of selenium. Slow growth, small size (failure to reach genetic potential for size and mass), Muscular Dystrophy, scoliosis, cardiomyopathy (Keshan disease), anemia, liver cirrhosis, muscular weakness, lowered immune capacity and neuromuscular diseases are also linked to selenium deficiency.

In young adults, selenium deficiency appears as anemia, chronic fatigue, Wilson's Syndrome, muscular weakness, myalgia, fibromyalgia, muscular tenderness, pancreatitis, infertility, Muscular Dystrophy, scoliosis and cardiomyopathy.

Cardiomyopathy is quite common in young athletes such as basketball and football players at the high school, college, university, and professional levels because of selenium deficiency, as are multiple sclerosis and liver cirrhosis.

Selenium deficiency in adults appears as reduced immune capacity, anemia, infertility, "age spots" or "liver spots," myalgia, fibromyalgia, muscle weakness, MS, ALS, Parkinson's Disease, Alzheimer's Disease, palpitations (irregular heart beat), cardiomyopathy, liver cirrhosis and increased risk for cancer (i.e. prostate, breast, colon, lung, etc.).

Selenium acts as an antagonist of mercury. Those at risk for chronic mercury toxicity (dental amalgams, industrial pollution, preservatives, etc.) should supplement with selenium prior to, during and after detoxification activities.

In a review of the anti-cancer properties of selenium, Dr. Gerhard N. Schrauzer (Head of the Department of Chemistry & professor emeritus, UCSD) states:

Selenium is increasingly recognized as a versatile anticarcinogenic agent. Its protective functions cannot be solely attributed to the action of glutathione peroxidase. Instead, selenium appears to operate by several mechanisms, depending on dosage and the chemical form of selenium and the nature of the carcinogenic stress. In a major protective function, selenium is proposed to prevent the malignant transformation of cells by acting as a "redox switch" in the activation-inactivation of cellular growth factors and other functional proteins through the catalysis of oxidation-reduction reactions of critical -SH groups or -S-S- bonds.

The growth-modulatory effects of selenium are dependent on the levels of intracellular glutathione peroxidase and the oxygen supply. In general, growth inhibition is achieved by the Se-mediated stimulation of cellular respiration (more oxygen/less cancer).

Selenium appears to inhibit the replication of tumor viruses in animals and the activation of oncogenes by similar mechanisms. However, it may also alter carcinogen metabolism and protect DNA against carcinogen-induced damage. In additional functions of relevance to its anticarcinogenic activity, selenium acts as an acceptor of biogenic methyl groups, and is involved in detoxification of metals and certain xenobiotics. Selenium also has

immunopotentiating properties. It is required for optimal macrophage and natural killer cell functions.

The school of pharmacy from the University of Georgia released a report in August of 1994 that concluded "that a human selenium deficiency is related to the clinical onset of full blown AIDS in clinically infected HIV patients." According to their report, HIV requires large amounts of selenium for replication. In selenium deficient patients, the virus competes with the patient for the limited amount of available selenium. The HIV patient actually dies of a chronic selenium deficiency encephalopathy, liver cirrhosis, or cardiomyopathy. Long-term HIV patients (20 years or more) that never developed full blown clinical AIDS had supplemented with large doses of selenium.

Si-Silica is found in igneous rocks at 281,500 ppm, shale at 73,000 ppm, sandstone at 368,000 ppm, limestone at 24,000 ppm, fresh water at 6.5 ppm, sea water at 3.0 ppm, soils at 33,000 ppm (found as SiO_2, the most abundant form of Si in nature, in silicates and clays), marine plants at 1,500 to 20,000 ppm, marine animals at 70,000 ppm, and in terrestrial animals at 120 to 6,000 ppm where it is mainly concentrated in hair, lungs and bone.

Silicon is the second most abundant element in the crust of the earth, exceeded only by oxygen. Compounds of silicon bond chemically to oxygen make up most of the earth's sand, rock and soil.

Silicon was first produced in its pure state in 1824 by the Swedish scientist Jons Jakob Berzelius (1779-1848).

The most important silicon compound is silica, or silicon dioxide (SiO_2). It exists in two familiar forms in nature: a crystalline form called quartz, small chips of which are found in sand, a a noncrystalline form called flint. Small gems and semiprecious stones such as amethyst, opal, agate and jasper are crystals of quartz with colored impurities.

Flint has been known for thousands of years. When struck with an acute-angle blow, it will flake in such a manner as to produce a sharp cutting edge. Some of the earliest prehistoric stone tools were made of flint.

Flint also allowed prehistoric man (Neanderthals) to start fires anywhere and at will by striking flint with iron pyrite or another piece of flint. Once they understood the fire starting properties of flint, man was able to move without carrying fire or burning embers with him - he could now start fire anywhere in just a few moments with dry tinder, flint and iron pyrite.

Silica as sand can be mixed with soda ash (sodium carbonate) and limestone (calcium carbonate) and when the mixture is melted it becomes glass - there are more than 1,000 forms of glass.

Plants accumulating the most silica are diatoms, horsetail, ferns, Cyoeraceae, Graineae, and Juncaceae, and the flowers of *Pappophorum silicosum*. Silicon supplementation increases the collagen in growing bone by 100 per cent. Tissue levels of silicon decrease with aging in unsupplemented humans and laboratory species. Dry brittle finger and toenails, poor skin quality, poor calcium utilization, and arterial disease characterize silica deficieny. High fiber diets contain high levels of silicon, which leads many investigators to believe that silicon helps to lower cholesterol. The recommended intake of silicon ranges from 200 to 500 mg/ day.

Sm-Samarium is a "light" rare earth and is found in igneous rocks at 6.0 ppm, shale at 5.6 ppm, sandstone at 2.7 ppm, limestone at 0.8 ppm, terrestrial plants at 0.0055 ppm (accumulates up to 23 ppm), marine animals at 0.04 to 0.08 ppm, terrestrial animals at 0.01 ppm in heart muscle and 0.0009 ppm in mammalian bone and liver. Samarium enhances normal cell proliferation and doubles the life span of laboratory species.

Samarium is the fifth most abundant of the rare earth

elements, it was discovered in 1879 by the French chemist Paul-Emile Lecoq de Boisbaudran, who correctly identified the element's spectral absorption lines in a mineral called samarskite, which has been named for a Russian army officer, Colonel Samarski.

The primary ores that samarium is extracted from are monazite and bastnasite. Monazite contains all of the rare earth elements; it is found in river sand in India and Brazil and in Florida beach sand. Extensive deposits of bastnasite are found in Southern California.

Sn-Tin is found in igneous rocks at 2.0 ppm, shale at 6.0 ppm, sandstone and limestone at 0.5 ppm, fresh water at 0.00004 ppm, sea water at 0.003 ppm, soils at 2.0 to 200 ppm (strongly absorbed by humus), marine plants at 1.0 ppm, terrestrial plants at 0.3 ppm (highest in bryophytes and lichens), marine animals at 0.2 to 20.0 ppm, terrestrial animals at 0.15 ppm with highest levels being found in lungs and intestines.

Originally the presence of tin in tissue was attributed to environmental contamination; however, careful and detailed studies by Schwarz demonstrated that tin produced acceleration of growth in rats and further met the standards for being an essential trace element. Tin has several chemical and physical properties similar to those of carbon, silica, germanium and lead.

Rats fed tin at 17.0 ng/gm show poor growth, reduced feeding efficiency, hearing loss, and bilateral (male pattern) hair loss, while rats fed 1.99 ug/gm were physiologically and anatomically normal.

Schwarz demonstrated tin to be an essential element in 1970. Tin has been shown to exert a strong induction effect on the enzyme heme oxygenase, enhancing heme breakdown in the kidney. There is also evidence for tin having cancer prevention properties. A federal study released in November 1991, showed that men in recent generations have poorer hearing at any given age than men in earlier generations. Men over age 30 lose their hearing more than twice as women of the same age. So much for having a "tin ear"!

Sr-Strontium is found in igneous rocks at 375 ppm, shale at 300 ppm, sandstone at 20 ppm, limestone at 610 ppm, fresh water at 0.08 ppm, sea water at 8.1 ppm, soils at 300 ppm, marine plants at 260 to 1,400 ppm, terrestrial plants at 26 ppm, marine animals at 20 to 500 ppm, and in terrestrial animals at 14 ppm, where it is most highly concentrated in mammalian bone.

Natural sources of strontium are the mineral ores celestite, which is a form of strontium sulfate, and strontianite, a strontium carbonate. Both strontium and the mineral strontianite were named in 1789 by the English scientist Dr. Adair Crawford, who first identified the element in the Scottish village of Strontian.

Strontium can replace calcium in many organisms, including man. There is considerable evidence for essentiality in mammals including man. Deficiencies of strontium are associated with certain types of calcium and boron resistant osteoporosis and arthritis.

Strontium-90, the man-made radioactive isotope of the fission atomic explosions and the greatest biohazard fear during the "Cold War," does not occur in nature and has a half-life of 28.8 years.

Ta-Tantalum is found in igneous rocks at 2.0 ppm, shale at 0.8 ppm, sandstone and limestone at 0.05 ppm, sea water at 0.0000025 ppm, and in marine animals accumulates up to 410 ppm.

Anders Gustav Ekeberg, a Swedish chemist, discovered the new element in 1802 near the Swedish town of Ytterby, which played an important role in the history of chemistry, particularly as a source of minerals for the discovery of rare earths.

Ekeberg named his new element for Tantalos, the father

of Niobe, who, in Greek mythology, was queen of the city of Thebes. For almost 50 years after Ekeberg's announcement of his new element, many chemist thought he had confused tantalum with niobium. Pure tantalum metal was not produced until 1903.

The principal ore of tantalum is the mineral columbite, which is widely distributed throughout the world, with large deposits in Africa, Thailand, Portugal and Canada. Tantalum is used for dental and joint prosthesis.

Tb-Terbium is found in igneous rock at 0.9 ppm, shale at 0.58 ppm, sandstone at 0.41 ppm, limestone at 0.071 ppm, terrestrial plants at 0.0015 ppm, marine animals at 0.006 to 0.01 ppm and terrestrial animals at 0.0004 ppm where it accumulates in bone.

Terbium is one of the least abundant of the rare earth elements. Carl Gustaf Mosander discovered the element in 1843 by isolating its oxide from the mineral yttria.

Terbium is recovered commercially from the mineral monazite, a mixture of rare earth elements combined with thorium and calcium. It is found in river sands from India and Brazil and in beach sand from Florida.

In its pure metallic form, terbium is silvery-white and is soft enough to be cut with a knife.

Tc-Technetium is not found in nature and all isotopes are radioactive. Technetium was the first new element to be produced in a laboratory. Technetium gets its name from the Greek word *teknetos*, which translates to "artificial."

While it is not found in nature in the earth's crust, technetium has been discovered in some stars. Technetium was discovered in 1937 by Emilio Segre and Carlo Perrier. The discovery was made in Italy from a small sample sent to them by the University of California at Berkeley. Technetium is poorly absorbed by mammals.

Te-Tellurium is found in igneous rocks at 0.001 ppm, terrestrial plants at 2 to 25 ppm, and in terrestrial animals at 0.02 ppm. Tellurium is a rare, silvery-white metalloid belonging to the family of elements that includes such nonmetallic elements as oxygen and sulfur. Sulfur and oxygen can combine with other metals to form sulfides; tellurium combines with gold to form a telluride.

Tellurium is one of the few elements that combines with gold. The compounds are gold telluride, and they are commonly found in gold-bearing ores.

Tellurium was discovered in Germany in 1782 by an inspector of mines, Franz Joseph von Reichenstein, an amateur scientist, who was experimenting with an ore he picked up in a gold mine in Transylvania. It was named in Berlin from the Latin word *tellus*, which translates to earth.

Th-Thorium is found in igneous rocks at 9.6 ppm, shale at 12 ppm, sandstone and limestone at 1.0 - 7.0 ppm, soils at 5 ppm, marine animals at 0.003 to 0.03 ppm and terrestrial animals at 0.003 to 0.1 ppm. Thorium is a radioactive, silvery-white metal that is very soft. Its oxide has a melting point of 3,300 C, one of the highest of any oxide, and when shaved into small pieces, it can be ignited in air to produce a brilliant white light.

Thorium was discovered in 1828 by the Swedish chemist Jons Jakob Berzelius, who named it for Thor, the Scandinavian god of war. He was not aware of its radioactivity as radioactivity was not known until it was discovered by Henri Becquerel and the Curies in 1897.

Thorium-232, the radioactive isotope of thorium that occurs naturally, is actually very weakly radioactive. Its half-life is a whopping 14 billion years, so that very little of it decays in a short period of time.

Thorium ores are as common as lead ore and approximately four times more abundant than uranium ores. Monasite sand, which is common as beach sand in Florida, can contain as much as 10% thorium, and this sand is used for the commercial production of the element.

Ti-Titanium is found in igneous rocks at 5,700 ppm, shale at 4,600 ppm, sandstone at 1,500 ppm, sea water at 0.001 ppm, soils at 5,000 ppm, marine plants at 12.0 to 80.0 ppm (accumulates in plankton), terrestrial plants at 1.0 ppm, marine animals at 0.2 to 20.0 ppm and terrestrial animals at 0.2 ppm.

Titanium is the ninth most abundant element in the earth's crust, and making up 0.6 per cent of the earth's mass. It was discovered in 1791 by an amateur English mineralogist, the Reverend William Gregor, titanium was named for the Titans of Greek mythology. The minerals rutile and ilemnite are the common sources of titanium.

Each jet engine from a Boeing 747 contains 10,000 pounds of titanium and its compounds.

Tm-Thulium is a "heavy" rare earth and is extremely rare; it is found in igneous rocks at 0.48 ppm, shale at 0.28 ppm, sandstone at 0.3 ppm, limestone at 0.065 ppm, terrestrial plants at 0.0015 ppm, and terrestrial animals at 0.00004 ppm. Thulium supplementation enhances the growth of normal cells in cell culture and has doubled the life span of laboratory species.

The Swedish chemist Per Teodor Cleve discovered the element in 1879 by isolating its greenish oxide from the mineral erbia. He named his new element for Thule, the ancient name for Scandinavia.

The main source of thulium is the mineral monazite, which consists of approximately seven thousandths of one percent thulium. Monazite, which contains all of the rare earth elements in addition to thorium and calcium, is found in the river sands in India and Brazil and in beach sand in Florida.

Thulium is a bright silvery metal that is soft that it can be cut with a knife.

U-Uranium is found in igneous rock at 2.7 ppm, shale at 3.7 ppm, sandstone at 0.95 ppm, limestone at 2.2 ppm, fresh water at 0.001 ppm, sea water at 0.003 ppm, soil at ppm (absorbed by humus, especially in alkaline soils), terrestrial plants at 0.038 ppm (*Astragalus spp.* is an accumulator plant), marine animals at 0.004 to 3.2 ppm, and animals at 0.013 ppm. All natural isotopes are alpha emitters and may also decay by fission. Uranium is accumulated by mammalian kidney and bone after ingestion.

Uranium is the last and heaviest of the natural elements. The average person associates uranium with nuclear reactors and the atomic bomb as a source of limitless energy. Once considered rare, uranium is now known to be commonly found in many minerals, including pitchblende, uranite, "yellowcake," and monazite sands. In the United States, the ownership and sale of uranium are strictly controlled by the U.S. Nuclear Regulatory Commission.

The use of uranium compounds to color glass and ceramic glazes dates back for thousands of years. In 1789, the German chemist Martin Klaproth, was the first investigator to recognize that pitchblende contained a yet unknown element. It was not until 1841 that the French chemist Eugene-Melchior Peligot first isolated and identified uranium. It was named after the planet Uranus. In 1896, the French physicist Henri Becquerel discovered that uranium was radioactive.

A typical sample of uranium consists of two isotopes, uranium-238 (99.2798 per cent) and uranium-235 (0.7171 percent). Uranium-238 is the dominant isotope of the element; its half-life of 4.6 billion years makes it the longest-lived of the three uranium isotopes.

V-Vanadium is found in igneous rocks at 1135 ppm, shale at 130 ppm, sandstone at 20 ppm, limestone at 20 ppm, fresh water at 0.001 ppm, sea water at 0.002 ppm, soils at 100 ppm (vanadium is absorbed by humus, especially in alkaline soils), marine plants at 2.0 ppm, terrestrial plants at 1.6 ppm (accumulated by the fungus *Armanita muscaria*), marine animals at 0.14 to 2.0 ppm, and in terrestrial animals at 0.15 ppm. Metallic vanadium (vanadyl sulfate) is absorbed from the intestinal tract very poorly at only 0.1 to 1.0 percent, vanadium chelates are absorbed at 40 percent, and plant derived colloidal forms at up to 98%.

Vanadium makes up 0.02% of the earth's crust, and is present in trace amounts in more than 60 different ores. The predominant source of vanadium is vanadinite. A Mexican professor of mineralogy, Andres Manuel del Rio, discovered vanadium in 1801. It was later named for the Scandinavian goddess Vanadis because of its many beautifully colored compounds.

Vanadium was proven to be essential in 1971. Vanadium stimulates blood sugar (glucose) oxidation and transport in fat cells and glycogen (animal starch) synthesis in liver and muscle, and inhibits liver gluconeogenesis (production of glucose from fat and protein) and absorption of glucose from the gut.

Vanadium enhances the stimulating effect of insulin on DNA synthesis. Despite low serum insulin, the blood glucose levels of diabetic rats fed vanadium was the same as the glucose levels of normal controls. Vanadium appears to function like insulin by altering cell membrane function for ion transport. Therefore vanadium has a very beneficial effect for humans with glucose and carbohydrate intolerance (i.e. hypoglycemia, hyperinsulinemia, narcolepsy, prediabetes, diabetes, depression, manic depression, bi-polar disease, "chemical imbalance," ADD, ADHD, violent behavior, autism, etc.) by making the cell membrane insulin receptors more sensitive to insulin.

Vanadium inhibits cholesterol synthesis in animals and humans; this followed by decreased plasma levels of cholesterol and reduced aortic cholesterol. Vanadium initiates an increase in the contractile force of heart muscle known as the "inotropic effect."

Vanadium has known anticarcinogenic properties. Feeding 25 ug of vanadium per gram of diet blocked induction of mouse mammary tumor growth. The vanadium supplement reduced tumor incidence, average tumor count per animal, and prolonged median cancer-free time without inhibiting overall growth or health of the animals.

Clinical Diseases Associated with Vanadium Deficiency

Slow growth
Increased infant mortality
Infertility
Elevated cholesterol
Elevated triglycerides
Hypoglycemia
Hyperinsulinemia
Narcolepsy
Prediabetes
Diabetes (adult onset, type II)
ADD, ADHD
Depression
Manic depression (Bi-polar disease)
Tourette's syndrome
Autism
Cardiovascular disease
Obesity

W-Tungsten is found in igneous rocks at 1.5 ppm, shale at 1.8 ppm, sandstone at 1.6 ppm, limestone at 0.6 ppm, sea water at 0.0001 ppm, soils at 1.0 ppm, marine plants at 0.0035 ppm, marine animals at 0.0005 to 0.05 ppm, and in terrestrial animals at 0.005 ppm. Tungsten accumulates in heart muscle and teeth at 0.00025 ppm.

When all of its impurities are removed tungsten is soft enough to be cut with a saw. It is believed that two Spanish brothers, Juan Jose and Fausto del Elhuar discovered tungsten in 1783, extracting it from the mineral known as wolframite. There is evidence, however, that the element was known before that time and was called wolfram. Many chemist, particularly in Germany, still refer to tungsten as wolfram - this explains the chemical symbol "W." The more widely accepted name for the element tungsten was taken from the Swedish words *tung stem*, which translates to "heavy stone."

The main ores of tungsten are wolframite and scheelite; about 75% of the world's tungsten deposits are thought to be in China.

Xe-Xenon is found in ineous rocks at 0.00003 ppm and in sea water at 0.000052 ppm. Xenon binds to mammalian hemoglobin and myoglobin producing an anesthetic effect.

Xenon is a heavy "noble" gas with a density that is five times heavier than air; like the other noble gases it exists as a monoatomic molecule that has no color, odor or taste.

Xenon was discovered by the English chemist Sir William Ramsay in 1898 and named by him. He derived the name for this new element from the Greek word *xenos*, which translates to "the strange one."

In 1962, Neil Barlett, an English chemist working at the University of British Columbia, made the first noble gas compound. He combined xenon and platinum hexafluoride which produced a solid, yellow-orange compound, which consisted of xenon, platinum and fluorine.

Y-Yttrium is a "heavy" rare earth element found in igneous rocks at 33 ppm, shale at 18 ppm, sandstone at 9.1 ppm, limestone at 4.3 ppm, sea water at 0.0003 ppm, soils at 50 ppm, terrestrial plants at 0.6 ppm (accumulates in ferns), marine mammals at 0.01 to 0.2 ppm, and in terrestrial animals at 0.04 ppm where it is found in mammalian bone, teeth and liver.

Yttrium is found only in small quantities in the earth's crust. Rocks brought back from the moon by the Apollo astronauts had a surprisingly high level of yttrium. Yttrium was first identified in 1789 by Johan Gadolin; he named it for the small Swedish village of Ytterby, near Stockholm. The greatest quantity of yttrium is extracted from monazite sand.

Yttrium is a silver-gray metal that is reactive enough to burn spontaneously in air when it is cut into tiny pieces.

Yttrium enhances normal cell growth and doubles the life span of laboratory species. Exposure of pregnant mice to yttrium leads to rapid placental transfer. Fourteen per cent of yttrium ingested by the pregnant female can be detected in the newborn mouse pups.

Yb-Ytterbium is a rare earth element found in igneous rock at 3 ppm, shale at 1.8 ppm, sandstone at 1.3 ppm, limestone at 0.43 ppm, terrestrial plants at 0.0015 ppm, marine animals at 0.02 ppm, and in terrestrial animals at 0.00012 ppm, where it accumulates at up to 0.3 ppm in bone, teeth and liver.

The French chemist Jean de Marignac discovered this element in 1878 as a part of the mineral known as erbia and was the first "rare earth" element discovered. It was named for the Swedish village of Ytterby. The main source of ytterbium is monazite sand which contains all of the rare earths, thorium and calcium and is found in river sand from India and Brazil and beach sand from Florida at three hundredths of one per cent.

Alloys are used in dentistry and to manufacture certain forms of stainless steel

Exposure of pregnant mice leads to rapid placental transfer; fourteen percent of ingested ytterbium can be detected in newborn mice.

Zn-Zinc is found in igneous rocks at 70 ppm, shale at 95 ppm, sandstone at 116 ppm, limestone at 20 ppm, fresh water at 0.01 ppm, sea water at 0.01 ppm, soils at 50 ppm, marine plants at 6 to 1,500 ppm, terrestrial plants at 100 ppm, marine animals at 6 to 1,500 ppm, and in terrestrial animals at 160 ppm.

Zinc accumulates in mammalian kidney, prostate, and eye. Zinc was known to be an essential growth factor for bread mold more than 100 years ago, essential for rats more than 50 years ago, and essential for humans 20 years ago.

Zinc deficiency produces a wide range of diseases including congenital birth defects and degenerative diseases of all age groups.

Congenital Birth Defects Associated with Zinc Deficiency

Down's Syndrome

Cleft lip and cleft palate

Brain defects (dorsal herniation, hydroencephaloceol)

Micro or anophthalmia (small or absent eyes)

Agnathia (small lower jaw)

Spina bifida (neural tube defects)

Clubbed limbs

Syndactyly (webbed toes and fingers)

Polydactyly (extra limbs and digits)

Atresia (failure to develop limbs. Digits, organs, openings, etc.)

Hernias (hiatal, diaphragmatic, umbilical, inguinal, etc.)

Heart defects

Lung defects

Urogenital defects (horseshoe kidney, small kidney, intersex malformations of the male and female genitals)

There are 1.4 to 2.3 grams of zinc in the adult human. The liver, pancreas, kidney, bone and skeletal muscle have the greatest reserves of zinc. Lesser amounts are found in the eye, protate gland, semen, skin, hair, fingernails and toenails.

There are no less than 70 metalloenzymes that require zinc as a functional cofactor. These metalloenzymes include carbonic anhydrase, alkaline phosphatase, lactic dehydrogenase, and carboxypeptidase. Zinc helps to bind enzymes to substrates by maintaining spatial and configurational relationships. Some enzymes bind zinc so tightly that even during severe zinc depletion they can still function.

Zinc participates in the metabolism of nucleic acids and the synthesis of proteins. Zinc is also an integral part of the RNA molecule itself where zinc provides the "metallic fingers" and participates in cell division and synthesis of DNA. The DNA-dependent RNA polymerase is a zinc-depndant enzyme, as is thymidine kinase.

Excesses of dietary copper and iron and high phytate diets (vegans) will reduce availability of dietary zinc. Heavy losses of zinc occurs in sweat, therefore, unsupplemented athletes are particularly at high risk for zinc deficiency with the following symptoms such as anorexia nervosa, muscle weakness, pica and cribbing, etc.

Symptoms and Diseases of Zinc Deficiency

Pica/Cribbing (geophagia, pagophagia, wool eating, hair eating, dirt eating, paint eating, etc.)
Loss of sense of smell
Loss of sense of taste
Infertility
Failure of wounds and ulcers to heal
Immune status failure
Poor growth (short stature)
High Infant mortality
Hypogonadism (small, poorly functioning ovaries and testes)
Perpetual prepubic state
Anemia
Alopecia (hair loss)
Acrodermatitis enteropathica (parakeratosis, celiac disease)
"Frizzy" hair
Diarrhea
Depression
Paranoia
Oral and perioral dermatitis
Weight loss (anorexia nervosa)
Benign prostatic hypertrophy (BPH, noncancerous prostatic enlargement)
Severe body odor ("smelly tennis shoe" syndrome)
Anorexia and Bulimia

Zr-Zirconium is found in igneous rocks at 165 ppm, shale at 160 ppm, sandstone at 220 ppm, limestone at 19 ppm, fresh water at 0.0026 ppm, sea water at 0.000022 ppm, soils at 300 ppm, marine plants at 20 ppm, terrestrial plants at 0.64 ppm, marine animals at 0.1 to 1.0 ppm, and terrestrial animals at 0.3 ppm.

Zirconium was discovered in 1787 by the German chemist Martin Heinrich Klaproth. The best known compound of zirconium is the mineral zircon. This mineral has been known since ancient times and is even referred to in the Bible. Zirconium derives its name from *zargun*, which is the Arabic name for zircon and translates to "gold color."

Zircon is a crystalline compound of zirconium silicate ($ZrSiO_4$). It is found in a variety of colors, and when the crystal is cut and polished, the stone is regarded as a semiprecious gem. Zircon has a very high index of refraction, which means that it has the property of bending light through large angles. Because the colorless crystals of zircon have a high brilliance they are oftentimes used as a diamond substitute in faux jewelry.

Essential Minerals and Elements Found in a High Quality Humic Shale (Plant Derived Minerals and Elements)*

Aluminum	Gold	Rhenium
Arsenic	Hafnium	Rubidium
Barium	Holmium	Samarium
Beryllium	Hydrogen	Scandium
Boron	Iodine	Selenium
Bromine	Iron	Silica
Calcium	Lanthanum	Silver
Carbon	Lithium	Sodium
Cerium	Lutetium	Strontium
Cesium	Magnesium	Sulfur

Chloride
Chromium
Cobalt
Copper
Dysprosium
Erbium
Europium
Gadolinium
Gallium
Germanium
Manganese
Molybdenum
Neodymium
Nickel
Niobium
Nitrogen
Oxygen
Phosphorus
Potassium
Praseodymium
Tantalum
Terbium
Thulium
Tin
Titanium
Vanadium
Ytterbium
Yttrium
Zinc
Zirconium

**Many of the minerals and elements listed are not "classically" considered to be "essential," however, they meet at least two or more of the criteria necessary to be declared an essential nutrient.*

Part 2

"In more primitive times man returned sewage, wastes, and dejecta (wood ashes) to the soil. Now he has become sanitary and discharges what came from the soil into the rivers, and eventually into the ocean."

D.C. Jarvis, M.D.
Folk Medicine

The Currency of Life

Chapter 6

"It is our duty, my young friends, to resist old age; to compensate for its defects by a watchful care; to fight against it as we would fight against disease; to adopt a regimen of health; to practice moderate exercise; to take just enough food and drink to restore our strength and not to overburden it."

Cicero,(106-43 B.C.)
Roman statesman

"Terra preta exists in two forms: terra preta itself, a black soil thick with pottery and terra mulata, a lighter dark brown soil with much less pottery. A number of researchers believe that although Indians made both, they deliberately created only the terra mulata. Terra preta was the soil created directly around homes by charcoal (wood ashes), kitchen fires and organic refuse of various types."

Bruno Glaser, *Chemist*
University of Bayreuh, Germany

The Currency of Life

It doesn't matter whether one is a devote of creationism or a student of evolution - our immediate and mutual problem is that the Earth, our planet, our environment is a limited finite resource for the raw materials that are necessary for the basis of all plant, animal and human life as we know it.

The sequence of events for the creation of all the elements of the periodic chart and life on Earth is the same for Biblical scholars, physicists, anthropologists, archeologists and geologists - the only real difference in the thinking of these groups is the time reference between events!

All living organisms procure their raw materials of essential elements for reproduction, development, growth, maintenance and longevity from a thin blanket of light, gas, water and solid matter on or just above the Earth's crust.

The Earth's atmosphere, a standard mixture of inert (nitrogen) and functional gases (oxygen), with the exception of local or regional pollutants, is universally the same around the Earth.

All water on Earth, our universal solvent and elixir of life, with the exception of the diversity of minerals and other elements in the aqueous solution or suspension, local or regional pollutants, water itself is universally H_2O.

Being found in the lowest crevices of the surface of the earth, the largest bodies of water on earth are the seas and oceans. The oceans are catch basins into which chemical and mineral substances of every kind have been dumped by the many moving forces in nature since the beginning of time.

Loose, transportable and soluble materials are either moved directly and swiftly, or indirectly and by varying degrees, downhill and downward into the sea. Particles are lifted and transported by the irresistible forces of wind, watercourse, and glaciers.

Highly soluble substances in soil are dissolved in water and are transported to the sea where they accumulate. In this way, "oceans have become a reservoir of accumulated mineral wealth" which makes the mineral resources of the land masses insignificant by comparison.

In contrast to the predictably and identical chemical analysis of the atmosphere's many gaseous elements and the simple universal chemical analysis of water, the Earth's plethora of mineral elements found on the periodic chart, are not distributed equally in the blanket over or in the crust (soil or parent rock) of the Earth. Mineral elements are found randomly in veins like chocolate in chocolate ripple ice cream, or like gold and silver.

The result of this disproportionate distribution of mineral elements in the crust of the Earth, there is in fact, a direct cause and effect of what appears on the surface to the casual observer to be a random pattern of the optimum location for plant (red wood trees) and animal populations (kangaroos) on Earth just as there is a disproportionate distribution of wealth.

Holy accounts of the formation of the Earth and the organisms that populate the Earth that are accepted by believers of the Jewish, the Kaleidoscope of Christian faiths and the Muslim faiths are brief ,however, the details need not be chronicled for the events to be in fact true any more than the details not being required when grandma says, "I baked you a dozen cookies" - you know she selected and ground the organic whole wheat berries into flour, sifted the flour, added filtered water, baking powder, salt, honey, yeast culture, butter, chocolate chips and walnuts; she then dutifully blended and mixed the basic elements into a cookie dough, she took a spoonful of the now complete cookie dough and plopped it onto a greased cookie sheet and baked them in the oven at 375 degrees F for 30 minutes into perfectly wonderful and chewy chocolate chip-walnut holiday cookies - although grandma never sat down and shared the details of her activities, we inherently knew in fact she did them!

The Biblical account of the Earth's formation (Genesis) goes like this:

"In the beginning God created the heaven and earth. And the earth was without form, and void; and darkness was upon the face of the deep. And the spirit of God moved upon the face of the water. And God said, Let there be light, that it was good: and God divided the light from the darkness. And God called the light day, and the darkness He called night. And the evening and the morning were the first day. And God said, Let there be a firmament in the midst of the waters, and let it divide the waters from the waters. And God made the firmament and divided the waters which were under the firmament from the waters which were above the firmament; and it was so. And God called the firmament Heaven. And the evening and the morning were the second day. And God said, Let the waters under the Heaven be gathered together under one place, and let the dry land appear: and it was so. And God called the dry land Earth; and the gathering together of the waters called the seas: and God saw it was good. And God said, Let the Earth bring forth grass, the herb yielding seed, and the fruit tree yielding fruit after his kind, whose seed is in itself, upon the Earth: and it was so."

Like grandma's cookies we don't need to know the intricate details of how it happened to appreciate the fact that the Earth or the delicious steaming chocolate chip-walnut cookies appeared miraculously before us to see, smell and savor the result of the effort.

The only scientific chemical theory of the origin of the Earth and its elements was crystallized in 1957 by E. M. Burbridge. According to his theory, all of the Earth's elements can be built up electron by electron from hydrogen gas; hydrogen atoms in space condense together by gravitational attraction into clouds of gas, which ultimately condense into stars and planets.

Burbridge's theory of the origin of the stars and the

Earth, to say the least is complex, detailed and controversial; some researchers support his theory of the condensation of hot gases with the subsequent transmutation of one element into another while others favor the theory of an accretion of cold gases.

The technique of radio-dating puts the Earth's genesis or "birth" at 4 to 5 billion years ago. Regardless of which theory is believed (and it is not an all or nothing choice as the biblical belief includes all elements of creation and formation), biblical or the "big bang," all must agree that the geochemical fractionation of the Earth's elements continues even today although at an almost imperceptible snail's pace and that the Earth is still not in a geochemical equilibrium (i.e. - erosion, earthquakes, tidal waves, volcanoes, etc.).

Radioactive dating is a powerful method of measuring relative geologic time. It has been employed in the estimate that the Earth is 4 to 5 billion years of age. However, even with the radioactive-dating techniques the embryologic stages of terrestrial development, including the accumulation of the Earth's great iron core and the genesis of the relatively light and movable land masses, have remained obscure and elusive because numerous events (i.e.- thermal and geochemical) that can reset the "radioactive clock."

As land masses float, migrate and relocate across the Earth's surface, the elements that reach the ocean's floor through erosion from land masses into creeks, streams and rivers into the ocean floor sink and recycle into the hot interior mantle and core; when land masses are forced into each other, mountain ranges are born. Molten elements find their way through the continental faults, frequently breaking through the surface and reaching the crust's surface as volcanic lava.

Three major segregations of the Earth's elements can easily be recognized; initially the primal Earth, heated by the radioactive decay process separated into three onion-like concentric layers:

We have limited indirect data on the Earth's core and

mantle, which in fact make up most of the Earth's solid mass; the Earth's crust on the other hand has been systematically and intimately probed, analyzed, gouged and extracted.

The Earth's crust is cooled and solid, whereas the inner layers of the mantle and core are in various states of molten (magma) minerals which are on occasion ejaculated onto the surface of the planet by volcanoes.

When the Earth's crust was initially cooling it separated into a series of minerals, crystallizing into igneous rocks in a definite and systemic order, the by products being liquid water and gaseous nitrogen which formed the great oceans and seas and nitrogen that makes up the majority of our atmosphere.

Over time, wind and water erosion wear off the mountain's surface which produces a mineral-rich dust and silt and sediment which are swept into valleys, forests, plains, creeks, rivers, lakes and oceans where they eventually are returned to the Earth's mantle. Periodic floods historically enriched the soils of flood plains and "bottom land" with life-giving mineral rich silt that accumulated over time to create "soil."

Soil, in its infinite number of forms is the last part of the geological genesis puzzle - it is basically the product of climate and the effects of living organisms on rocks; its physical nature and chemical composition is determined by the make up of the parent rock in a particular location and by the natural forces attacking them.

As a rule of thumb, regions with similar climates have like types of soils, but each type of soil has numerous variations related to the underlying rock, topography or vegetation.

Soil structure is comprised of three distinct layers:

A) Humus or decomposed plant material - this is the "organic" layer of the soil ("top soil"); usually the mineral elements are rapidly lost by the leaching effects of water, rain, irrigation, "mining" by plant growth (wild and cultivated) and acid rain.

B) Sand and various accumulations of some of the mineral elements leached from layer A.

C) The Subsoil, gravel and parent rock.

Soil is a dynamic "living" environment, an ecosystem unto itself, the health of which we are dependent upon for our own health and longevity. Frances Moore Lappe said it very well, "If you eat, you're involved with agriculture."

Coarse inorganic particles with a diameter greater than 0.0002 cm contribute from 5 to 90% of the dry weight of most soils and may be separated into gravel, sand and silt depending upon particle size and character.

Colloidal inorganic particles have a diameter of less than 0.0002 cm; they can be separated by mass or size in a water column. Inorganic colloidal particles usually comprise less than 10 to 80% of the dry weight of soils and are responsible for a soils color, texture and ion-exchange properties.

The soil solution, or water held in soil capillaries, which contains dissolved matter can be extracted by centrifugation and may compromise as much as 50% of healthy soil by weight. The soil solution is important as a media for the propagation of microorganisms and as an efficient medium for the rapid growth of plant rootlets.

The soil atmosphere is comprised of various gasses in equilibrium with the soil; it can be measured by use of a vacuum pump and may constitute up to 50% of healthy soil by volume.

The actual organic matter in soil is very difficult to separate from its colloidal inorganic matter in the soil; it is usually found as 1.0 to 50% of the dry weight of soil and rarely up to 90%. Organic matter in the soil primarily originates from plant debris and dead microorganisms (i.e.- bacteria and fungi).

The living organisms in the soil are of infinitely greater numbers and varieties than those species found on the surface of the soil. Soil organisms for the most part are unicellular, however, worms can be important in excavating minerals from sub soils and bring them to the Earth's upper layers in their manure or digestive "casts."

Worms also carry plant debris (with their mineral content) from the surface of the Earth into the humus layer where microorganisms make up 0.1 to 0.2% of soil by weight.

Soil microorganisms, although small in percentage of total weight of the soil are indispensable for soil formation, soil health and for the regulation process of pH (acid balance), nitrogen fixing (fertilization) and oxidation potentials.

From Dust to Dust

Our Earth is anemic! A potentially apocalyptic mixture of mining, deforestation, intensive farming, irrigation and acid rain has shifted, eroded or leached our life giving and life-sustaining raw materials from the formerly mineral rich crust of the Earth.

Unfortunately, we were given a finite amount of raw materials (minerals) in the Earth's crust and without daily infusions of mineral rich meteors, volcanic eruptions (i.e. - Mt. St. Helens, eastern Washington; Mt. Pinatubo, Philippines, etc.), flooding with highly mineralized silt or "rock flour" or "Glacial Milk", dust (finely ground rock flour) or wood ash (plant minerals) we are forced to make do with what we have - a declining mineral reserve in the soil.

There are those who would propose to re-mineralize mountain ranges, forests, farms and yes, whole continents to get minerals into our crops and therefore into our human food chain; but put into economic perspective these dreams and proposals are not sustainable. To re-mineralize the Earth is technologically possible, however, as a realistic economically sustainable agricultural program, however, it is a non-starter.

To re-mineralize the Earth for one growing season we would have to grind up the equivalent of Mauna Loa, the colossal Hawaiian mountain, each year and redistributing the resultant rock dust several times each year to coincide with soil preparation and planting programs.

To comprehend the enormity of this task, one has to appreciate that Mauna Loa is the most massive mountain in the world and is also the largest volcano; Mauna Loa rises 13,677 feet above the surface of the Pacific Ocean - an additional 17,000 feet drops from the water's surface to the ocean floor making it technically taller (almost one mile taller) than Mt. Everest.

Mauna Loa's total mass is 100 times larger than that of Mt. St. Helens in Washington State and the lava that forms the massive dome could cover the land masses of the Earth with four feet of additional mineral dust. The cost of such a Herculean effort would result in your hamburger reaching an eye-popping price of $275 per pound and corn $35 per ear - this sticker shock would make $5 per gallon gasoline look cheap!

When 23 year old Charles Darwin sailed the H.M.S. Beagle to the coast of South America in 1833, he recorded a fine, red dust accumulating on his ship each day and correctly deduced that the dust originated in West Africa.

This African dust in its westerly flight across the Pacific Ocean travels all the way to the Amazon and the rainforests where it is essential to annually replenish the rain leached mineral poor soils of the rainforests.

Man has always realized the enormity of the great and tireless power of the Earth's winds for energy and travel, but their importance to the biological vitality of the Earth and the mineral value of our food is far beyond what we have ever suspected!

There are many wind currents, east to west, that transport great loads of mineral dust across predictable routes, "linking ecosystems hundreds and even thousands of miles apart."

Billions of tons of mineral rich dust from the deserts of Asia and Africa annually fertilize oceans and rainforests halfway around the world.

Michael Garstang, professor of meteorology, at the University of Virginia in Charlottesville says, "During the violent Amazonian rainstorms, the particulates that originate in African deserts are literally sucked out of the sky."

Garstang and his colleagues calculate that 13,000,000 tons of African and Asian mineral-rich dust enter the Amazonian soils each season to enrich and fertilize the rain leached and mineral depleted tropical soils!

The wind-borne African dust adds essential and critical minerals to help maintain and support the rainforest's survival and productivity.

"While the Amazon Basin teems with life the soil itself lacks reserves of nutrients, especially phosphates, which spur plant growth.

The historical record shows that the Amazon Rainforest has periodically shrunk to a fraction of its present size, then bounded back again, and the researchers now believe that it expands and contracts as the supply of nourishing African dust waxes and wanes with mirror changes in the Saharan Desert."

The principal minerals found in the coarse inorganic fraction of soil are directly related to those minerals present in the local parent rock.

Minerals that are resistant to weathering (i.e.- quartz) are especially abundant in soils while minerals that weather quickly are rare or absent. It is therefore possible to calculate the relative age or maturity of a soil covering igneous rocks from its content of primary minerals (i.e. - feldspar, mica, amphiboles and pyroxenes); these relatively soluble minerals are common in young soil and less abundant in mature soils and absent from senescent soils. Soils covering sandstone often contain 90 to 99% quartz; those soils overlying limestone are made up of as much as 80% calcium carbonate.

It is obvious that minerals are not equally distributed

in soils. The scary part is that fields where our food crops are grown do not contain a uniform blanket of minerals, if they contain any nutritional minerals at all, they occur in veins much like the chocolate swirls found in chocolate ripple ice cream - at best depending solely on getting minerals from food grown in soil is an extremely risky crap shoot!

Trace Elements

Trace elements are defined as those elements present in soils in amounts of less than 0.1% by weight. Sixty percent of all trace minerals are found in the coarse inorganic fraction of the soil including Ba, Be, Co, Cr, Cu, Ga, La, Li, Mn, Mo, Ni, Pb, Rb, Se, Sr, V, Y and Zr.

Rare Earths

The term, rare earths, refers to any of a large series of very similar oxides of metals obtained from widely distributed but relatively scarce minerals. The Rare Earth metals are often divided into three groups, according to the method of separating them:

1) the cerium metals

(lanthanum, cerium, praseodymium, neodymium, illinium, samarium).

2) the terbium metals

(europium, gadolinium, terbium).

3) the yttrium or ytterbium metals

(dysprosium, holmium, erbium, thulium, yttrium, ytterbium, lutetium).

Beryllium, hafnium, scandium, thorium and zirconium are also included as Rare Earths by some geochemists.

Rare Earths added to laboratory animal's diets as a supplement to the well recognized major and trace minerals have doubled the expected life span of several different species.

These Rare Earths, known to be so vital to animal health and longevity (and most probably our human health and longevity) are no longer found in our food supply in any consistent or significant amounts - the only warranty to adequate Rare Earth intake for we humans is daily supplementation!

Basic Soils

Basic soils tend to be rich in minerals whose ionic radius is close to that of magnesium, i.e - Co, Cr, Cu, Fe, Mg, Ni, Se, Ti, V and Zn.

Acid Soils

Acidic soils containing feldspar that have ionic radius' close to silica, calcium or potassium, i.e. - Al, Ba, Ca, Cs, Hf, K, La, Na, Nb, Pb, Rb, Sr, Ta, Tl, Y and Zr.

Limestone soils are rich in elements which form insoluble carbonates, i.e. - Ba, Ca, Mg, Mn, Pb and Sr.

Colloidal inorganic particles are referred to as clay;

clay minerals are primarily aluminosilicates, many of which swell in water and act as ion exchangers. The hydrous (water) oxides of aluminum, iron and manganese are responsible for the natural colors of most clays, i. e. - blue, gray, red, orange, black; they also function as scavengers for phosphate and some trace minerals and Rare Earths.

Manufactured Soil

A common denominator for all of the "old ones" in the "Blue Zones" of the world is the fastidious attention they devote to the soil that their vegetable gardens, orchards and grains are grown in. In all instances this means the daily injection of mineral nutrients (glacial milk, wood ash, peat ash, rice straw ash, kelp ash, charcoal, etc.) and organic soil conditioners (kitchen wastes, manure and agricultural byproducts) into ancient growing sites that in some cases are thousands of years old.

In many cases, the successful formula to their longevity, supporting crops is a serendipitous mix of location, raw materials available and political events.

Terra Mare & Terra Preta

Roman culture has been thoroughly investigated and written about by cultural and anthropological scholars. The enormous Roman contribution to European civilization is obvious and agreed to by all who are familiar with the languages that developed over almost half of the European continent; the letters of the modern alphabet, the grand and massive architecture of our governmental buildings, our practice and steadfast devotion to the letter of the law and legal procedure, our republic style of governmental systems of checks and balances and the legend of Rome as a world state and the messenger and implementer of universal peace.

The Romans, themselves, first appear in history as a people who were traders and farmers who settled on a collection of low hills on the left bank of the Tiber River about 15 miles from its mouth.

The original settlement became a bustling trading center, and by 753 B.C. it could be considered a small city-state governed by a king.

All of the romantic stories of Rome overshadowed the fact that until well after Rome had ascended to the status of a world class political power, Romans, were in fact simple barbarians.

Even Pyrrhus, the Epirote, who encountered the Romans almost 100 years after the time of Alexander the Great, regarded them as barbarians and seemed surprised that they employed what was an advanced form of tactical thinking in regards to their military operations.

The Roman's conquest of the Greek cities of southern Italy, and their amazing and rapid expansion which established their power over the eastern Mediterranean in the short space of 50 years, surely was regarded by the "civilized populations" of the region as a feat equal to a Gaulish invasion!

Culturally, Italy lagged behind the Aegean countries throughout most of its history. The first Neolithic populations of Italy came from the east, either in boats by sea or by following and hugging the bountiful coastline, and were part of the Mediterranean phalanx of the Neolithic colonization of Europe.

The culture and practices of these original settlers were relatively simple, and there were no significant cultural advances after they set up house keeping in Italy.

The Neolithic period in Italy was also considerably shorter than it was in northern Europe, as Italy provided a considerable supply of mineral wealth, which attracted foreign miners and salt traders. Merchants from the Aegean and Beaker Folk from Spain had reached Italy by 1200 B.C., however, they seemed to have had little influence on the local people.

By 1500 B.C., Bronze Age invaders occupied the Po Valley. These people originated in central Europe (Hungary), and are thought to have spoken an Indo-European language. They constructed fortified villages by which they overpowered and eventually absorbed the older Neolithic population. Their villages were occupied for greater periods of time and were characterized by mounds of a gray, greasy soil called terra mare, which the Italian peasants constantly dug and spread on their fields as fertilizer.

Terra mare was a mix of wood ash, charcoal and organic compost consisting of manure, plant debris, kitchen waste and the organic byproducts of daily living.

According to Peter Stahl, an anthropologist from the State University of New York, Binghamton, many investigators believe that, "what the ecoimagery would like to picture as a pristine, untouched Urelt primeval world, in fact has been managed by people for millennia." The phrase "built environment," Erickson argued, "applies to most, if not all, Neotropical landscapes."

According to Wim Sombroek, author of Amazon Soils (1966), "Every Ecology 101 student knows that Amazonian soils are fragile and impoverished. If farmers cut down the canopy of trees overhead to clear cropland, they expose the earth to the pummeling rain and sun, which quickly wash away its small store of minerals and nutrients and bake what remains into something resembling brick - a 'wet desert,' as these ruined areas are sometimes called." The certainty of destroying the land, environmentalists claim, makes large-scale corporate agriculture impossible in the rainforest. What Sombroek observed was a big surprise - large patches of "terra preta do indio (Indian black earth).

Amazonian Indians literally "created the ground

beneath their feet." According to Susana Hecht, a geographer from the University of California, at Los Angeles, investigators of upland Amazonia took most of their soil samples along the regions modern highways, which indeed passed through areas with lifeless soil. These original samplings gave a skewed view of Amazonian soil nutritional values, however, a few investigators found zones of something recognizably different and considerably more fertile, "in part, because of the original empty-Amazon model."

Beginning a little more than 2,000 years ago, the central and lower Amazon, were disrupted by violent cultural change. Azawak-speaking peoples migrated into the area from the south and west, sometimes apparently driving Tupi-speaking groups north and east. Sedentary villages were established and the production of terra preta appeared to begin in earnest at the same time.

Terra preta exists in two forms: terra preta itself, a black soil thick with fragments of pottery, and terra mulata, a lighter dark brown soil with much less pottery. A number of researchers believe that although Indians made both, they deliberately created only the terra mulata.

Terra preta is blacker than the blackest coffee and the man made soil is filled with fragmented and broken pre-Columbian pottery. According to Charles Mann, a National Geographic reporter (2008), "It was as if the (Amazon) River's first inhabitants had thrown a huge, rowdy frat party, smashing every plate in sight, (and) then buried the evidence."

Terra preta was the soil created directly around homes by charcoal (wood ash) kitchen fires and organic refuse of various types. Just before the time of Christ (360 B.C.), the central Amazon had numerous large settled villages when and where terra preta manufacturing began.

Terra preta is rich in essential minerals, including phosphorus, calcium, zinc and manganese, which are typically missing in tropical soils.

Earlier inhabitants left no trace of terra preta; the new

villages quickly developed thick deposits of "Indian black earth."

Hecht, believed that, these fertile sites were originally "seen as anomalous and insignificant." However, in the 1990s, investigators began studying these unusual sites of "terra preta do Indio" - rich, fertile "Indian dark earth" that anthropologists are convinced were created by early humans.

Throughout Amazonia, farmer's prize terra preta for its enormous power to stimulate productivity; some have worked it for as many as 20 years with minimal need for additional fertilizer. The ceramic fragments found in terra preta indicate that the manufactured "soil" retained its nutrients for a millennium.

Terra preta is sold in great quantities by merchants as special growing "soil" for gardens. Woods has estimated that manufactured terra preta might represent as much as 10% of the total usable soil in the Amazon Basin, an area the size of France! A recent, much more conservative, estimate is that terra preta covers only 0.1 to 0.3% of the Amazon basin, a few thousand square miles - a few thousand square miles of manufactured farm land was sufficient to feed the millions of people in the Mayan heartland!

Most large terra preta sites of manufactured soil are found on the low bluffs at the edge of the floodplain. Typically, they cover five to fifteen acres, however, some encompass more than seven hundred acres. The layer of manufactured black soil is typically one to two feet deep, but can be as thick as six feet.

According to a study by Dirse Kern, of the Museu Goeldi in Belem, terra preta is "not associated with a particular soil type or environmental condition," indicating clearly, that it was not produced by natural events.

Another clue to the human origin of terra preta is the broken ceramics with which it is usually mixed. "They practiced agriculture here for centuries," said Glaser. "But instead of destroying the soil, they improved it, and that is something we don't know how to do today" in tropical soils.

Typically, terra preta has more "plant-available" phosphorus, calcium, sulfur, nitrogen and trace minerals than is common in the rainforest; it also has much more organic matter, better retains moisture and nutrients, and is not rapidly exhausted by agricultural use when managed well. The key to terra preta's long-term fertility, Glaser says, "is charcoal (wood ash): terra preta contains up to 64 times more of the wood ash than the surrounding red earth."

Organic matter "sticks" or "adsorbs" to charcoal, rather than being washed away or attaching to other non-available compounds. "Over time, it partly oxidizes, which keeps providing sites for nutrients to bind to." But simply mixing charcoal into the ground is not enough to create terra preta.

Glaser argues, "High nutrient inputs - excrements and waste such as turtle, fish and animal bones - are necessary." Special soil microorganisms are also likely to play a role in its persistent fertility, in the view of Janice Thies, a soil ecologist, who is part of a Cornell University team studying terra preta. "There are indications that microbial biomass is higher in terra preta than in other forest soils."

Despite the presence of charcoal, terra preta is not a byproduct of simple slash-and-burn agriculture. Slash-and-burn does not produce enough charcoal (wood ash) to manufacture terra preta - the carbon mostly is released into the air in the form of carbon dioxide, instead Indians appear to have made terra preta by a process that Christoph Steiner, a University of Bayreuh soil scientist, has dubbed "slash-and-char." Instead of completely burning organic matter to ash, ancient farmers burned it incompletely to make charcoal, then, stirred the charcoal or wood ash back into the soil.

One must remember that pure "wood ash" is not carbon, but rather plant minerals as the carbon of the wood was burnt or released as carbon dioxide into the atmostphere.

Indians, yet today, are still making terra preta in this way, according to Hecht, the UCLA geographer. Hecht spent years with the Kayapo', in Central Amazonia, watching them create "low biomass" fires "cool enough to walk through" of pulled weeds, cooking wastes, crop debris, palm fronds and termite mounds. Hecht wrote, "To live among the Kayapo, is to live in a place where parts of the landscape smolder."

In an early test at recreating terra preta, Steiner, Wenceslau Teixeira of the Brazilian Agricultural Research Enterprise, and Wolfgang Zech of the University of Bayreuh applied a variety of treatments involving charcoal and fertilizers for three years to rice and sorghum plots outside Manaus. In the first year, there was little recognizable difference amongst test and control plots (except that in the control plots nothing grew). By the second year, Steiner declared, "the charcoal really made a difference." Plots with charcoal alone grew little, but those treated with a combination of charcoal and natural fertilizers yielded as much as an 880% increase in yield than with fertilizer alone!

Chapter 5

"The number of humans surviving to 'old age' (at least double the age of reproductive maturity) quadrupled at about 30,000 to 50,000 years ago - something equally as dramatic as the taming of fire happened."

Dr. Joel Wallach & Dr Ma Lan
HELL'S KITCHEN

"Man is also digging iron, tin, copper, zinc and other minerals from the ground, making them into automobiles, tin cans, buildings, and so on. Eventually these are worn out, discarded, piled up in junk heaps, there to rust, corrode, burn, dissolve, and wash away finally to the sea. Vast quantities of materials are destroyed by combustion as fuel, or for disposal of wastes. All of the coal, most of the petroleum, and much of the products of the forests are eventually consumed by fire. Their smoke and dust go into the air, their ashes are leached out by rain, the portable materials going to the sea."

D.C. Jarvis, M.D.
Folk Medicine

Human Aging: fire power

Fire is far older than man. In the beginning fire was flung into the forests and grasslands by volcanic eruptions, lightening strikes, spontaneous combustion ignited by the friction of dry branches rubbing against each other and heat generated by decomposing plant material.

These original untamed wildfires produced a mineral-rich plant ash on the crust of the earth that impregnated the primitive "soil." The process mixed and kneaded the ash, a fine particle sized mineral rich nutrient mix, into the deep accumulated organic mulch that had built up over the years, decades, centuries and millennia.

The human is one of the most efficient converters of the "solar income" found in food into mechanical work or movement. Humans need only 50% of the calories required by a horse to exert the same level of physical energy. Human metabolism is very efficient!

Anthropologists theorize that our large brains are the result of a constant stream of high protein, high fat food supplies, "as we ate more meat our brain got larger and it allowed us to figure out how to get more meat."

Our larger and more functional brains allowed us to develop other methods to tap into the seemingly endless reserves of "solar income" trapped by plants - fire!

By burning plants that we couldn't eat, including trees and underbrush, humans and their cultures quickly stretched far beyond the creative limits and immediate needs of their digestive system and their metabolic processes.

The ability to tame or kindle a fire at will catapulted humans farther than our earthly competitors - humans controlled fire, something that no other species would ever do!

Fire, as a tool, separated humans from other tool-using animals - animals metabolically used the sun's solar income by eating plants and other animals, they could use sticks, rocks, fiber, mud and water - only man had fire! Man tamed fire and employed it as a tool for many thousands of years before he learned how to start and kindle fire at will.

Fire, the new technique of tapping into stored energy or "solar income" protected us from the otherwise uninhabitable frozen environment of the Ice Ages and allowed us to control the temperature of our microenvironments or dwellings. Humans were no longer controlled by the environment - we had fire power!

Early human remains from nine individuals that were discovered in an Ethiopian fossil cache were dated back to 4.3 million years ago. These prehistoric humans, *Ardipithecus ramidus,* were surrounded by a collection of the oldest dated stone tools. Plant and animal fossils identified at the same site revealed that these very early humans lived and flourished in a low lying woodland and grassland heavily populated with monkeys, mole rats and wild cattle.

Anthropologist had long believed that primitive man "tamed" fire some 500,000 years ago; however, a recent study of burnt antelope bones from caves in Swartkrans, South Africa, show that early man, *Australopithicus robustus* and *Homo erectus,* had built camp fires and had cooked meat on these fires about 1.5 million years ago - about one million years earlier than had been previously thought.

The cooked antelope bones were discovered and described in 1988 by Bob Brain, a South African paleontologist from the University of Cape Town. Brain originally theorized the bones had been cooked by humans because the degree of charring indicated temperatures of more than 1,100 degrees F - heat levels that could have only be achieved by a human campfire as heat produced by a grass fire does not exceed 700 degrees F.

Many technologically ignorant humans, including *Homo erectus* (Java Man some 250,000 years ago), found that starting fire from raw cold fuel was a difficult and frustrating job. Early on, when fire was originally "captured," it was fed and maintained for as long as possible, an ancient technique which is still practiced in many areas of the world today.

Fire can easily be maintained and transported by the use of wet wood, lichens, dry fennel stalks, etc. In some cultures hearth fires are maintained for generation after generation, oftentimes for the life of the dwelling.

The first evidence we have for fire starting by humans is associated with the early Paleolithic Period of Europe approximately dated at 25,000 to 30,000 B.C. Flints in the classic "strike-a-light" hand held shape and chunks of iron pyrite were discovered together in charcoal fire beds.

Iron pyrite (fool's gold) is only found in very few places on earth, therefore most early fire starting methods fall into the category of the fire drill (a bow used to spin an arrow shaft that is inserted into a baseboard), fire saw and fire plow (a pointed stick that is rapidly pushed back and forth in a groove created in a log or board). Humans eventually learned that they could start fire at will with less work by generating sparks that were directed into fine dry grass "tinder."

With fire, humans were able to smelt metal, make tools, "fire" pottery, bake bricks, produce weapons, keep themselves warm, cook and eat food that was otherwise inedible (grains), keep predatory animals at bay, destroy our enemies, develop specialties and unwittingly, we humans, with the wood ash (plant mineral) by-product that was generated by fire, produced the mineral fertilizer and mineral supplements ("culinary" ashes), that would nurture and sustain we humans for thousands of years to come!

Early humans who had not yet learned to put their wood ashes from their heating and cooking fires into primitive gardens lived a life that was short, hard, miserable, filthy, fearful, brutish and violent. They were often on the verge of starvation.

They subsisted primarily in family units or family bands. During their waking day, they were driven by an eternal, internal, intrinsic and relentless salt and mineral hunger (pica) as were all living creatures. The hunger for salt and minerals didn't begin with the appearance of potato chips, these behaviors began with the appearance of the first animals and the first humans.

One isolated group of tiny people, dubbed the "Hobbit," *Homo floresiensis*, existed on the Indonesian island of Flores, 370 miles east of Java. They were the size of a *Homo sapiens* pygmy or midget only three feet tall with the body of a three year old, however, their brain was smaller than a grapefruit - a small human with a brain that was smaller than the brain of a chimpanzee.

There is some evidence that these tiny, tribal and carnivorous humans accepted gourds filled with food that the modern human Floresians offered to them, until the 1500s, when Dutch traders arrived.

The "Hobbit" were clever enough to employ fire, make tools (points, blades, awls and tiny barbs) and hunt - cooking fire charred bones of the Stegodon (dwarf elephant), Komodo Dragon (dinosaur), a wide variety of rodents and other animal species were collected from garbage dumps.

Early skeletons of the south Pacific "Hobbit" were dated as far back as 95,000 years ago, the more recent ones were dated at 13,000 - 18,000 years; however, the primitive "Hobbit" crafted stone tools dating back to 800,000 B.C.

The island of Flores was populated by hoards of an extinct dwarf elephant ((Stegodon), monster rats and giant lizards (including the Komodo Dragon), all of which were the primary food of the "Hobbit."

There is no evidence that the "Hobbit" learned to use the ashes from their heating and cooking fires to put in their food, salt or gardens - they disappeared leaving only a small fossil record. Only six skeletons have been found, suggesting the Hobbit skeletons were minerally poor and their skeletons simply didn't survive the ravages of the millennia.

The small stature of the Hobbit demonstrates very

clearly that humans, like other life forms are not exempt from natural laws, in this case the "island rule." The island rule states that "a combination of selective forces - geographic and temporal isolation, scarce resources and the absence of predators - will occasionally result in the development of giant and dwarf species." The Hobbit simply followed the same historical course as the isolated desert Bushman of Southern Africa.

Humans were territorial, they hunted and gathered in naturally productive and fruitful areas that had large quantities of small game, edible insects, their favorite plants and either salt or clay deposits for a source of minerals, a virtual Garden of Eden. There were endless fights and mini-wars between competing family bands and tribes over access to these flora and fauna rich Edens.

Their offspring had a very low survival rate, and those that did survive were often deformed with congenital birth defects (Down's Syndrome, heart defects, cleft palate, cleft lip, spina bifida, muscular dystrophy, clubbed hands and feet, etc.) caused by pervasive maternal nutritional deficiencies.

Injuries took their toll; fractures healed all askew or didn't heal at all, leaving the victim to remain deformed and dependant upon the good graces and surpluses of the rest of the band. If the injuries were catastrophic, the victim was oftentimes eaten by his fellows. Revered relatives were often eaten when they died so as to acquire and perpetuate their spirit (mortuary cannibalism).

On the other hand, those humans who learned to put wood, peat or kelp ashes from their heating and cooking fires into their food and primitive gardens, were taller, their bones stronger, they were more fertile, had lower rates of infant mortality and they lived longer!

Harder mineralized skeletons resulted in their bones surviving the ravages of rodents and scavengers, decomposition and various destructive forces of the millennia - full skeletons were now surviving into the 21st century.

Between 200,000 and 40,000 years ago, Neanderthals dominated the landscape of western Asia and Europe. Archeologists and anthropologists have found over 10,000 complete skeletons of these ancient peoples. They were the first humans to bury their dead and care for their sick and infirm. Their stone tools, however, were still crude and lacked the standard shapes that would indicate that they were designed for a specific function.

African fossilized skeletons from 100,000 years ago had more modern skeletal features (humans continued to put the ash byproduct of heating and cooking fires into their food and gardens) than did their Neanderthal counterparts - they did, however, make the same crude stone tools.

The bone evidence of their food prey indicated that their hunting skills were minimal and they only killed and ate small safely killed animals, including rats and rabbits. They had not yet reached the capability of killing pigs, buffalo and larger more dangerous species such as the elephant (mastodon, mammoth and the dwarf Stegodon). They could not yet catch fish - their living sites on the sea coasts and lake shores are devoid of fish hooks and fish bones.

Human developmental history (including physical emotional, spiritual and creative) appears to have found its footing, took hold and "gained traction" about 50,000 years ago marking a time that Dr. Jared Diamond calls the "Great Leap Forward." The first real signals of this human leap forward include an increase in height and the universal appearance of standardized tools and jewelry.

Chapter 7

"How readily we manipulate our soil. We rearrange and restructure it. We pump it full of chemicals, we flood it, we drain it. On it's health the fate of empires has rested. Yet we avoid it. In our cities, rivers of concrete keep us from its touch. Naked it tends to offend the eye. But a close look reveals that the soil is an essential bridge between the rock below and the life above. It is dynamic and vital, and far too easily - and frequently abused."

Boyd Gibbons
National Geographic

"Living organisms procure their raw materials of essential elements for reproduction, development, growth and maintenance and for longevity from a thin blanket of matter and gas on or just above the Earth's crust."

Dr. Joel D. Wallach & Dr. Ma Lan
RARE EARTH'S: forbidden cures

Our Food is Anemic

Marked human development occurred about 50,000 years ago in southwestern Europe, where numerous artifacts are associated with the skeletons of Cro-Magnons. Soon after, the garbage dumps unearthed at archeological sites become more and more complex, pointing to biologically and behaviorally modern humans.

Cro-Magnon garbage heaps yielded stone tools, bone tools, and bone fish hooks. Tools were produced in diverse and distinctive shapes so modern that their functions as needles, awls and engraving tools are straight forward and easily identified. Tools became more complex, moving beyond simple hand held scrapers to multi-piece tools (stone axes) and weapons such as harpoons, spear throwers and bows and arrows.

These new weapons allowed the human hunter to kill larger and more dangerous game from a safe distance. The creation of ropes and thread for nets, twine and string permitted the invention of nets, lines and snares which allowed for the addition of small mammals, fish and birds to our human diet, which then promoted the expansion of human habitable territories.

Rubble from houses and scraps from sewn clothing point to an improved capacity to survive freezing environments. Modern jewelry and tenderly buried skeletons showed a new aesthetic and spiritual progression for humans - humans were now talking to God!

Of all the Cro-Magnon creations that have been preserved, the most remarkable is their artwork, including their famous cave paintings, statues and musical instruments.

The impact of the life-sized painted bulls and horses in the Lascaux Cave of southwestern France or the rhino, lion, horses, mammoth, panther, owl, bear and buffalo paintings of the limestone Chauvet grotto in southern France on a visitor is dramatic - you realize these ancient people were modern, not only in their skeletons but also in their abstract minds!

The last Chauvet artist produced a painting between 24,000 and 32,000 years ago. The artists work was "signed" with a negative print of his hand, which was produced by blowing red ochre onto a non-arthritic hand that was held palm down against the cave wall. Other artists also signed their work with a positive print of their hand by putting the ochre on their hand and then placing their palm print on their painting.

No human bones have been found in either of the caves, however, the Chauvet grotto has been a treasure trove of bones from 14 different animal species including rodents, reptiles, birds and bears. The bear bones dominate - they have recovered 3,700 of them.

It is important to note that there were no grains or fruit seeds found in the caves, clearly indicating that the Cro-Magnon artists were primarily hunters and carnivores and that hunting dominated their lives.

At 40,000 years ago, Cro-Magnons "moved into the neighborhood" of Europe with their modern skeletons (signaling the use of the ash by-product of their heating and cooking fires as a supplement mixed with salt to extend and cut the more valued salt and directly into their food as "culinary ash"), tools and more clever weapons.

Classical anthropologists believe that the Cro-Magnons used their advanced technology and superior weapons to kill, infect or displace the Neanderthals - a theorized event that left little or nothing behind in the form of evidence of hybridization between the Neanderthals and Cro-Magnons or a straight forward and ruthless genocide.

We don't believe the Cro-Magnons fought, captured, enslaved or slaughtered the Neanderthals, because they would have eaten them and left their charred, cracked and scraped bones in their garbage heaps with the rest of the debris of hunting, butchering and cooking. They would have created art work that depicted the great heroic battles, heroes, the slain Neanderthals and victories.

We believe the Neanderthals just failed to learn and employ a basic survival technique that the Cro-Magnons had learned, which caused them to be "edged out" in a similar fashion as the prehistoric Bushmen allowed themselves to be "edged out" of the isolated and idyllic Cape of South Africa and chased into the Kalahari Desert by the more advanced gun toting Dutch explorers from the Dutch East Indies Tea Company in 1462; and in a similar fashion as the island of Flores "Hobbit" allowed themselves to be "edged out" by the 16th century Dutch.

Neanderthals were primarily hunters and they developed the nutritional deficiencies of pure carnivores who had failed to develop the habit of using wood, peat or kelp ashes to mix with salt and season food and/or failed to put the ashes into their primitive or crude "gardens." One bad hunting year or a drought covering several years could have significantly diminished their numbers or totally wiped them out.

The number of humans surviving to "old age" (at least double the age of reproductive maturity) quadrupled at about 30,000 years ago - something equally as dramatic as the taming of fire happened here which we will cover in due course.

Anthropologists looked at 750 fossilized dental and jaw fragments of early humans spanning over millions of years, from the Australopithecines to Neanderthals and early modern humans. Old age was defined as at least double the age which reproductive maturity was reached, which is also the point when the third molars usually erupt in the teen years.

In calculating the ratio of old-to-young hominids, Rachel Caspari of the University of Michigan, at Ann Arbor and Sang-Hee Lee of the University of California, at Riverside found a trend of increased longevity across the human family. With "modern" humans, older adults finally outnumbered younger ones for the first time at the 30,000 year mark.

The leap in longevity is thought to have been critical to the development of modern human culture, as elders passed down knowledge and helped to weld together complex societies.

This "hand-me-down" knowledge, included, how to cook and preserve meat, how to use wood ashes to extend and cut what they perceived as the more valuable salt with wood ashes and to employ the use of "culinary" ashes in the preparation of certain foods and the value of putting wood ash into their primitive gardens.

The results and benefits of incorporating wood ashes (plant minerals) into their food, either directly as salt extenders, or "culinary ashes" or indirectly as a garden fertilizer produced stronger, taller, healthier, more fertile, more creative and longer liver humans - we had not yet left the main road and humans were in fact accumulating good habits, becoming healthier, more fertile, living longer and honing better survival skills.

Chapter 8

"Aetios, noted pregnant women to crave various and odd foods, some salty and some acid; some, he said, 'crave for sand, oyster shells and wood ashes.'"

Dr. Joel D. Wallach & Dr. Ma Lan
RARE EARTHS: forbidden cures

"In humans and animals alike, the body definitely wants potassium and if necessary will go to great lengths to get it. Take children for an example. It does not always please mothers when children eat dirt, but perhaps that is because they do not realize that instinctively children find the potassium needed for their bodily growth in the dirt."

Dr. D.C. Jarvis, M.D.
Folk Medicine

Pica, Salt Hunger, and Basic Drive

The universal human drive to survive was overtly and gainfully occupied by a search for salt and minerals. Killing and eating small animals and insects almost daily and eating the occasional and highly seasonal plant foods (grass seeds, etc.) were just a means to the end.

"Food" as we think of it (meat, fish, birds, insects, cheese, seeds, nuts, fruit, etc.) kept man alive while he was searching for the more critical salt and minerals.

"Pica" is a term that describes a seeking, a craving behavior dominated by licking and chewing frenzies, that have their genesis in mineral deficiencies - interesting enough neither vitamin deficiencies, protein deficiencies or calorie deficiency initiates this "pica" behavior, nor will supplementing vitamins or eating sugar, carbohydrate, fat or protein quench it!

Historically, the consumption of salt to satisfy a pica behavior was of value because salt was not processed and did often times contain trace minerals and rare earths.

Today, salt consumption, although contrary to popular belief, is not in and of itself harmful; it does present the problem of allowing our bodies to think we are getting minerals (the equivalent of the "empty calorie diets," i.e. - processed food calories without vitamins).

Farmers and husbandrymen use the salt hunger of animals to ensure the consumption of trace minerals by incorporating trace minerals into salt blocks containing 85% salt - anything less than 85% sodium chloride in a salt block will be ignored by the animals even if they have major mineral deficiencies!

"Cribbing" is a name given to a particular form of pica in domestic animals. A good husbandryman knows when a horse or cow "cribs" (chews or gnaws on a corn crib, wooden feed box, fence, stall rail, hitching post or barn door), the animal really has a craving for minerals. Mineral starved animals, when first presented with minerals, will at first eat large amounts of supplemental minerals until they are satisfied, then they will automatically reduce their level of consumption to a maintenance level.

"Salt appetite" is very striking in both pregnant animals and pregnant humans. Bizarre cravings are legendary in the pregnant human. From antiquity, the description of cravings or "pica" in humans records its major incidence to pregnant women. The Hawaiian King Kamehameha's mother, Queen Kekuiapoiwa had cravings for eyeballs, although she specifically wanted chief's eyes, she was given the eyes of sharks to eat.

We have seen a hundred pregnant sheep in Montana lined up along an embankment eating clay. This is a form of pica known as "geophagia." Earth eating, or geophagia, is a very common behavior in minerally deficient pregnant women.

Pica, or perverted appetite or irresistible cravings with the eating of bizarre or unsuitable nonfood substances (or fattening nonfoods or snack foods) has been a curiosity for philosophers, doctors and priests for thousands of years.

Pica as a symptom of mineral deficiencies is universal in the world and has been reported in animals and humans of all age groups. In modern times the easy availability of candy, sugared-high calorie snacks, soft drinks and junk foods has led to obesity when people feel the deep cravings of pica.

A doctoral thesis on pica by Agustus Fridericus Mergiletus (1701) begins with the definition of pica: "The malady pica is called "kitta" in Greek. Its derivation comes from the name of the common magpie because the bird ("pica" is the Latin Name for "magpie") itself is believed to suffer from some malady ....because it flits from tree to tree constantly seeking food or because it enjoys all sorts of foods."

A catalogue of bizarre instances of pica is found in Mergiletus' thesis. In men, he recorded one individual who ate leather, wood, nestlings, live mice; a second consumed woolen garments, leather, a live cat, and some mice; a third ate cats' tails and decomposed human bodies with maggots!

In Mergiletus' female subjects, he recorded women who ate human flesh including one particularly horrible lady - "she lured children with sweets, killed them and pickled them for her daily fare (sounds like a female version of Jeffrey Dahmer). The murders were only discovered when the women's cat stole a pickled hand of a child and carried it over to the neighbor's house."

The most common description of pica by Mergiletus were of women's desire for mud and mortar scrapped from the walls (just like modern children who eat caulking and lead paint - we have often said that children who eat lead paint are screaming for minerals for their mineral starved bodies - give them minerals and they won't eat lead paint); girls who ate their own hair; girls who ate cotton, thread from their own clothes, raw grain and lizards.

Mergiletus also described pica in animals including cats that ate wood ash and pregnant hunting dogs that ate unusual objects.

Cooper (1957), in her classic report on pica, refers to several ancient and medieval writers who emphasized the occurrence of pica in pregnant women, i.e. - Aetios noted pregnant women to crave various odd foods, some salty and some acid; some he said "crave for sand, oyster shells and wood ashes." Aetios recommended a diet including "fruits, green vegetables, pig's feet, fresh fish and old tawny fragrant wine."

Boezo (1638) noted that pica occurred most often in pregnant women. Boezo saw pica as a physiological problem, and is the first to mention iron preparations as a treatment for pica - he suggested, "one and one half scruples of iron dross taken for many days as wonderfully beneficial for men and women."

Boezo also noted, "The case of a virgin who was accustomed to devour salt in great quantities from which chronic behavior she developed diarrhea and wasting (Addison's disease?)."

Christiani of Frankfurt (1691) reported a woman who ate 1400 salt herrings during her pregnancy. LeConte (1846) suggested that animals eating earth do so because of "want of inorganic elements."

In modern times, the substances frequently reported as eaten as a result of pica behavior in humans includes paper, metallic gum wrappers, ice, dirt, coal, clay, corn starch, chalk, baking powder, pebbles, wood, wood ashes, plaster, paint, chimney soot, hair, human and animal feces (kitty litter box) and cloth.

Because of social constraints on our public behavior, most people under public scrutiny who display pica eat sugar, salt, snack food, soft drinks when they crave minerals - many minerally deficient individuals smoke, drink alcohol or use street (or prescription) drugs in an attempt to satisfy a nagging underlying craving.

Ice eating (pagophagia) is also common, especially for obese iron deficient children and adults.

Worms have been reported as a cause of pica - ankylostomiasis, ascariasis, oxyuriasis and others have been blamed. Parasites of course can cause anemia and malnutrition by direct blood sucking from the host or by competing for food in the gut. The resulting anemia is in fact perceived by the body as an iron deficiency resulting in pica.

Pica is more frequently seen in the poor and the obese; however, David Livingston observed that "both slaves and the gentry developed pica in Africa." In Africa, pica is viewed by tribal peoples as a magical superstitious behavior.

Henrock (1831) attributed pica to "paucity of good blood and lack of proper nutrition." Waller (1874) reported that David Livingston observed many cases of clay and earth eating (geophagia), a frequent form of pica in pregnant women.

Orr and Gilka (1931) and de Castro (1952) recognized that "edible Earths might be rich in sodium, iron and calcium." Gelford (1945) reported that pica was common in Kenya amongst African tribes (Kikuyu) living mainly on a vegetarian diet; but absent in those people eating diets rich in animal flesh, blood and bones (Massai).

Richter (1955) reported Kirkam and Birch's analysis of 20 samples of edible clay from Africa:

Clay Minerals	Percent
Silica	47.76
Aluminum oxide	22.03
Sodium oxide	4.87
Potassium oxide	2.88
Iron oxide	4.98
Manganese oxide	0.32
Calcium oxide	2.97
Magnesium oxide	1.08
Phosphorous pentoxide	0.13

Dickens and Ford reported that 25% of all children ate earth. Cooper (1957) reported a 21% rate of pica in American children referred to the Mother's Advisory Service in Baltimore.

Lanzkowsky (1959) reported that 12 children with pica had a hemoglobin that ranged from 3 g% to 10.9 g% with a mean of 7.89% =/- 2.64. The institution of iron (i.m. - iron dextran) "resulted in a cure for pica in one to two weeks." Again, if children have sufficient nutritional minerals they will not eat lead paint - they only eat lead paint because of pica.

McDonald and Marshall (1964) reported on 25 children who ate sand. They divided the group in half; they gave one group iron and the other group saline (salt solution). After three to four months 11 of the 13 children given iron had lost their pica behavior compared with only 3 of the 12 in the saline group.

Reynolds et al (1968) reported that 38 people with anemia exhibited pagophagia (ice eating) as the most common form of pica; twenty two of 25 had their symptoms of pica disappear after correcting the iron depletion.

Woods and Weisinger (970) reproduced pagophagia experimentally in rats by withdrawing blood. The pagophagia in the anemic rats was cured when the anemia was cured. It is of interest to note that pica or cribbing behaviors are not produced by vitamin deficiencies!

Two thirds of the 153 pregnant women studied by Taggart (1961) developed cravings. The most common craving was for fruit, pickles, blood pudding, licorice, potato chips, cheese and kippers; a craving for sweets, vegetables, nuts and sweet pickles came in second place.

Charles Mann (2008) reported that to satisfy pica, a traditional dietary supplement used by pregnant Haitian women takes the form of gray clay pigeon-like "cakes" made of clay, salt and lard.

Phosphate appetite was described by LeVaillant (1796) as the anxious search by cattle in phosphate deficient South African pastures for discarded dog bones (osteophagia); they also chewed on wood (pica) and each others horns.

Bone chewing (osteophagia, a form of pica) has been reported in many wild species of herbivores including reindeer, caribou, red deer, camels, giraffe, elephant and wildebeest.

We have seen elephant eating bones, limestone roadbeds and large termite heaps as ready and available mineral supplements. A search for calcium rich edible clays and soils and territorial disputes over limited supplies led to wars in tribal Africa.

It was demonstrated that calcium deficient weanling rats will consume large amounts of a lead acetate solution (even though the solution tastes bad) when compared with calcium fed controls. The Oriental diet is extremely low in calcium leading them to habitually and preferentially eat bones (when Dr. Ma Lan and I were courting, she ate the bones and gave me the fillets of the fish that we caught) softened and partially leached of calcium with vinegar.

There is no evidence of a specific pica behavior unique to a magnesium deficiency. Magnesium deficient animals will crave and eat common salt. Magnesium tastes bad enough that animals will die of magnesium deficiency initiated seizures rather than consume a pure magnesium supplement. It has been suggested that recovery from a magnesium deficiency can be a very unpleasant process, enough so that the bad taste of magnesium supplements normally required for recovery exceeds the unpleasant features of the deficiency!

A natural potassium deficiency is highly unlikely as all grains, fruits and vegetables tend to be rich in potassium - a potassium deficiency can, however, be common in those individuals taking diuretics for high blood pressure or weight loss.

Potassium deficient rats are hyper alert and lick everything including their metal cage, lab equipment, each other and urine puddles. It is of interest to note, that even with a severe potassium deficiency, laboratory rats have a strong craving for sodium chloride (salt)!

Chromium and vanadium deficiencies are manifested by an intense thirst for liquid (high fructose corn syrup laden soft drinks being the usual first choice and water the last for minerally deficient humans) and hunger for carbohydrates (i.e. - soft drinks, coffee and tea with added sugar, alcohol, pasta, deserts, bread, etc.).

The "munchies," cravings for alcohol and "candy cravings" (especially chocolate) are sure signs of chromium and vanadium deficiencies.

The preteen and teen age infatuation with snack foods, drugs, tobacco and alcohol appear to be the result of pica - because they are so minerally deficient they are seeking something, anything to put in their mouth that will satisfy an irresistible craving for minerals.

Chapter 9

"To the Printer of the London Chronicle":

SIR, I have often heard it remarked, that our Colonies in North America were unhealthy and unfavourable to long life; and more particularly so upon their first settlement. In opposition to this groundless notion, I here send you two paragraphs taken from the Pennsylvania Gazette of July 16, and the New-York Gazette of August 27, giving an account of the deaths of the first-born of the city of Philadelphia, and the province of Pennsylvania:

PHILADELPHIA, July 16. "At Kennet, in Chester county, the 5th instant, died John Key, in the 85th year of his age, and the next day was interred in the burial place belonging to the people called Quakers, in that township, attended by a large number of reputable people, his neighbours and acquaintance. He was born in a cave, long afterwards known by the name of Penny-Pot, near Race-street; and William Penn, our first proprietor, gave him a lot of ground, as a compliment on his being the first child born in this city. -- In the early part of his life his conversation was very engaging, and his company much sought after by those of his own age; in his decline he was much esteemed for his peaceful disposition. His constitution was very healthy till about 80, when he was seized with the palsy, and continued weakly till his death. --About six years ago he walked on foot from Kennet to Philadelphia in one day, which is near 30 miles. --It has been said that people in this province are short-lived; but when we consider how few children were born here 75 years ago, and observe how many old people there are still alive among us (who were born here) we shall rather think no quarter of the world can shew a greater number of aged persons than this province can, in proportion to the children born."

PHILADELPHIA, Aug 24. On the 10th instant, at Brandywine Hundred, in New-Castle county, died Emanuel Grubb, in the 86th year of his age, and the next day was interred in St. Martin's church-yard, at Lower-Cichester, in Chester county, attended by a large number of his relations, neighbours, and acquaintance. -- He was born in a cave, by the side of the Delaware River, not far distant from where he always lived, and died, and was the first child born of English parents in this province. His constitution was remarkably healthy during his whole life, having never been afflicted with any sickness till a few days before his death. His strength and activity were surprising in a man of his age; he could mount and ride a horse with as much dexterity as a lad of 20. -- A few months ago, he rode from his own house to this city, and back again, which is upwards of 40 miles. -- His memory was equally surprising, and not in the least impaired, til his death; he could remember transactions of a late date equally well with those which happened in his younger days. He was exceeding temperate in his living, seldom making use of spirituous liquors; and for his peaceable and friendly disposition, was highly esteemed by all who knew him. This instance, among many, is a proof of the longevity of people born here.

It is worthy of observation also, that Governor Hutchinson, in his valuable History of the Massachusett's Bay, Vol. II. Pp. 148 and 216, says,

"July 20, 1704, died at Marshfield, Peregrine White, aged 83 years and eight months, the first-born in Plymouth colony."

"Jan. 14, 1716, died at Salem, Elizabeth Patch, the first-born female in the old colony of Massachusett's Bay, so that she must have lived 86 or 87 years; and April 14, following, died at Newport, in Rhode-Island, Mary Godfrey, aged 87, being the first child born there. -- The longevity of the first-born in each of the three colonies, is worth noting."

As a well-wisher to mankind in general, I thought it worth while to send this to your useful paper, in order to allay the apprehensions of those, whose inclinations, business, or necessities may induce them to settle in that part of the British Empire. I must add at the same time, that I have myself lately traveled over the greater part of that extensive continent; and can with truth say, in spite of all that hath been boldly and positively asserted to the contrary, that I could not discover among the whole people, one grain of disaffection to their brethren in Britain, nor did I meet with a single person who had ever formed the most distant idea of throwing off their allegiance to the mother country. This it is doing them but bare justice to declare; and is all the return I can at present make them for the kindness and hospitality with which, purely on account of my being an Old England-Man, I was universally treated. I am, Sir, your constant reader, F + S.

The London Chronicle, December 15, 1767

Benjamin Franklin

The Energy Crisis

It was a manmade ecological shift and the resultant Industrial Revolution that interrupted the historically successful renewable system for obtaining plant minerals that had been developed and had met the needs of human populations for millennia.

In 1268 Norman castles and great manors of noblemen had chimneys to draw the wood and coal smoke up and out of the fireplace, it would be another 200 years before this inefficient luxury was installed in the humble houses of the common people.

The heating and cooking fire of the commoner filled a hole in the middle of the floor or sat on a raised stone hearth in the middle of the main room to avoid setting the wooden walls on fire. The fire produced smoke which filled the room until it seeped through the gaps in the walls or roof - the dusty ash byproduct of the fuel's combustion were collected and taken out each morning, mixed with salt (3:1 to 10:1) to cut and conserve the precious salt, used as "culinary" ashes for the baking of grain dishes and the balance was tossed outside as kitchen waste, added to the compost pile or mixed directly into the garden.

From an indoor air quality standpoint, the majority of Englishmen had not advanced much beyond the conditions suffered by *Homo erectus*, who, over hundreds of thousands of years earlier, had huddled over open wood fires inside large huts constructed of sticks and branches.

The 13th century Englishmen were still getting their daily supply of minerals, either directly (wood ashes mixed with salt or mixed directly in their food), or indirectly, by placing the wood ashes into their gardens. Beginning in 1285, during the reign of Edward I, various commissions were established in London to address the problem of coal smoke, which early environmentalists complained, "had infected and corrupted" the air.

During the summer of 1306, bishops, barons and knights from all over England ventured from their country estates and manors and traveled to London town. They arrived to take part in a new political experiment called parliament. When they arrived in London they were met with an awful odor - fumes and smoke from burning coal. Blacksmiths and other tradesmen had begun burning coal in place of wood, filling London's air with sooty smelly smoke.

By the summer of 1306 enough coal was being burned by blacksmiths, brewers (20,000 wagon loads of wood were used each year to distill beer and whisky), and other industries that required large quantities of fuel, that there was an organized resistance against the practice, which led to a royal ban of coal use in the city limits of London and other cities.

Despite new laws threatening steep fines and the destruction of furnaces, coal use continued to increase. Some sources reported that one transgressor of the coal ban law was, "hanged, tortured or decapitated."

The reason for London's rising coal use was obvious. The population of London and of Great Britain generally, had been increasing, and as a result the forests were in a severe state of decline. Forests near London were consumed first simply because of easy access; they were burned for firewood, cut for building, or simply burned to clear land for crop production or pasture for livestock.

Wood ash supplies for garden fertilizer, cutting salt and culinary uses declined. The people did not like to use coal ash or "clinkers" for fertilizing their gardens, culinary ashes in food or cutting salt because they imparted an undesirable burned petroleum smell and taste. The reduced supply of wood ashes caused a general decline in the health and immune defenses in the populations of Great Britain and Europe.

As supplies of energy from living forests declined and became scarce, and more costly, the demand for energy from coal rose significantly. The coal merchants, watching the burgeoning cities and the shrinking forests surely thought coal was nearing a boom in sales.

As luck would have it, the energy crisis was solved, not by coal, but rather by a plague that devastated Europe's populations.

In October 1347, the crew of a trading ship that docked in Sicily brought the Bubonic Plague to Europe. The "Black Death" was already wiping out the populations of China, India and the Middle East; in its first European rage, continuing until 1351, it would kill almost one third of Europe's population - in fact 25 million souls were lost.

Some modern scholars speculated that the plague was particularly deadly because the general population had already been weakened by years of bad weather, bad harvests, reduced supplies of wood (and therefore ashes) and famine.

At the time, most residents of Europe viewed the plague as evidence of the wrath of God! After careful consideration, the medical staff and faculty of the prestigious University of Paris determined that the plague was caused by "an unusual alignment of the planets that had occurred on March 20, 1345."

In England, the plague would break out again and again and again, for at least three additional charges before 1400, and Europe's population would continue to be ravaged by disease until 1500. By 1500, only 3 million people lived in England, about half the number that had lived there before the plague's assault. As deserted and abandoned farms and lands were reclaimed by the forests and trees became large enough to provide for the needs of the decimated population, coal sales went into the tank - the coal market literally dried up, and wood ashes were back!

In the late 1500s, the English suffered an energy crisis again, when their population grew and again, because of an increased demand for and consumption of wood, the forests shrank.

The English learned to tolerate what had been thought of as intolerable - they became the first western culture to mine and burn coal on a massive preferential national scale. The coal burning public and businesses filled the air of London and other cities with the most polluted and foul air in the history of humanity.

The English went on to power an Industrial Revolution with coal and transform the world of industry, agriculture, human health and the fate of the planet Earth itself - the energy produced from coal was a double edged sword and had devastating unintended consequences.

The nobles led popular demonstrations with the populous denouncing the use of coal in the city - King Edward I banned the use of coal for political expediency. The original bans were ignored, so more desperate laws were passed to punish first offenders with "great fines and ransoms." Second offenders had their furnaces destroyed.

In 1661, John Graunt, a little known London draper, theorized that by making tables out of London mortality data and analyzing it, he could create more useful information. His resulting observations, published in 1662, resulted in Charles II, recommending Graunt's appointment to the prestigious and newly formed Royal Society - adding that, "If they found any more such tradesmen, they should be sure to admit them all without further ado."

Graunt's analysis confirmed that infant and childhood mortality was higher than earlier believed, and that thirty per cent of London's deaths were children under the age of four or five years old. The records also showed that lung related deaths reached between 20% and 25% of the total deaths.

Graunt recorded that, "Seasoned residents lived nearly as long in London as elsewhere, yet new-comers, and children do not, for the Smoaks, Stinks, and close Air are less healthful than that of the Country; otherwise why do sickly Persons remove to the Country Air?"

Benjamin Franklin

Benjamin Franklin, as a result of the unintended consequences produced by some of his scientific endeavors, would actually shorten the lives of Americans and individuals in other industrialized nations.

Franklin was born in Boston on Sunday, January 17, 1706. Boston was by then an incorporated town for 76 years. Boston was no longer a simple, isolated religious outpost - it was a bustling, growing port city.

Boston boasted more than 1,000 permanent houses, a thousand seagoing ships registered at its port and 7,000 permanent residents - the population would double every twenty years.

Even as a child, Franklin was a creative, yet practical inventor. One of his first inventions was a set of flippers for his hands and feet to improve his swimming speed. He made two oval palettes, with holes for his thumbs, and "I also fitted to the soles of my feet a kind of sandals."

Early in life Franklin became infatuated with kites. While flying his kites, Franklin would strip, wade into a pond or lake, floated on his back, and used the kite and wind power to pull him across the body of water. "Having engaged another boy to carry my clothes round the pond," he recalled, "I began to cross the pond with my kite, which carried me quite over without the least fatigue and with the greatest pleasure imaginable."

Franklin was originally slated by his father to be a minister, and to that end he was sent to the Boston Latin School at the age of eight to prepare for entry into Harvard.

Franklin did well at Harvard, moving up from the middle of his class to the number one slot, which resulted in his being advanced to a higher grade level. Because Franklin's father couldn't sustain the tuition cost, Franklin was forced to drop out of school.

Young Franklin was described as skeptical, puckish, curious and irreverent, "Dr. Franklin, when a child, found the long graces used by his father before and after meals very tedious," his grandson stated. "One day after the winter's provisions had been salted, 'I think, Father,' said Benjamin, 'if you were to say Grace over the whole cask - once for all - it would be a vast saving of time.'"

At age ten, with only two years of schooling, Franklin went to work full time in his father's candle and soap shop. It was not the most fun job that a ten year old kid could have; he spent his working hours skimming rendered tallow from boiling tubs of "stinking" fat; trimming wicks, adding wood ashes to the soap and filling candle molds was considered a mindless repetitive activity by young Franklin. His father took him on long walks to visit various tradesmen to find a trade or art that might better interest him.

As it turned out, his knowledge of many crafts and skills allowed him to become a first rate tinker and inventor. Franklin at age twelve years went on to sign on for nine years of indentured service as an apprentice and to acquire the training and the experiences of a publisher, printer and newspaperman.

Franklin was directed to produce poetry based on news stories, the stories were well received, to which Franklin wrote, "(the praise) flattered my vanity." Herman Melville would write that, "Franklin was everything but a poet."

Benjamin Franklin's four year old son died of smallpox in 1736, causing him to become an advocate of vaccination for smallpox.

The print industry was a natural course of life for Franklin, "From a child I was fond of reading," he recalled, "and all the little money that came into my hands was ever laid out in books." Books became the most important influence in his life. The love and respect of books was one of the common traits shared by the Puritanism of Mather and the Enlightenment of Locke, worlds that would blend in the character and personality of Benjamin Franklin. "Often I sat up in my room reading the greatest part of the night, when the book was borrowed in the evening and to be returned early in the morning, lest it should be missed or wanted," admitted Franklin.

In 1743, Franklin proposed the formation of the American Philosophical Society, which was to be an American version of the Royal Society think tank of England. It would be housed in Philadelphia, and its members would include illustrious scientists and thinkers from other cities.

The members would exchange their studies by post, and abstracts would be distributed to the members quarterly. The subjects to be investigated were to be practical rather than theoretical and included "newly discovered plants, herbs, trees, roots, their virtues, uses, etc....improvements of vegetable juices, such as ciders, wines, etc.; new methods of curing or preventing diseases, ...improvements in any branch of mathematics...new arts, trades, and manufactures... surveys, maps and charts...methods of improving the breeds of animals... and all philosophical experiments that let light into the nature of things."

In 1747 Franklin proposed a volunteer military force that would be independent of Pennsylvania's colonial government - the Pennsylvania Militia was born.

Franklin didn't realize it, but his charter of the Militia Association, in its spirit as well as wording, conceived and preceded the writing of the Declaration of Independence three decades later:

> *"Being thus unprotected by the government under which we live, we do hereby, for our mutual defense and security, and for the security of our wives, children and estates...form ourselves into an Association."*

In 1748, at age 42, Franklin retired and sold his printing business to David Hall, his trusted foreman; the agreement provided him with half the businesses profits for eighteen years, which amounted to 650 British pounds per year (the average colonial income at the time was 25 pounds per year). Now, he calculated, he would have "leisure to read, study, make experiments, and converse at large with such ingenious and worthy men as are pleased to honor me with their friendship."

Franklin gave up his print shop to focus and engage his energies on science, then politics, then diplomacy and statecraft. As Poor Richard (one of Franklin's pen names) declared in his almanac that year, "Lost time is never found again." His intellectual curiosity and infatuation with the orderliness of the greater universe drew him to science.

Franklin didn't have any formal academic training in science or math to be considered a great theorist of the likes of Einstein; his interests of what he fondly called his "scientific amusements" caused some educated contemporaries to dismiss him as a mere tinker. However, even during his life he was held up as the most famous scientist alive - as Harvard professor, Dudley Herschbach stated, "His work on electricity was recognized as ushering in a scientific revolution comparable to those written by Newton in the previous century or Watson and Crick in ours."

An example of Franklin's practical application of science was his 1740s invention of an iron wood-burning stove that could be built into fireplaces to maximize heat output into the house while at the same time minimizing, fuel requirements, smoke and drafts - using his understanding of convection currents and heat transfer, he produced an original and unique stove design.

The resulting byproduct of the daily use of the "Pennsylvania Stove" - wood ash (plant minerals), were still available to mix with food as "culinary ashes," cut salt at the rate of ten parts ash to one part salt as a condiment and the balance mixed into homemade lye soap and into the compost to fertilize the garden.

During a visit to Boston in the summer of 1743, Franklin and others were entertained one evening by a traveling scientific showman from Scotland called Archibald Spencer. Spencer featured amazing demonstrations of science that were designed to amuse the host's guests. He revealed Newton's theories of light and exhibited a device that measured blood flow - both were interests of Franklin's.

Dr. Spencer performed electricity parlor tricks, such as creating static electricity by rubbing a glass tube and drawing sparks from the feet of a boy hanging by silk cords from the ceiling. "Being (entertained and educated) on a subject quite new to me," Franklin recalled, "They equally surprised and pleased me."

One hundred years earlier, Galileo and Newton had described, explained and demystified a force known as gravity, however, another awesome force of the universe, electricity, was no more understood than it had been by the prehistoric people who had tamed fire. There were individuals, like Dr. Spencer, who used the wonders of electricity as a parlor trick to entertain admiring audiences; however, no one as yet, had put the power of electricity to the task of real work.

The Abbe' Nollet, court scientist to France's King Louis XV, connected 180 soldiers and then 700 monks and "made them jump as if one of the court's entertainment by sending a pulse of static electricity through them." Franklin however, was the ideal person to convert electricity from the status of a simple parlor trick into a functional, practical and working science.

Franklin's initial experiments involved collecting an electric charge and then studying its various properties. He employed his friends to draw charges from a spinning glass tube and touch each other to see if sparks flew. These early experiments resulted in the discovery that electricity was "not created by the friction of rubbing the tube, but collected only."

Many of Franklin's originally coined terms such as

battery, charged, neutral, condense and conductor are still used today in the fields of electricity and the greater subject of energy. "He has written equally for the uninitiated as well as the philosopher," the 19th century English chemist, Sir Humphrey Davy noted, "and he has rendered his details as amusing as well as perspicuous."

Franklin's discovery that the creation of a positive charge was accompanied by the generation of an equal negative charge became known as the "conservation of charge" and the "single-fluid theory" of electricity. The concepts were easily formulated in Franklin's "book keeper" mind. His observations were a scientific breakthrough and discovery of historic greatness - "As a broad generalization that has withstood the test of 200 years of fruitful application," Harvard professor I. Bernard Cohen declared, "Franklin's law of conservation of charge must be considered to be of the same fundamental importance to physical science as Newton's law of conservation of momentum."

In a practical progression of his electrical storage experiments, Franklin lined up a series of parallel glass plates separated by metal - charged them up, wired them together, and discovered a new electrical device - "what we call an electrical battery."

Franklin was able to use the "electrical battery" to turn the iron fence surrounding his house into the first electrified security fence; he created an electrical toy spider that would hop like a live one; he electrocuted turkeys with his electrical battery for the entertainment of his guests before the birds were roasted for dinner with electricity, thus inventing the first electrical execution device and first electrical cooking device.

This early Franklin experiment, in which he killed and cooked turkeys with electrical devices, was perhaps the very first close call humanity had with an epidemic of obesity, type II diabetes, the metabolic syndrome, arthritis, osteoporosis and many other chronic degenerative

diseases, for with the use of electricity there were no wood ash byproducts that had been produced for millennia by the burning of wood. No wood ashes to mix with salt, no culinary ashes - no plant minerals with which to nourish our bodies or to fertilize the garden.

For millennia, lightening was universally considered to be a supernatural phenomenon or an expression of God's wrath. During one 35 year period of time during the 1700s, in Germany alone, "386 churches were struck by lightening and an excess of 100 bell ringers were killed by heavenly bolts. In Venice, 3,000 people were killed when tons of gunpowder stored in a church was struck."

Franklin noted that, "The lightening seems to strike steeples of choice and at the very time the bells are ringing; yet they continue to bless the new bells and jangle the old ones whenever it thunders. One would think it was now time to try some other trick."

Franklin concluded that the "water vapors in a cloud can be electrically charged and when these electrically charged clouds pass over a high tree, lofty towers, spires, masts of ships ...draw the electrical fire and the whole cloud discharges." His proposal led to some practical advice - "Dangerous therefore it is to take shelter under a tree during a thunder gust."

Before he even tried his lightening experiments himself, Franklin detailed his thoughts in two famous letters to Collinson in 1750, which were presented to the Royal Society in London and then widely published. The basic concept was to use a tall metal rod to draw some of the electrical charge from a cloud, just as he had done with a needle to draw off the charge of an iron ball in his workshop.

Franklin correctly surmised that the "lightening rod" could, render safe one of the greatest natural dangers faced by humans. "Houses, ships and even towns and churches may be effectively secured from the stroke of lightening by their means," he predicted.

Franklin had been waiting for the steeple of

Philadelphia's Christ Church to be finished to perform his first lightening rod experiments; because of construction delays, he became impatient and in his typical zeal, he developed the idea of using instead a kite. To that end he enlisted the efforts of his son William to help fly the silk kite. A sharp wire was attached to the top of the kite, and a brass key was attached near the base of the wet string, so that a wire could be brought near it in an effort to draw sparks.

Initially clouds passed over the kite to no effect. Franklin almost fell into despair until he saw several of the strands of the string straighten out and stiffen. He put his knuckle to the key and drew an electrical spark.

Franklin was literally moments away from discovering a commercially viable source of clean household energy - electrical appliances and the end of the dusty ash byproduct of heating and cooking fires! However, the onset of the American Revolution and the birth of a new nation siphoned off his creative juices and energies.

It would take an additional 150 years before Edison's work produced the practical generation of electrical power and the flurry of invention of patented electrical appliances that would replace wood fueled heating and cooking fires and eliminate once and for all the health and life supporting kitchen and heating byproducts of wood ash - plant minerals!

Chapter 10

"Every basket is power and civilization. For coal is a portable climate. It carries the heat of the tropics to Labrador and the polar circle; and it is the means of transporting itself whithersoever it is wanted. Watt and Stephenson whispered in the ear of mankind their secret, that a half-ounce of coal will draw two tons a mile, and coal carries coal, by rail and by boat, to make Canada as warm as Calcutta; and with its comfort brings its industrial power."

Ralph Waldo Emerson, 1850

The Fuel Revolution

After having tamed fire 1,500,000 years earlier, humans had created many unique ways to use the power of fire to change natural materials into everything from metals, pottery, bricks, and glass, to salt, soap and ale. However, in all those hectic and creative millennia of baking, boiling, melting and smelting, it didn't quickly come to them that fire held another power - the power of movement and motion.

For the average human, the back-breaking work of transporting loads from one farm to another, or from one market to another was performed only with the power of muscle, water and wind.

This fact of work powered only by humans, animals, water or wind limited the production and growth that a culture could expect to accomplish in each century. There was only so much mechanical lifting, turning and pulling that humans and animals could do and only so many hours in the day.

In the 1700s, a machine was invented that allowed humans to grow beyond the historical constraints and limits by turning "solar income" fuels into enormous amounts of mechanical torque, lift and forward motion!

This invention was the steam engine and the fuel was coal. The steam engine would soon become the center of the Industrial Revolution, causing it to be called, "The most important invention in the creation of the modern world."

Coal, "motivated" the steam engine and its inventors, who were searching for a solution to the problem of coal mine flooding as the mine shafts were driven below the water table. Wood had become scarce, and as a result, coal had become a necessity of life and the problem of mine flooding had to be solved.

To keep the mines dry, operators employed gravity by digging tunnels or "watergates" from the valleys up into the mine; others used various means of power including windmills, windlass, chain of buckets and simple buckets carried on the backs of diggers. The greatest amounts of water in the largest mines was raised by horse power, however, the cost of maintaining 50 to 60 horses and their teamsters was too burdensome for even the largest mines.

By 1700, coal production was ten times greater than it had been in 1550. England was now mining five times more coal than all other nations combined, she was now totally dependent on coal as a fuel for home use and for powering industry. Even if England optimized her wood fuel production from her forests, ceased the use of wood for building and manufacturing, the forests could no longer replace the dependency on coal - wood fuels were once and for all gone in England.

The flooding of the mines remained a threat to England's very existence as a world power - as a result, in 1660 Charles II created the Royal Society. The Royal Society was an independent group commissioned to study and promote the theory and application of science.

The original members of the Royal Society were the great philosophers, thinkers and scientists of the day, including Sir Issac Newton, Gottfried Leibnitz, Christopher Wren, Samuel Pepys, John Evelyn and Robert Boyle - "Religion, nationality, profession - all were subordinated to a degree perhaps never before found in history."

One of the more important and practical concerns of the illustrious group was coal, yet coal was still a mystery to them. In the 17th century, people still believed that coal was a living organism and still alive much like peat moss.

The Royal Society members, although initially confused about the origin of coal, they agreed for certain to one thing - England's coal supply was threatened by mine flooding. They focused all of their attention on pumping technology, and on atmospheric pressure.

Scientists had only recently begun to appreciate that the atmosphere had weight and volume and it fills vacuums with a powerful force. They learned and appreciated the fact that the force of air opposing a vacuum could be put to work, however, producing and controlling the vacuum was problematic.

Denis Papin, a French Huguenot living in England, found the solution - steam! Papin had previously proven his knowledge of steam by demonstrating to the members of the Royal Society his steam pressure cooker which he named the "Digester" or Engine for softening bone so they could be completely eaten.

Between 1690 and 1695, Papin invented a small contraption consisting of a moveable piston within a brass cylinder. When he heated water that filled one end on the cylinder, the resulting steam vigorously drove the piston upward. When he removed the flame, the steam condensed and produced a vacuum - the piston was then vigorously pushed back toward the vacuum by the outside atmospheric pressure.

Papin didn't believe his first steam piston could be built large enough to be of practical use. The inventor who actually put the steam piston to work, was not a member of the Royal Society or London's scientific elite, rather it was Thomas Newcomen, a simple ironmonger or "tinker" from a small rural town.

The members of the Royal Society tried to downplay the importance of Newcomen's steam engine, leading many historians to believe that Newcomen's lack of credentials was the problem. One historian went on to say, "to the small scientific world of London, whose center was the Royal Society, it seemed inconceivable that such a man could excel the brightest intellects of the day in the power of invention."

Newcomen's steam driven device was similar to the Papin piston, however, it was much larger and sported a separate boiler in which to generate the steam. After the steam was let into the bottom of the cylinder, cold water was added to condense the steam; the resulting vacuum forced the piston in a downward stroke. As the piston moved up and down, it rocked an overhead beam. The opposite end of the beam moved the rod of a vacuum pump in a similar fashion to those driven by horse power.

The first practical Newcomen steam engine was "quietly and without ceremony" installed at a coal mine in 1712. The engine was called a "fire engine," and the men who fed coal into the engine's boiler and kept the engine's fire alive were called "firemen."

Newcomen's steam engine was an immediate success and much revered by mine operators - one engine did the work of pumping more efficiently and more economically than 50 horses!

Those historians who know Newcomen's story, write

of him and his work with an almost religious reverence, calling his steam engine, "the most wonderful invention which human ingenuity had yet produced," and credited him with giving "to the whole world ...The art of converting fuel into useful power for the benefit and convenience of humanity."

By the 1760s, hundreds of Newcomen engines (because they used atmospheric pressure rather than steam pressure were often called atmospheric engines) were pumping water from mine shafts throughout England and Scotland; some of Newcomen's engines were built to gigantic proportions for the day, reaching cylinder diameters of more than six feet and lengths of ten feet.

Initially the Newcomen engine was used only by coal mine operators because it was a fuel hog, and coal was for all practical purposes free at the mouth of the shaft.

In 1736, James Watt, the son of a Sottish carpenter was born. He was the only one of five children born to his parents to survive to manhood; however, Watt was very frail and suffered from continuous migraines that kept him in bed for weeks at a time.

According to a 19th century biographer, Watt's fragile health left him with "an almost feminine delicacy and sensitiveness, which made him shrink from the rough play of robust children"; as a result, he was home schooled during his early years, he spent his time playing with his father's carpentry tools and intently watching steam pouring from tea kettles.

Watt excelled in math and studied the art of constructing mathematical instruments. It was as an instrument maker, only 20 years old, that he was asked to fix a small working model of a Newcomen engine that had been reverently kept at Glasgow University.

The Newcomen model, like the full sized engine, was extremely wasteful, requiring enormous amounts of coal to keep it going. Watt observed that as steam was injected into the system and then cooled with water, heat was wasted in the cyclical process of reheating and cooling the cylinder.

Watt revolutionized the Newcomen steam engine by installing a separate condenser; the cylinder would be attached to another container that was surrounded with cool water, after the cylinder filled with steam, the steam passed into the cooler container where it condensed. In this way, the cylinder itself would always remain hot and ready for the next injection of steam!

According to Dr. Joseph Black, a good friend, of Watt's, "This capital improvement flashed upon his mind at once, and filled him with rapture."

Watt, after suffering many challenges ("of all things in life, there is nothing more foolish than inventing"), eventually found the perfect partner, the Birmingham industrialist, Mathew Boulton, and one of the most successful partnerships in history was started.

Boulton was a manufacturer and an industrial visionary. Together, Boulton and Watt formed the Lunar Society - members included Joseph Priestly who had discovered oxygen, sulfur dioxide and carbon monoxide; Joseph Wedgewood, the pottery giant; and Erasmus Darwin, inventor, poet and grandfather of Charles Darwin.

Boulton built his financial empire with buckles, rather than coal, iron or textiles. He employed 1,000 workers in his Soho manufactory, where they made precision crafted goods, with a range from buckles, buttons and filigree to classic scientific instruments including clocks, thermometers and telescopes. Boulton's manufactory became so famous that it drew tourists, including Catherine the Great.

Boulton had a serious interest in steam engines because the water wheels that powered the Soho facility could not be depended upon for a continuous source of power. He had unsuccessfully tried his hand at inventing and designing steam engines, he even exchanged letters on the subject of engine design with his good friend Benjamin Franklin.

In 1773, Watt moved to Birmingham and began working on improvements on his steam engine at Soho.

Boulton provided skilled artisans, financial backing and best of all emotional encouragement to Watt.

The all important cylinder was produced by John Wilkinson, the pioneering iron founder. In 1776, while the American Revolution was in full swing, James Watt installed his first two engines, one to pump water out of a mine shaft and the other to inflate and drive the bellows in Wilkinson's iron foundry.

While Watt improved the steam engine in many ways, his finest moment was in getting the Newcomen engine to extract four times the work force or "horse power" out of a lump of coal. The steam engine's new fuel efficiency moved it out of the darkness of the coal mine and into the business world to find a home in the world's factories.

England's coal industry had become relatively large by the 1700s just to meet the domestic and non-iron industrial requirements of the nation; it would expand again tenfold by 1830; and double again by 1854. Between 1842 and 1856 the number of English coal mines quadrupled again.

The steam driven Industrial Revolution's impact on human endeavor has been compared to the discovery and taming of fire, the invention of the wheel, and to the tasting of the apple from the Tree of Knowledge.

Not until the 1800s would it be scientifically established, and commonly accepted, that coal itself, not only the plant fossils held within, was plant material and prehistoric.

By 1790, "potash fever" swept through the young, American country; trees were burned by the tens of thousands simply for the ash which was exported to Great Britain for fertilizer and culinary ashes. The first U.S. Patent, Patent Number 1, was awarded for "the production of wood ash and the use of wood ash as fertilizer."

Coal was not just another simple fuel, and "no mere article of commerce." Coal represented man's victory over the elements of nature - it became the foundation of civilization itself:

"With Coal, we have light, strength, power, wealth and civilization; without Coal we have darkness, weakness, poverty, and barbarism."

For centuries, Britain led the world in coal production, and as a result, the Industrial Revolution started there; Britain became the most powerful country on the planet, it created the first "industrial society," one that no one could have imagined - the genie was out of the bottle!

In the United States, coal transformed an empty wilderness into an industrial superpower at warp speed. Without coal we would have wallowed longer in the poverty wracked, backbreaking hand labor of backwardness and the ignorance of the pre-industrial world; however, given more time, we might have discovered a more graceful, a more gentle and a more friendly path to modernization.

Michael Faraday, the scientist, acclaimed by all the world, had little formal education and had taught himself everything. Since the 1820s his had been a career of "marvelous discoveries in many different fields, that of induced electricity appearing as the most remarkable of all."

"With his horseshoe magnet and disc rotating between its poles, Faraday, had demonstrated before the Royal Society in 1831 (some 41 years after Franklin's death), how mechanical energy could be converted into electrical energy - thus presenting to the world, the first miniature model of the dynamo (generator)."

Faraday published a two volume collection of his experiments and theories called, *Experimental Researches in Electricity* - Thomas Edison, as a young boy devoured Faraday's written works on electricity and formed his views on electricity based on the work of Franklin and Faraday.

Faraday's "dynamo" seemed to provide the answer to the problem of a cheap supply of electric current. This early dynamo, powered by steam engines, was gradually improved over time by many inventors and tinkers - by the 1860s light houses along England's coast were lit by giant arc lights.

In 1876, at the Philadelphia Exposition, Moses G. Farmer exhibited three arc lights powered by his privately built dynamo. In 1877, a newspaper reported that Paul Jablochkoff, a former Russian officer of engineers had invented "electric candles" which were introduced as street lamps in Paris.

Coal, steam and electricity now had a toe hold in the daily life of human culture - it was clear that wood as a fuel for the hearth and industry was no longer viable, because the maximum rate of re-growth of trees could no longer keep up with the growing demand for fuel and power.

Unfortunately at this point in history, territorial expansion, financial empires, industrial growth and mass transportation (i.e. - roads, canals, railroad, trans- Atlantic ships, etc.) were the driving force in all industrialized nations - the race was on! As a result of all the excitement generated by new sources of power and business growth, no one paid any attention to the human price that would be paid over the horizon of time.

Wood, the source of the seemingly endless flow of wood ashes (plant mineral nutrition) that had supported human development in the fields of agriculture, nutrition, intellect, art, industry, health, longevity and science had begun to be pinched off - we had moved from wood to coal as the common fuel, we had moved from wind, water and muscle power to steam and electricity to run our machines, farms and industries in almost a single breath.

Part 3

"We do not want to be like the immortal Struldbruggs in Swift's novel Gulliver's Travels, who kept on growing older, more ill, and more miserable, and acquired an additional Ghastliness in Proportion to their number of Years.'"

Sally Beare
50 Secrets of the World's Longest Living People

The Age Beaters

Chapter 11

"If I had known I was going to live so long, I'd have taken better care of myself."

Eubie Blake
Celebrate ragtime pianist
1883 - 1983

The Age Beaters

At the date of publication of *IMMORTALITY*, there are 210,000 to 300,000 centenarians worldwide out of more than seven billion people. In 2006, the U.S. Surgeon General said that, "of the 2.2 million deaths in America each year, that 1.8 million are diet related" - this statement agrees with the 1968 observation of Dr. Wallach that, "Every animal and every human being that dies of natural causes dies of a nutritional deficiency disease."

The gerontologists and geneticists of today agree that all humans have the genetic equipment and therefore the genetic capacity to live well beyond 100 years of age. Most of these "experts" on aging believe the true maximum lifespan of humans is 120 years of age, however they really don't know for a fact that humans have a maximum life span of 120 because there has not been a controlled study with 1,000 humans fed a perfect Calorie Restricted diet, a perfectly supplemented diet and perfect intake of antioxidants - their belief is their theory!

At the beginning of the 20th century when we were switching from horses to cars, there were those "experts" who believed that if we drove cars 50 miles per hour that our hearts would explode; it was believed before Roger Bannister broke the four minute mile, that it was humanly impossible to run that fast, yet one year after his miraculous feat that broke the four minute mile, 300 more runners broke the four minute mark; it was said that the sound barrier couldn't be broken by a manned flight; it was believed that we would never get a man to land on the moon and return to earth and so on - who is to say we can't live to be 150, 175 or 200 - we believe we can!

Dan Buettner, author of the *Blue Zones*, believes that there are only four places on earth where people successfully live to be over 100 years of age. His is quite the simple view as there are in fact literally an infinite number of places on earth where people commonly live beyond 100 years of age and if all humans were to employ the four basic principals of IMMORTALITY almost all could live beyond 100 years of age just as an entire colony of rats on a perfect longevity diet with Calorie Restriction can live to be five years of age instead of three years.

Our purpose here is to share with the reader the wide variety of peoples and cultures all over the world who can and do live beyond 100 years of age because they all employ either knowingly or unknowingly the four principals of healthful longevity and yes - even Immortality.

The Tibetans & Chinese

Since before written history, wood ashes (plant derived minerals) were the most universally available mineral nutritional supplement and mineral based fertilizer. Wood ashes were predictable; they were a fine particle-sized mineral dust and an immediately available source of plant food (fertilizer) and mineral supplement that was produced everyday in the human's daily life as a simple byproduct of cooking and warming our homes.

Wood ash was an unintended, passively produced by product, a cottage industry in even the most humble of dwellings. Wood ash was produced and employed in their daily lives by Neanderthals 200,000 years ago.

The systematic cultivation and fertilization of land to commercially produce food was first written about in 4000 B.C. in China. Chinese farmers used "organic material, wood ashes and silt reclaimed from streams and rivers that had been eroded from the hills and mountains to fertilize gardens and field crops."

Wood ashes were universally available and contained a wide variety of "plant derived minerals" that were easily available to cultivated garden plants and directly available to humans as a source of nutritional minerals when mixed with table salt and applied to our food as a condiment and mixed with our food as "culinary ashes."

"culinary ashes" were of great and absolute importance to human survival, health, fertility and longevity. Wood, peat and kelp ashes were added to human and animal food since before written history.

The "munchies," pica and cravings didn't begin with the first potato chip or Hershey bar - the munchies began with the first man as a "salt craving." From the first man to the modern man, we were and still are dependent on plant source minerals.

Food preparation, in its earliest and simplest form, was raw meat or meat crudely "cooked" in fire. Food was immediately eaten or preserved by being rolled in wood ash or "salted."

Salt was a valuable and cherished substance and it was traded ounce for ounce for gold and slaves. As a result, salt was not squandered by simply eating it, it was mixed, "cut" and diluted with wood, peat or kelp ashes. And so with the simple act of "extending" salt with "culinary" ashes, humans, from the beginning of time, unknowingly acquired the 60 essential minerals daily as a food supplement.

About 5,000 years ago, one of the world's early civilizations began along the banks of the Yellow River, as the Chinese stopped their hunting and gathering, drove and dragged their Neolithic tools into the virgin soil of the flood plains - the hunters became farmers.

Over the millennia, the Chinese extended farming as far north as the rain fall permitted. Beyond the rain fall line only barbarian nomads who herded goats and camels could survive. The northern boundary of Chinese civilization was in fact determined by the Chinese deferring to the climate; the Great Wall was China's way to codify the natural border between wet and dry, settled and unsettled.

Climate not only determined the borders of Chinese civilization, but also stimulated the formation of one of its most important identifying features - a powerful, centralized government, designed, in a manner like that of the Roman Empire.

Even south of the Great Wall, rainfall is so unpredictable that China has always been squeezed between the double-edged disasters of drought and flood, and many millions have starved or drowned.

Chinese mythology describes the first dynasty as being founded about 2200 B.C. by Yu the Great, who provided some relief from the natural disasters. Yu the Great was "part god, part hydraulic engineer" - he brought an equilibrium between the earth and the waters and made cultivation predictable by constructing dams, canals and irrigation ditches, and also as legend has it, "by dancing a special flood control dance."

For thousands of years, China's emperors, had the

responsibility, of constructing, and maintaining enormous water projects. To this end the emperors mobilized huge armies; the stakes were high, failure to control flooding and droughts raised doubts as to whether the emperor's heavenly appointment to rule the people had ended.

Success resulted in long dynasties, the crops flourished and taxes flowed to the emperor's coffers. The emperors succeeded more than they failed, so China grew to such impressive levels that their degree of modern civilization would shock the West.

Marco Polo wrote and published his famous China travel book in 1300. The book described the amazing feats and wonders of wealth, food, farming, canals, huge bustling cities and successful government in an attempt to educate and entertain his fellow Europeans. Polo's descriptions seemed so outrageous to the Western mind he was condemned as a liar.

One of the unusual practices in China was described by Polo as:

"Throughout this province (of northern China) there is found a sort of black stone, which they dig out of the mountains, where it runs in veins. When lighted it burns like charcoal, it retains fire much better than wood; insomuch that it may be preserved during the night, and in the morning be found still burning. These stones do not flame, excepting a little when first lighted, but during their ignition give out a considerable heat.

It is true there is no scarcity of wood in the country, but the multitude of inhabitants is so immense, and their stoves and baths, which they are continually heating, so numerous, that the quantity (of wood) could not supply the demand. There is no person who does not frequent a warm bath at least three times in a week, and during the winter daily, if it is in their power. Every man of rank or wealth has one in his house for his own use; and the stock of wood must soon prove inadequate to such consumption; whereas these stones may be had in abundance, and at a cheap rate."

The Tibetans were the inspiration for the Pulitzer Prize winning book, by James Hilton, *The Lost Horizon*. Tibet's "Old People" are found on Chang Tang or the northern plateau, elevation 15,000 feet, which consists of salt lakes fed by glaciers from the eastern slopes of the Himalayan Mountains.

This mountain culture has about 500,000 people who are devout Buddhists. The Tibetans are a mix of nomadic herdsmen, merchants of salt, farmers and great cavalrymen on camel or horse.

Tibet makes up almost 10% of China's land mass and was founded in the 7th century by King Songtsan Gambo. The Chinese government sent an army into Tibet in 1950 and established a military governor to prevent Tibet from establishing an independent nation. Since 1965 the region has been administered and known as the Tibetan Autonomous Region (T.A.R.) of China.

The herdsmen build their corrals, huts and roads out of salt bricks carefully cut from dried salt lakes on top of the plateau; they hunt Marco Polo sheep, antelope, gazelle, wild asses and yak.

The yak, which translates to "wealth," provides meat, sausage, milk, cheese, yogurt, butter, wool, skins and animal power for plowing, riding and to transport freight.

The staple diet of the Tibetan consists of "tsampa," a smelly hand-mixed paste of lightly toasted barley flour, yak butter, salt and black tea. The tsampa mainstay is supplemented with turnips, cabbage, potatoes, trout, omelets and beans.

Tibetans routinely drink 30 to 40 medium sized cups of black or green tea daily because the high elevation has an extremely low humidity, requiring a high fluid intake. Each cup of tea is flavored with a chunk of rock salt the size of a Concord grape and two pats of yak butter.

The Tibetan capital city of Lhasa (translates to "Place of the Gods") was the inspiration for James Hilton's legendary city of Shangri-La. The city is found at an elevation of 12,000 feet, where temperatures can fluctuate as much as 80 to 100 degrees F each day.

In the center of old Lhasa is the holiest shrine in Tibet - the Jokhang built in 650 A.D. The Jokhang is the "Mecca" to the Tibetan Buddhists - many of the faithful would trek through the mountains for years to come and pray at this holy site.

In the mountains west of Lhasa is Drepung, a gigantic monastery that houses 10,000 monks, 25,000 serfs and assistants working 185 estates and tending over 200 pastures.

The Potala, "high heavenly realm," is a sprawling mountaintop palace of the Dalai Lama (translates to "ocean of wisdom" and represents the living prophet of the Buddhist faith and the inspiration for the ancient living sage in James Hilton's, *The Lost Horizon*) built into the mountain 700 feet above Lhasa.

The Potala is famous for its 1,000 rooms, 10,000 altars, 20,000 statues of Buddha and the eight gold gilded tombs of past Dalai Lamas.

South of Lhasa, there are tens of thousands of acres of terraces fed and irrigated by mineral rich "Glacial Milk" which originates from the Himalayan glaciers and wood ash (from heating and cooking fires) enriched compost. The vegetables, fruit and grains that are grown in this mineral rich essentially manufactured soil take up these plant minerals and are consumed by the Tibetans.

The Yao People of Bama

In 2008, China is being challenged by what they call the "Gray Tide." The annual growth rate for the numbers of Chinese seniors over age 80 years is approximately five percent bringing their numbers to mind boggling 11 million in 2008.

Wangang, which translates to "thousands of mountains" is a remote area of Bama county in the semi-tropical district of

Guangxi in the southwest of China. The Panyang River falls rapidly some 4,500 feet to the isolated valley below.

Wangang is inhabited by the legendary and long lived Yao people who have tilled their fields and terraces for thousands of years. The World Health Organization has recently designated Bama an official "hometown of longevity," and a research institute has been established in order to discover the reasons for the Yoa people's good health and longevity. In 1991 Bama County was ranked by the United Nations as being in the world's top five long lived cultures.

The octogenarians in Bama have the dubious pleasure of "looking up to their elders, the nonagenarians, who in turn defer to those centenarians aged a hundred and over."

Wangang typically has large numbers of centenarians that number 34 per 100,000. It is not uncommon for households to contain five generations of the same family.

The Yao typically buy their own coffin at age 61 and use it as a sitting bench and grain storage locker until the need arises to use it for their own burial.

Yao centenarians typically participate in their share of chores by climbing the mountain paths to work the fields and terraces and actively engage in social activities, particularly folk singing.

The Yao people of Bama irrigate their terraces with the mineral laden waters of the Panyang River, and they fertilize their gardens with compost consisting of kitchen waste, wood ash, plant debris and animal manure.

The Yao people have an extremely low incidence of chronic disease such as coronary artery disease, cancer and diabetes. There are no sudden increases in the rates of killer diseases after the age of 40.

Only 10% of those individuals over 90 years of age suffer from coronary heart disease; in one study, not a single malignant tumor could be found.

Hair analysis found that the Yao people had high levels of trace elements in their tissues.

Diet, is regarded by gerontologists, to be the most important factor of longevity in Bama. Three low calorie vegetable, seed, fish, eggs and meat - based meals are eaten daily.

The Yao people consume large quantities of lima beans, mung beans, soy beans, tofu, corn, brown rice, pumpkin, tomatoes, green leafy vegetables, amaranth, peppers, banana, guavas, grapes and pear.

The people of Bama regularly drink "snake wine" - fermented rice or corn wine bottled with snakes that are preserved in the alcohol.

Mahjong, chess, calligraphy and folk singing are favorite pastimes that have been practiced by the Yao for 1,000 years.

Bama Recipes*

Sweet Potato and Salad:

1 medium sweet potato
Mixed green leafy vegetables (romaine, arugula, watercress, spinach, mixed greens, etc.)
1 cooked sliced beet
2 thinly sliced tomatoes
1 medium avocado, sliced
1 handful basil or cilantro leaves, chopped
10 black olives, sliced
Sesame seeds
Olive oil/vinegar dressing or lemon wedges

1. Scrub the sweet potato with water and bake for 35 minutes at 375 F or until done.

2. Mix other ingredients except for the sesame seeds; add the olive oil/vinegar or lemon juice but do not toss.

3. Heat sesame seeds in a dry pan for 2 to 5 minutes, then add to the dressed salad and toss.

Sweet Potato and Carrot Soup:

2 to 3 medium sweet potatoes
4 to 5 large carrots
2 Tblsp extra-virgin olive oil
1 tsp cumin**
1 pinch of ground cardamom seed**
1 1/2 pints chicken or vegetable stock

1. Peel and chop the sweet potatoes and carrots.

2. Heat the olive oil in cast iron pan and add vegetables.

3. Add tsp cumin powder and a pinch of ground cardamom seeds, stir in, and sweat the mixture for a few moments.

4. Add enough stock to cover the vegetables and simmer until they are soft (approximately 5 minutes).

5. Pour into a blender or food processor and blend - if the soup is too thick - add more stock.

6. Return to the pan for a few seconds after blending and heat - soup serves two!

Grilled Polenta with Spinach:

2 1/2 cups water
1 cup polenta flour
3 Tblsp grated Parmesan cheese**
Sea salt and freshly ground pepper
Tblsp extra-virgin olive oil
14 oz spinach
1 clove garlic, chopped

1. Bring the water to a boil in a heavy pan. Pour the polenta slowly, in a steady stream, whisking it at the same time. Turn the heat down as low as possible, and simmer gently for a few minutes, until it is the same consistency as oatmeal. Stir in the Parmesan cheese, a pinch of salt and pepper to taste. Transfer to a small, shallow dish and leave to cool and harden.

2. Cut the polenta into wedges, brush a little olive oil on both sides, and grill for a few minutes on each side until it becomes slightly golden.

3. At the same time, steam the spinach for 1 to 2 minutes until just wilted. Heat the olive oil in a pan on medium heat, add the garlic, cook for just a few seconds, toss spinach into the pan for a few seconds. Serve the polenta and a few extra shavings of the Parmesan cheese. Serves 1 - 2.

**Sally Beare, 50 Secrets of the World's Longest Living People. 2006.*
*** Added by the chief; this ingredient is not part of the Bama diet.*

Li-Ching-Yun

Li-Ching-Yun reportedly lived to the age of 256 years, he outlived 23 wives and had 180 descendents! Li of Kaihsien, in the Province of Szechwan, China, was born in 1677; he sold herbs for 100 years; and died in 1933 at the age of 256 years (and was the inspiration for the 200 year old leader of Hilton's Shangri-La).

Professor Wu-Chung-Chien, the Dean of the Department of Education, of the Minkuo University reported that he had found records showing that Li was in fact born in 1677 (the Chinese have the most extensive and the most accurate of all census records in the history of man), and that on Li's 150th birthday (1827), he was congratulated by the Chinese Imperial Government. Fifty year later, in 1877, Li was sent a second official birthday congratulations, for his 200th birthday. Fifty years later, at the age of 250 years, Li lectured to 1,000 medical students in Beijing on the art of living a long and healthy life.

Li's advice for a long and healthful life was to, "Keep a quiet heart, sit like a tortoise, sleep like a dog." The "Sit Still and Do Nothing" approach to health has many proponents, and there is a time-tested practice that has been found over and over to reduce the risk of illnesses, retain beauty and youth and to engender longevity - meditation and prayer.

Meditation has been shown to lower blood pressure, relax one's muscles, raise the circulating levels of DHEA (the "youth hormone"), lower age-inducing cortisol levels, and generally support the rejuvenating processes in the body.

According to several studies, meditation reduces one's risk of cancer by 55% and heart disease by 80%. In a study of more than 2,000 people who meditate, there was a 50% decrease in the use of medical facilities, for those over 40 years of age the reduction was 70% (this included visits for heart disease, respiratory disease and gastrointestinal problems).

Being religious definitely increases one's longevity. In a meta-analysis of 42 studies which examined 125,826 people (American Psychological Association in the year 2,000), it was demonstrated that regular attendance at a place of worship (church, synagogue, mosque or temple) added eight years to the average lifespan and improved general health.

London Times, May 8, 1933

Telegrams in Brief - A telegram from Chungking in the Province of Szechwan, China states that Li-Ching-Yun, reputed to be the oldest man in China, and presumably the world, has died at Kiah-Sien, at the alleged age of 256. - Reuters

"Here, since endless centuries, man has tamed the impossible mountainside into terraces, he has quarried the rock, he has fed his sheep among the thin woods, he has cut his boughs and burnt his charcoal, he has been half domesticated even among the wild fastnesses. This is what is so attractive....Life is so primitive, so pagan, so strangely heathen and half savage."

D. H. Lawrence, 1921

"Diet probably plays an important role. Barbagia is not like the rest of the Mediterranean. They don't eat a Mediterranean diet."

Dr. Antonio Cao, Geneticist
Akea study

Sardinians

Dr. Paolo Francalacci, an evolutionary anthropologist from Stanford University, said, "Eighteen thousand years ago, during the period called the Glacial Maximum, humans could survive in Europe only in two refuges, one in Iberia and one in the Balkans."

As the glaciers receded and the climate began to warm, humans began to re-enter Europe. They traveled westward from the Balkans and eastward from the Iberian Peninsula. Sardinia, itself was populated almost entirely by a genetically homogeneous Iberian peoples. They originally survived by hunting, gathering and fishing.

Farming showed up in Sardinia 6,000 to 7,000 years ago, brought by Neolithic bands of peoples from the Levant, where farming had been recorded 3,000 years earlier.

About 14,000 years ago, Earth was thawing from an Ice Age. As the ice melted, a small group of "genetically related" people in Iberia migrated from the Pyrenees Mountains to the Mediterranean Sea. They traveled east along the sea coast, passing through what would become the "French Riviera," Tuscany, then crossing the sea to Corsica and finally established villages in the Sardinian coastal foothills.

The Nuraghic peoples, tribal bands from the Bronze Age appeared in Sardinia - the Nuraghi people were named for the stone towers commonly found throughout Sardinia. The Phoenicians and Romans appeared with their armies and occupied the Sardinian coasts and the southern lowlands. Sardinians, who had originally settled the entire island of Sardinia, were squeezed into the central hills.

Gianni Pes, a medical statistician, traced the personal histories of 1,000 Sardinian centenarians. He personally did physical examinations of 200 individuals.

While examining his data, he noticed an unusual

concentration of male centenarians in mountainous Barbagia, Sardinia in the administrative district of Ogliastra.

The word Barbagia, comes from the Latin "*Barbaria,*" land of the Barbarians. They had little or no interest in the tedium of farming. "Even if ancient Sardinians knew of farming techniques, it didn't take," Francalacci said. "They carried on largely as hunter-gatherers and later as shepherds."

Like most island nations, Sardinians, Buettner says, "developed an intense wariness and distain for visitors. Newcomers had always meant subjugation, exploitation, and taxes. So they turned inward, developing an intense dedication to their families and community and earning a reputation for toughness. One Barbagia proverb said it all about foreigners: Furat chie benit dae su mare (He who comes from the sea is here to steal)."

In one particular Sardinian village, he found seven centenarians out of a population of 2,500 - one out of 357!

Dr. Michael Poulain, a Belgian demographer created the Extreme Longevity Index, an index that codified the birth and death data of all centenarians born between 1880 and 1900. He focused on areas that had the greatest numbers of documented centenarians and circled them on maps with blue ink which resulted in the use of the term "Blue Zone" to indicate longevity sites throughout the world.

The Blue Zone sites in particular showed extreme longevity in men. Typically women centenarians are recorded at a rate 400% greater than men, however, in Barbagia, Sardinia, the rate was one to one!

Statistically, male longevity is the story in Sardinia! In the Sardinian Blue Zone, 47 men and 44 women have made it past their 100th year out of 17,865 born between 1880 and 1900 - a rate of 100 year olds that surpasses America's rate by a factor of 30!

As time passed in Sardinia, the native Sardinians developed their own unique culture and environment. Many villages retained their pre-Roman names. "In this region," says Francalacci, "the names of the Sardinian villages such as Ollolai, Illorai, Irgoli, Ittiri, Orune, to name a few, sound very exotic to a continental Italian ear like mine."

Nurra, a region north of Alghero, is thought by linguists to be derived from the word *nur*, which translates to "a heap of stones" in the Nuraghian language. The Bronze Age towers that are commonly found scattered throughout Sardinia are referred to as nuraghi.

The early Sardinians, did not hold on to their ancient Nuraghic dialect, because the Romans had occupied them over sufficient time, they learned to speak Latin. "It suggests that the Sardinians' lifestyle in the Blue Zone hasn't changed much since the time of Christ," Francalacci said.

Francalacci continued, "The laws of evolution dictate that a species will not evolve in a comfortable, isolated environment where reproduction is easy. By contrast, a species will evolve quickly in a tough environment where individuals of different backgrounds and conditions interact. Similarly, in a place like the Sardinian Blue Zone, there is less pressure to adapt (and change). The people there maintained not only their pure genetic features, but also their economic isolation and traditional social values, such as the respect for elders as a source of experience, the importance of the family clan, and the presence of unwritten laws - all of which proved to be effective means for avoiding foreign domination over the centuries."

Prior to 1950, "Sardinia had looked more like a backwater than a centenarian's Shangri-La. Poor hygiene, poor water quality, and a scarcity of water led to rampant infectious diseases. Dysentery, plague, tuberculosis, malaria, and diarrhea killed many young Sardinians. As English traveler William Henry Smyth wrote in his 1828 *Sketch of the Present State of the Island of Sardinia*, 'it is surprising that with such inconvenient residences, and uncleanly habits, the natives should remain so generally healthy as they do."

As D. H. Lawrence traveled through Sardinia in 1921

in search of a simple lifestyle, he embraced Barbagia. "Here, since endless centuries, man has tamed the impossible mountainside into terraces, he has quarried the rock, he has fed his sheep among the thin woods, he has cut his boughs and burnt his charcoal, he has been half domesticated even among the wild fastnesses. This is what is so attractive...Life is so primitive, so pagan, so strangely heathen and half savage."

Dr. Gianni, Blue Zone demographer, said, "Consider, for instance, the genes of inflammation. We studied several tens of gene variants related to inflammation but we didn't find any evidence of their role in survival of Sardinians. The same for genes related to cancer, and those related to cardiovascular disease. I suspect that the characteristics of the environment, the lifestyle, and the food are by far more important for a healthy life."

Villages in the center of Sardinia's Blue Zone (Fonni, Gavoi, Villagrande Strisali, Talana, and Arzana) around the Gennargentu Mountains have progressed over the centuries from small collections of shepherd huts into modern communities that are home to thousands of people.

The traditional Sardinian diet consists of fava beans, eggs, pecorino cheese, sheep and goat cheese, vegetables (squash, zucchini, onions, olives, tomatoes, potatoes, eggplant, etc.), bread, pasta, almonds, raisins, minestrone soup, olive and mastic oil and boiled meat (goat meat, roast lamb, ham, chicken, etc.) - adults drink a liter of Sardinian flavonoid and resveratrol rich red Cannonau wine every day. Fish is not commonly found in their diet. The Sardinians cook and heat their homes with wood stoves, the resultant wood ashes are then mixed with plant debris, kitchen waste and animal manure to create a compost, that is then mixed into the gardens and terraces as a fertilizer.

Campodimele

Campodimele is known as Europe's "village of Eternal Youth." Campodimele, translates to "meadow of honey," is an isolated hilltop village that sits halfway between Rome and Naples in the south of Italy.

It is said that it is a rare thing for a villager to die before their 85th birthday, many reach their nineties, and is not unusual for them to pass the age of 100 years without ever having to visit a doctor.

The 1995 census revealed that there was forty-eight 90 year-olds, three 99-year-olds and a centenarian of 104 in the population of 840.

The village is a rat warren of cobblestone streets and stone houses surrounded by plantings of grapes, herbs, chili peppers and protected by a medieval wall. Outside the walls are planted with olive groves, orchards and groves of fruit and nut trees and terraces dense with vegetables and grain. The meadows beyond are used to graze cattle, pigs, goats and sheep. Red and white wines are daily staples.

Meals are based on whole grain breads and pasta, beans, fruit, olive oil, garlic, onions, tomatoes, Porcini mushrooms, eggplant, meat, eggs, snails, goat cheese, butter, arugula, lettuce and wine.

Campodimele Recipes*

Pasta and Bean Soup

1-2 cloves garlic, chopped small
3 tomatoes, chopped small
2 Tblsp extra-virgin olive oil
5 cups pork or vegetable stock
1 cup beans (fagioloi or cannelloni beans, presoaked or canned)
1 pinch chili pepper
4 oz pork, small pieces
4 oz fettuccine, break into short strips
2 Tblsp Parmesan, grated
Basil leaves

1. Cook the garlic and tomatoes gently in the olive oil, with lid on to retain moisture.

2. Add the stock, then the beans, and a pinch of chili pepper. Put in the raw meat and simmer until the beans are cooked. If using uncooked beans, cook for 45 minutes to 1 hour, add more liquid if necessary. If using canned beans, add them to step 3 when the pasta is almost ready.

3. Add the fettuccini and cook until it is done (al dente), following the cooking time on the package.

4. Serve with a drizzle of olive oil and the grated cheese. Garnish with basil leaves. Serves 2.

Gnocchi with Porcini Mushrooms

5 oz gnocchi
1-2 Tblsp extra-virgin olive oil.
1 1/2 oz dried porcini mushrooms, soaked in a small amount of warm water.
1 pinch thyme
1-2 cloves garlic, chopped small
Sea salt
2 tsp parsley, chopped
1 small pinch ground chili pepper
2 Tblsp, Parmesan or goat's cheese

1. Put on a pan of water to boil for the gnocchi. Meanwhile heat the olive oil and add the porcini mushrooms with a pinch of thyme. Cook for a minute, then add the garlic and a pinch of salt. Cook for an additional 2-3 minutes, then, add the parsley and a pinch of chili pepper, stir for a minute and remove from the heat.

2. When the pan of water is boiling, add the gnocchi and cook for a couple of minutes until they float.

3. Drain gnocchi and serve with the mushroom sauce, a small amount of cheese, and an extra dribble of olive oil. Serves 1.

Mixed Salad with Sesame Seeds

4 oz green beans
4 oz broccoli
1 bunch lettuce (romaine, butter lettuce, bibb lettuce, arugula, wild organic greens, etc.)
10 black olives
4 oz feta cheese
Sesame seeds**

Dressing

1 tsp mustard
1 tsp vinegar (balsamic, white wine, or apple cider)
1 clove garlic, chopped
2 Tblsp extra-virgin olive oil
Sea salt and freshly ground pepper

1. Make the dressing by shaking the mustard with the vinegar to dissolve it, then add the garlic and olive oil. Add salt and pepper to taste.

2. Cut the beans and broccoli into bite-sized pieces and steam for only 3 to 4 minutes, so they remain crunchy.

3. Mix the greens together and add the black olives. Crumble in the feta cheese.

4. Gently roast the sesame seeds for a few minutes in a dry sauce pan over low heat, stir to prevent burning.

5. Pour the dressing over the salad, and then immediately add the sesame seeds. Toss and serve. Serves 2.

Fettuccine with Asparagus

5 oz (1 bunch) asparagus (thin/baby)
7 oz fettuccine
2 Tblsp extra-virgin olive oil
1 clove garlic, chopped small
2-3 Tblsp parmesan cheese
Sea salt and freshly ground pepper

1. Steam the asparagus for 5-10 minutes, until tender but still reasonably firm. At the same time boil the pasta.

2. Heat the olive oil with the garlic, toss together with the asparagus.

3. Serve the asparagus with the fettuccine, with some parmesan grated on the top. Add salt and pepper to taste. Serves 2.

**Sally Beare: 50 Secrets of the World's Longest Living People. 2006.*
*** This is not part of the original Campodimele recipe.*

Symi

The classical Mediterranean diet is legendary for its health benefits and the Greek island of Symi is a well known success story - "may you live to be one hundred and more." According to Sally Beare, "Even when they are old, Symiots are young - men in their seventies and eighties, are well toned and vigorous, flirt openly with any woman who catches their eye, which is hardly surprising , as the women on Symi are also well toned and vigorous, with beautiful skin and hair."

Up into their nineties, men and women are still working their herds and flocks, collecting herbs, fermenting yogurt and working their gardens. The population on the island of Symi is only 2,700. Epidemiologists have recorded that Symi has the best health record and highest longevity for the region. Experts believe that the most important piece of the Symiot health and longeviy secret is their diet and their very unique cooking style.

The Symiot diet consists of fish, olive oil, tomato sauces, goat's cheese, Greek yogurt, red meat, vegetables, salads, fruit and red wine.

Vegetables include artichokes, green beans, stuffed grape leaves, potatoes and Greek salads (add olive oil, lemon, herbs and garlic). Symiot fruit include figs, pomegranate and grapes.

The Symiots eat garlic with just about everything - tsatsiki (a yogurt dish), fish, Greek salads, meat dishes, and vegetables are all impregnanted with the "stinking rose."

Capers are a classical ingredient in the Symiot version of the Greek salad. The zingy taste of capers adds zest to the salads, rabbit and fish dishes. Capers, eaten with the stalk and leaves are believed to encourage longevity.

Agapios Monachos, a Cretan monk wrote of the caper in the 15th century, "It cures the spleen, destroys the vermin, heals the hemorrhoids, increases the vitality of the sperm, cures liver ailments and cramps, mobilizes the urinary bladder, facilitates menstruation, and prevents rheumatism," and he recommended starting each meal with a single caper.

Thyme bushes are scattered all over the hillsides of Symi; sage basil, peppermint and spearmint are grown as potted plants at the front door and windows. Thyme is used with ham and as a preservative for fruit.

Marjoram goes into Greek salads and marinades; rosemary is steeped in wine, olive oil and mint and is used to flavor cheese and lamb dishes.

Fresh whole grain wheat bread is a dietary staple, it is typically dipped in olive oil and is eaten with goat cheese, soups, stews, fish, and salads or eaten by itself as a breakfast dish.

Symiots prepare soups with beans, tomatoes, garlic, herbs, and lamb. Organ meats, rabbit, goat and lamb are commonly used in stews or roasted with garlic and herbs including rosemary.

Feta cheese produced from ewe's milk and live yogurt are commonly eaten in Symi.

Meals in Symi are laced with red or white wines, ouzo, raki and retsina. Retsina is flavored with pine resin to create a zesty and hardy dinner wine.

Symi Recipes*

<u>Rustic Bread with Olive Oil and Sesame Seeds</u>*

Approximately 1 Tblsp yeast
4 fluid oz tepid water
5 cups whole-wheat flour (or other whole grain flour)
2 tsp sea salt
2 Tblsp extra-virgin olive oil
1-2 tsp sesame seeds

1. Dissolve the yeast in 1 cup of tepid water

2. Mix the flour and salt together and put in a pile on a clean, dry surface. Make a well in the middle and add the dissolved yeast water, a small quantity at a time. Each time the yeast water is added, swirl the yeast into the flour, using circular movements until the yeast is totally mixed in.

3. Keep adding water and mixing together until you have a moist dough. Knead the dough for five minutes until it is springy - the Symiots claim that, when done, it should feel "like a woman's breast." If the dough is too dry or too sticky, you can add more water or flour as required.

4. While kneading the dough, add the olive oil one tsp at a time.

5. Shape the dough into a round shape and place on a baking sheet. Score the top with a knife - this helps it to rise. Cover with a dishtowel and set aside in a warm place for 40 minutes to 1 hour, until it is approximately double its original side.

6. Remove the loaf from the sheet, punch the air out of it, and knead for a few minutes. Reshape into a loaf and allow it to rise a second time for 20-30 minutes.

7. Sprinkle the top of the loaf with sesame seeds, and bake at 435 degrees F for about 25 minutes until brown on the outside.

8. Serve warm with a small bowl of extra-virgin olive oil for dipping.

**Sally Beare: 50 Secrets of the World's Longest Living People.*

Fish Soup*

Fish stock: Fish for boiling, including the heads and bones (turbot, halibut, or monkfish heads and bones are preferred).

5 cups of water
1 medium onion
2 ribs of celery
1-2 carrots
2 bay leaves
6 peppercorns
A few stalks of flat-leaved parsley
1 tsp sea salt

For the soup:

2 Tblsp extra-virgin olive oil
1 medium onion, chopped
2-3 cloves garlic, chopped
3 stalks fennel, chopped small
1 pound of fish for boiling, filleted (fresh sardines or monkfish).

2 cups of white wine
2 large tomatoes, chopped small
1 Tblsp tomato paste
Juice of 2 lemons
Sea salt and freshly ground pepper
1 large pinch of saffron
1-2 large potatoes, peeled and sliced thick
A few sprigs of parsley

1. For the fish stock, put all of the ingredients together in a large pan of water, and boil for about 1 hour, until the liquid is reduced by half. Strain, throw out the solids, and keep the liquids.

2. To make the soup, heat the oil gently in a heavy-based pan, and sweat the onions (cook them gently with the lid on, so that they stay moist in their own juice), garlic, and fennel - keeping the heat low. Add a spoonful of the fish stock.

3. Put in half of the fish and stir it around in the vegetables.

4. Add the wine, turn the heat up, and cook for about 10 minutes, or until the wine has reduced by half.

5. Add the tomatoes, tomato paste, and lemon juice, and continue cooking for several minutes.

6. Cover with the fish stock and simmer for about 20-30 minutes, until the liquid has reduced by half.

7. Taste and add salt, pepper, and more lemon if desired.

8. Add a large pinch of saffron.

9. Put in the sliced potatoes and the rest of the fish, and cook for approximately 10 minutes.

10. Garnish with parsley and serve. Serves 3.

**Sally Beare: 50 Secretes of the World's Longest Living People.*

Baked Fish in Wine

1 large fish for baking (use one whole fish such as salmon, trout, or small monkfish).
Sea salt and freshly ground pepper
2-3 Tblsp parsley, chopped
1-2 large cloves garlic, chopped
1 lemon
5-6 red tomatoes (ripe)
2 medium onions, sliced
1 green pepper, 1 red pepper, 1 yellow pepper, cut into strips
1 cup extra-virgin olive oil
1 large glass white wine

1. Clean and wash the fish

2. Put a little salt on both sides of the fish, stuff the belly cavity with the parsley and garlic, and squeeze the lemon over the fish. Refrigerate for 1 hour.
3. Put half of the tomatoes, onions, and peppers in a small baking dish in a single layer, put the fish on top, then make a second layer of the vegetables on top of the fish. Pour the oil over it.

4. Bake at 400 degrees F for 15 minutes, then baste the mixture with the juices. Add the wine, and bake for another 15 minutes. Serves 2-3.

**Sally Beare: 50 Secrets of the World's Longest Living people.*

The Georgians

The Georgians, as well as the Abkhazians, Azerbaijanis and Armanians are found at the timber line of the Caucasus Mountains which have peaks of 12,434 to 13,274 feet above sea level.

They live in simple stone houses without electricity, their blood pressure is typically 104/72 at age 100; women continue to have children after age 52, they typically drink an eight ounce glass of vodka or "applejack" with breakfast and have a large glass of red wine with lunch and dinner. Almost all of the "old people" are from rural backgrounds or occupations such as farmers, shepherds and/or hunters.

This group of centenarians, from the Caucasus Mountains, are found between the coasts of the Black Sea and the Caspian Sea, and mountain villages at or above 4,500 feet above sea level. This region supports over 500,000 people 4,500 to 5,000 of whom are reported to be over 100 years of age. They make up more than 25% of the regions centenarians.

The oldest known person from the Caucasus region was identified in 1973 as Shirali Mislimov - at age 167 he still worked in the village tea plantation in the small Azerbaijani village of Barzavu on the Iranian border.

Those in the Caucasus region believe that those individuals under 80 years of age are still considered a youth; from 80 to 100 years one is considered middle age and only those over 100 years of age can be considered a senior.

The strength and vigor of the peoples of the Caucasus region are so legendary, that in the mid-eighteenth century Johann Blumenbach used their region's name to represent all of the "white" peoples of Europe - Caucasians.

Many married couples claim to be married for over 100 years, although the Guiness World book of records says that 80 years of marriage is the official record.

In a study that looked at 15,000 individuals over the age of 100, only the married individuals attained advanced age and still have an active sex life after the age of 100 years.

Mejid Agayev celebrated his 140th birthday February 12, 1975. Agayev was the oldest living citizen in the Azerbaijani village of Tikyaband that bragged of having 54 people over the age of 100 years.

Work delegated to centenarians included weeding fields, feeding livestock, shepherds, picking tea, washing laundry, house work, cooking and baby sitting.

Women over 100 years of age had an average of 4 to 15 children during their child bearing years.

The staple diet of the Caucasus region includes chicken, mutton, beef, goat milk, cheese, butter, yogurt, bread, tomatoes, cucumbers, green onions, garlic, fruit, pita bread, boiled corn meal mush (abusta), red pepper, tea, red wine and salt. The total caloric intake per person ranges from 1,500 to 1,900 - 70% from vegetables and dairy products, a small daily portion of meat and most food is eaten raw or boiled - nothing is fried.

The terraced fields and gardens have been irrigated with a highly mineralized "Glacial Milk" and fertilized with a wood ash (from heating and cooking fires) enriched compost for over 2,500 years.

The Indians of North America, Mexico, Central & South America

The Indians of North America, Mexico, South America and Central America share a common history and similar cultural evolutions.

They had trade routes reaching from what would become Canada, the United States, Mexico, Central America and South America. They traded salt, cacao, dried fish, meat, grain, quetzal feathers, pyrite (for fire starters), tools, jewelry, obsidian and jade.

Central to this transcontinental trade was a pre-Columbian city state known as Takalik Abaj. Takalik Abaj, located near the western coast, of what is now Guatemala, was a hub for trade, information and goods.

Archeological evidence points to Takalik Abaj being ruled by the Olmec culture (known as the "rubber" people and the traders of cacao) and then the last Mayan King.

In almost every Indian culture, there was and in many cases, there still are, clusters of long lived people living as they did hundreds or even thousands of years ago.

Like all long lived people, these seemingly primitive tribes, through the accident of choices of where to live and what and how to eat produced healthful centenarians.

In all cases these cultures have daily practices that provide Calorie Restricted diets without malnutrition and have discovered some form of highly efficient antioxidants.

"Culinary" ashes were used by pre-Columbian Indians. In the 13th century, the use of culinary ashes was identified from the analysis of the contents of garbage dumps in North America and reported by anthropologists.

In 1588, Thomas Harriat (1560-1621), tutor to Sir Walter Raleigh, was appointed "geographer" for his second Virginia expedition - he soon published in *Hakluyt's Voyages* on North Carolina Indians and how they raised corn. He described mountain spinach five foot high and how the Indians made a "fine broth from the seeds, and from the stalks of the herb, they produced a kind of "salt" by burning it to ashes, they then season their broth with it. This is the only "salt" they know, and they enrich their fields by burning weeds after drying in the sun. This they (unknowingly) do to save them selves the labor of carrying it away, rather to enrich better the ground."

The Navajo

The diets of the Navajo Indians have changed significantly since the pre-Columbian times. Archeological data suggests that their early diet, was the standard fare of hunter gatherers and consisted only of indigenous plants and wild game until A.D. 1200, when a northern Athabaskan tribe of Navajos migrated to the southwest and learned farming from the Pueblo Indians.

Corn, laced with "culinary" ashes, became a staple in the Navajo diet. Two centuries later, the Spanish brought sheep and cattle, and the Navajo became shepherds.

Today the Navajo Nation numbers more than 151,000 and is the largest Native American tribe. In recent decades, many processed foods have been introduced into the Navajo diet as a result of government rationing, food distribution programs and the growth of trading posts and food stores, yet the tradition of "culinary" ashes being added to their food remains in the more rural areas.

Juniper ash proves to be a good source of dietary calcium, iron and a moderate source of magnesium. One teaspoon of juniper ash provides the equivalent calcium levels found in one cup of milk; it supplies 28% of the RDA for iron and nine percent of the RDA for magnesium. The woody branches contain more calcium and silica, whereas the twigs and needles (the growth part of the tree) contained the highest levels of trace minerals.

Typical Navajo recipe that includes "culinary ashes":

Shaped Corn Griddle Cakes

Mix one cup juniper ashes with water and strain through a grass brush into basin of corn flour, using about three and one half cups of the liquid. Add one half cup clear water to this greenish dough and knead until thick. Shape with moist hands into round cakes less than an inch thick and four inches in diameter. Bake on a fry griddle, rubbing it (the griddle) with a cloth between bakings, and moisten cakes on both sides when done.

Even today, the corn based foods of the Navajo contain "culinary" ash, which is mixed with boiling water and added after straining, to the blue corn flour "to make it blue." Blue corn contains an anthocyanin pigment that turns a distinct greenish-blue color in the alkaline medium created by the addition of wood ash. The wood ash was also used daily to make a "tea" and was used medicinally for stomach and intestinal ailments.

Of the three major types of plants used to make culinary ashes listed in the Navajo culture, juniper (*Juniperus monosperma*), commonly called cedar is used most frequently. The small branches and needles are most favorably used as they produce the finest particle ash (minerals that are left when the wood and needles are burned).

Green juniper branches are gathered, placed on a grill or screen and set alight. The ash is colleted in a pan placed underneath the grill. Juniper being absent, ash was also made from dried tumbleweed or greasewood.

The three sources of "culinary" wood ashes were all good sources of essential minerals. Iron concentration was higher in the greasewood. Wood ash in general, although variable in analysis, tends to be rich in potassium, calcium, iron, copper, zinc, trace minerals and rare earths.

When wood ash was not available, a special traditional clay was mixed with salt and/or the Navajo food. Unfortunately in the 1940s, urban Navajo cooks used electricity and gas to cook and heat with and so began replacing "culinary" ashes with the more available baking soda - thus began the transition from the slim wood ash using Navajo shepherds to the obese and diabetic baking soda using urban Navajo.

An Average Mineral Analysis of Wood Ash (1926)

Mineral	Percentage of Dry Weight
Potassium	16 - 40
Phosphoric acid	2
Calcium carbonate	32
Magnesium oxide	2 - 5

A Multiple Sample Analysis of Wood Ash (mg/G)

Mineral	Amount
Calcium	271 - 307
Iron	2.2 - 3.7
Magnesium	16.5 - 46.5
Potassium	15 - 83
Copper	0.05 - 0.15
Zinc	0.10 - 0.92
Sodium	1.0 - 13.9
Chromium (ug/G)	0.04 - 0.005
Phosphorus	7.3 - 19.4
Silica	1.1 - 17.6
Aluminum	2.4 - 7.4

(March 1998)

The Pima

The Pima Indians are a band of Native Americans who live on the invisible border dividing the state of Arizona and Mexico. The Pima band on both sides of the border are from the identical genetic pool; yet the Pima Indians on the Mexican side of the border have no almost no type II diabetes and have only a ten percent obesity rate compared with the rate of 22% diabetes and the 70% obesity in the Arizona Pima!

With a small population of 12,000 individuals, the Arizona Pima ran up a $7 million annual Federal cost for pharmaceutical treatments; additionally $3 million was spent annually for dialysis charges for diabetic Pimas. As a result of the epidemic rate of diabetes and obesity, the Arizona Pima Indian's life span is shorter than the average American life span by 15 to 19 years.

The Pima Indians from Arizona live in government provided trailer homes that use natural gas or propane, electric stoves and microwave ovens for cooking and heating - they use automobiles, pickup trucks and tractors; and they buy food and government Native American "commodities" from the grocery store like every body else.

The Arizona Pima's transition from subsistence farming, wood stoves and their traditional diet to the American lifestyle began in the 1940s, and by 1960, the epidemic of obesity and type II diabetes, seemingly targeting the Arizona Pima had started in earnest.

By contrast the Pima Indians living south of the Arizona border, in Mexico, are still subsistence farmers, they still cook and heat their traditional homes with wood and they are still putting their wood ash byproduct of daily living into their gardens and their corn tortillas.

Trace Mineral Analysis of a Juniper Ash Sample (ppm)

Analyte	Amount	Analyte	Amount
Aluminum	9.41	Mercury	0.006
Antimony	0.062	Molybdenum	0.041
Arsenic	< 0.01	Neodymium	0.048
Barium	1.42	Nickel	0.078
Beryllium	<0.005	Niobium	< 0.01
Bismuth	0.011	Osmium	< 0.005
Boron	0.759	Palladium	< 0.005
Bromine	0.22	Phosphorus	8.69
Cadmium	< 0.005	Platinum	< 0.005
Calcium	698.0	Potassium	536
Carbon	107.0	Praseodymium	0.048
Cerium	0.064	Rhenium	< 0.01
Cesium	0.055	Rhodium	< 0.051
Chloride	620.0	Rubidium	0.121
Chromium	0.011	Ruthenium	0.067
Cobalt	0.041	Samarium	0.055
Copper	0.258	Scandium	0.12
Dysprosium	0.029	Selenium	0.060
Erbium	2.11	Silica	67.9

Trace Mineral Analysis (continued)

Europium	0.010	Silver	0.045
Fluoride	0.29	Sodium	26.1
Gadolinium	0.036	Strontium	2.44
Gallium	0.017	Sulfur	5.96
Germanium	0.099	Tantalum	0.018
Gold	0.021	Tellurium	<0.01
Hafnium	0.028	Terbium	< 0.01
Holmium	0.01	Thallium	0.011
Indium	0.02	Thorium	< 0.005
Iodine	2.15	Thulium	0.023
Iridium	< 0.005	Tin	0.009
Lanthanum	< 0.005	Titanium	0.486
Lead	0.016	Tungsten	< 0.01
Lithium	0.036	Vanadium	0.085
Lutetium	0.013	Ytterbium	0.021
Magnesium	1760.0	Yttrium	0.011
Manganese	3.12	Zinc	1.87
		Zirconium	0.028

Tarahumara

Another "Blue Zone" in the Western Hemisphere that is considered to have a reputable longevity record is the hot, arid Sierra Madre Mountains of northern Mexico. The areas most famous residents are the Tarahumara Indians, iconic as the world's only "jogging nation." Their tribal name, Tarahumara, roughly translates to "foot runners," and jogging is their main mode of travel - "*Run, don't walk,*" is their national motto.

The Tarahumara warriors and hunters are legendary for trailing deer for two or three days until the deer collapses from exhaustion or blindly falls over the edge of a cliff.

Foot races are the national pastime of the Tarahumara; in 1928 two Tarahumara men, Jose Torres and Aurelio Terrazas, participated in the Olympic marathon competition held in Amsterdam - they lost first place by two minutes, claiming they would have run faster if they had known the race was so short.

Another Tarahumara sport is a kickball game that is played on fields ranging in length from two to 12 miles and can last from six hours to days.

The hostile climate and poor soil fertility make the existence of the Tarahumara culture an "ecological marvel." Their main crops are corn, pumpkins and beans, plus goat meat provide only a 1,200 to 1,800 calorie diet - they did not speak Spanish; in 1970 their total population was only 40,000.

The Tarahumara love to celebrate and are famous also for drinking and eating feasts called *tutuguri*. These events are described by the *National Geographic* as "a cacophony of chanting, fiddles, rattles, guitars, stomping dances, shouts, raucous laughter, and howling dogs. Both men and women dropped out of the dancing lines to drink corn beer (rarely drank anything stronger) and soon were staggering about in a stupor." It is estimated that a minimum of 200 pounds of corn are required by each family for the annual party.

Following the Jim Fixx running craze in America, legends of the Tarahumara health and longevity prospered, although, reliable records are few and far between.

The Vilcabamba

Ecuador's star-shaped "Sacred Valley of Longevity" (Vilcabamba) is actually five valleys that converge and sit between two Andean Mountains at 12,434 feet above sea level. The western skyline of Vilcabamba is dominated by the summit of Mandango, the tallest mountain whose glaciers supply the mineral rich "Glacial Milk" that is used to irrigate the terraced fields.

The "Glacial Milk" originating from the high peaks of Podocarpus National Park pours into the Rio Yambala which converges with the Chamba River, the waters of which are also used for irrigation.

In 1971, a census revealed nine people over 100 years of age for every 819 people or an astounding one centenarian per 100 people - this gave Vilcabamba a centenarian population almost 400 times that of the United States. Vilcabamba has a historical record of good health and longevity dating back to the Incas, these claims are backed by religious (Roman Catholic churches) and civil records dating back to the 18th century.

Popular interest in Vilcabamba was ignited in 1956 during a press conference in New York City when Javier Pereira, age 167, was introduced by the syndicated newspaper feature, *Believe It or Not*.

Miguel Carpio, at age 123, was the oldest living Vilcabamban found at the census - he still smoked, drank red wine and "chased women."

The staple diet of the Vilcabamba Indian includes corn, beans, goat meat, chicken, eggs, milk, cheese and a soup, known as repe that is made from bananas, beans, white cheese, salt and lard. Their average total calorie intake is 1,200 to 1,800 calories per day.

"Dr. Weston A. Price, (while working in the high Andes of Peru) chanced to notice that each individual carried a little bag, of which all seemed to be particularly careful. Out of curiosity he looked into the bags and discovered that they contained kelp. When he asked where they had got kelp so far from the ocean, they said calmly that they got it from the ocean. This surprised him since it took a month to make the trip to and from the coast. What did they use the kelp for? 'To guard the heart, they explained to him.'"

D.C. Jarvis
Folk Medicine

The Titicaca

Gucilaso de la Vega, whose father was Spanish and whose mother was an Inca princess, recorded (1609) the legend of the beginnings of the Titicaca peoples:

"Our Father, the Sun, seeing that men lived like wild animals, took pity on them, and sent to earth a son and daughter of his, in order that they might teach man the knowledge of our Father, the Sun, and that they might know how to cultivate plants and grains and make use of the fruits of the earth like men and not beasts. With these orders and mandate, our Father the Sun placed his son and daughter in Lake Titicaca."

Thus as legend holds, the first Incas came to Earth on an island in Lake Titicaca, to start what was to become the most advanced civilization in pre-Columbian America.

Titicaca is found in the Andean highlands of Peru at 12,506 feet above seas level. The main city of Titicaca is Puno (population 32,000); the people of the Altiplano (high Plains) are divided into the pure Indians and the "mestizos" who are a mix of Indian and Spanish.

The treeless hills that form the Altiplano surrounding Lake Titicaca are covered with "pata pata," the stone terraces built by the Incas to provide level farming areas, and as catchments for the mineral rich "Glacial Milk" from the great Andean Mountain, Mt. Cardillera Real with which they irrigated their crops.

Because of the extreme elevation of the Altiplano, maize or Indian corn wouldn't grow in the Titicaca region, instead the Incas grew tubers never before seen by the Spanish; "They supplement the lack of bread with some roots they call "papas" (potatoes) and which produce under the earth," noted Father Acosta. When introduced into Europe by the Spanish, the potato became more valuable than all the gold in the world. The Inca also invented a freeze drying technique to save harvested potatoes for the winter, described in 1609 by a Spanish Friar:

"To keep potatoes from rotting, they leave them out for many months to freeze. After they have been repeatedly frozen, they tread gently on them, to press out the moisture they contain. When they have been well squeezed, they are placed in the sun until they are thoroughly dry. In this manner, the potato keeps for a long time, and it changes its name to chunci."

The original Indians of the Lake Titicaca region are the Aymara; the Quechua, who still speak the language of the Incas, were descendants of Inca slaves after the Inca occupation in the 12th century.

The grinding of the massive glaciers of the Cordillera Real, the towering Andean Mountain that reaches over 20,000 feet produces a mineral rich "Glacial Milk" that is used to irrigate the terraced fields that the Titicaca grow their grains and vegetables in and the wind up in Lake Titicaca itself.

When Francisco Pizarro arrived in 1532, the Inca Empire was in the midst of a great civil war, making it easy for a small band of Spaniards to conquer a kingdom of over 3,000 miles in length, reaching from Ecuador to Chile. In the early days of the Inca culture, the word Inca referred only to the king and not to a race or nation.

The ancient ancestors of the Titicaca worshipped many gods; today they have settled on a patchwork of ancient gods and Catholicism that was injected by the Spanish.

Lake Titicaca itself is over 3,200 square miles in surface area, 122 miles long and 47 miles wide - when viewed from a plane the outline of the lake looks like a jaguar ready to pounce on a rabbit, thus the name Titicaca (translates to "Rock of the Puma" or Jaguar). The effluent or Rio Desaquadero from Lake Titicaca flows from the "head of the rabbit."

The Incas used irrigation ditches to channel water from the lake itself as well as from the "Glacial Milk" to water and remineralize, along with the wood and animal manure ash (plant minerals) enriched compost, their well manicured terraces.

Like all Alpine habitats, the Lake Titicaca area has very little variety when it comes to wildlife. Father Acosta noted in his early writings that the lake held only two kinds of fish, a large catfish and a minnow.

The catfish made up a major source of animal protein for the local Indian tribes. In 1939, trout were released into the lake and to no one's great surprise, the trout flourished.

Within two years the Indians began landing lake trout weighing more than 25 pounds - the highly mineralized waters of Lake Titicaca produced a bounty beyond anyone's wildest dreams.

The Isla de Sol, the mythical birthplace of the Incas is located 40 miles into Lake Titicaca. Manco Capac and Mama Ocllo appeared approximately 1,100 A.D.

The Incas, much like the Romans, were at the same time conquerors and lawmakers, engineers and very firm taskmasters - "their totalitarian state was a benevolent dictatorship." Whenever the Incas conquered a culture, they basically left it intact, requiring only a tax in the form of salt and that the conquered people worship the Sun god. No one went hungry or naked but nothing was left to free will.

When the first Aymaras came to Lake Titicaca, they found other Indians, the Urus, already living on floating islands made of Tartara reeds. "Whole villages of Urus, were to be found on the lake living on their rafts of Tartara," wrote the Jesuit Father Jose' de Acosta in 1590. The Uru still live long healthy lives today and still refuse to give up their Tartara islands.

The quinoa, a grain of Titicaca begins to ripen in late April or May, it is used as Europeans use wheat; barley is also grown. At 15,400 feet, the barley never ripens to seed heads so the Indians use it for cattle feed. The Titicaca shepherds live and work at 17,000 feet.

The Inca "Cattle" were in fact llamas or New World camels that feed on moss and lichens.

"There is nothing in Peru of greater value and utility than the cattle of the land, which our people call "sheep of the Indies, but the Indian in their tongue call llama," wrote Father Acosta.

When the Spanish discovered the Maya in the 1500s, they noted that everyone drank liquid chocolate.

The Incas also built 10,000 miles of stone roads to provide rapid communication around Lake Titicaca. Messengers were stationed every 1.5 miles and ran messages in relay, much like a human pony express - these warriors could relay messages over 150 miles per day. Inca nobles also used the roads to reach the Isla del Sol to worship the Sun god.

The Costa Rican Nicoya

A Costa Rican man at age 60 has twice the chance of reaching age 90 as does a man living in the United States, France or even Japan. It is also known that when a Costa Rican man reaches 90 years of age, he can expect with high probability that he will live another 4.4 years.

Vital information of every person born in Costa Rica has been collected since 1888, so conformation of age is quite easy!

Costa Rica spends only 15% of what the United States does on health care, yet its citizens live considerably longer - longer and healthier lives than people in any other country on Earth! Specifically the greatest concentration of Costa Rican centenarians was found in a cluster of villages scattered around the Nicoya Peninsula.

The Nicoya have a higher fertility rate than other centenarian groups, they are taller, weighed less and had slightly higher blood pressures, yet most smoke.

An examination of the life expectancy and mortality rates showed that one region in the northwest of the country, including the 80 mile long Nicoya Peninsula that was significantly different from any other (in that area, people die of cancer - particularly stomach cancer - at a rate 23% lower than in the rest of Costa Rica).

Specifically the oldest of the old in the Nicoya Peninsula were found only in the middle segment of the peninsula - they were not found in any significant numbers in the southern or northern segments or along the Pacific Coast.

The Nicoyan diet consists of corn, beans, cheese, pork, eggs, lard, garden vegetables, yams, garlic, onions, nanpi' and a plethora of fruit (papaya, mango, chico zapote, oranges, lemon, banana, jobo (Spondias), guayabo (*Psidium guajava*), caimito (*Chrysophyllum cainito*), papaturro (Coccoloba), maranon and anona), much of it grown in and around their yards.

The Chorotega Indians, the original inhabitants of the Nicoya, thrived before the Spanish arrived in 1522. They lived in simple thatched-hut communities ringed by vegetable gardens, fruit trees, which then are ringed by milpas or fields of corn and beans.

The Chorotega were subsistence farmers who employed slash-and-burn agriculture, they grew maize and many varieties of beans.

The corn is dried, then, soaked in water with wood ash and lime; the corn is then ground, made into dough, patted into tortillas and served with beans and squash.

A University of California Press report - *Nicoya: A Cultural Geography*, dated 1958 and written by Philip Wagner, an anthropologist, read:

"The day of the country people begins before sunrise, when the women rise to prepare coffee. The family meets about dawn to take its cup of black coffee, or coffee with milk, heavily sweetened, and perhaps to eat a cold tortilla. The time from dawn to eight o'clock is for chores and beginning the day's work. At eight there may be a complete breakfast with rice and beans and eggs. In seasons of heavy work the men take with them to the fields tortillas with gallo pinto (rice and beans cooked in pork fat). Work may end on very hot days at twelve, or at two in the afternoon. The workers come home from the fields or the woods and wait about an hour for their meal.

The midday meal often begins with a pot of soup in which there are a few bits of meat, fat, boiled plantains, tisquisque or yucca, and perhaps a few greens. After the soup come rice and beans, usually accompanied by fried eggs (cooked in lard). On occasion there may also be some vegetables: pipidin or ayote (*Cucurbita moschata*) or calabaza (*Lagenaria*), cabbage, the flower of pinuela (*Bromelia penguin*) or some other wild product. Meat sometimes appears on even the poorest table, and there is usually cuajada, a milk curd. Tortillas come with this meal and afterward the men sip heavily sweetened black coffee, made from local berries or from the mashed seeds of nanju (*Hibiscus esculentus*).

The evening meal is simpler, since the custom is to spend the afternoon in idleness, and appetites are less hearty. Rice and beans, tortillas, and perhaps eggs are served just at dusk."

The Costa Ricans take daily "sun-bathes" for 15 to 30 minutes each day by exposing their faces, arms and legs.

The Nicoyan water supply percolated up through the Nicoya limestone bedrock and contains high levels of calcium, magnesium and other minerals. "The water is so hard and has such high levels of calcium and magnesium that it had to be diluted by 50% with distilled water just so it could be tested."

Nicoyans typically cook on a wood-burning fogon, the traditional Chorotega clay oven. The wood ashes are saved to fertilize the garden and to add "culinary ashes" to the soaking corn kernels to make tortillas.

"The Hunza soil is almost a manufactured soil. Every solitary thing that can serve as food for vegetables, field crops and fruit trees are diligently collected, stored and distributed in rationed equality for every square foot of the hundreds of terraces. Sunken compost pits are conveniently located, and into them go ashes from cooking and heating fires, inedible parts of vegetables, pulverized animal bones, dead leaves, rotten wood and the collected manure of animals."

Dr. Allen E. Banik and
Renee Taylor
Hunza Land

"'Glacial milk' is the exclusive water source used for drinking and irrigation purposes (the fields are flooded, when the water soaks into the soil, a thick layer of mineral silt or 'rock flour' is left on top of the soil-this silt is plowed into the soil before it is planted)."

John H. Tobe
HUNZA

"How is it that man can be such a magnificent physical creature as the Hunza? These people are long lived, vigorous in youth and age, capable of great endurance and enjoy a remarkable freedom from disease in general."

Sir Robert McCarrison
The King's Personal Physician (1920)

"The serendipitous irrigation of their terraced fields with the common denominator of a highly mineralized Glacial Milk and the fertilization of their fields with an organic compost rich with the recycled colloidal minerals found in wood ashes from their heating and cooking fires is the secret of the Hunza's long and fruitful lives."

Dr. Joel D. Wallach & Dr. Ma Lan
RARE EARTHS: forbidden cures

HUNZA

"Land of milk and honey."

Doctors practicing in Hunza today have concluded that the main cause of premature death amongst the Hunzakut people is from accidents, from landslides or falls from the shear rock walls. Infant mortality from infectious diseases have been reported; however, the average individual surviving past one year of age lives beyond the age of eighty, in excellent health and significant numbers live into their nineties and past 100 years.

According to Dr. Alexander Leaf, "The Hunzakuts eat an average of 1,900 calories daily, which are composed of 50 grams of protein, 36 grams of fat and 354 grams of carbohydrates."

Adding to their already Calorie Restricted diet was the fact that by late spring of each year the Hunzakut's food reserves ran low, producing what they call "Starvation Springtime." Meals are reduced to a frequency of two to three meals a week.

The original research into the secrets of the Hunza

health and longevity was done by Dr. Robert McCarrison, personal physician to the King of England. His extensive work was published in 1927.

During the 1890s, Robert McCarrison completed his medical studies at Oxford University. In 1901 at the age of 23, he traveled to India, and became a regimental officer in the Foreign Department in 1902. He was recognized for identifying the sand fly as the carrier of the Three Day Fever of Citral. In 1904, McCarrison was appointed to the post of army surgeon to the nine villages of the Gilgit Agency, where he served until 1911.

Soon after his appointment, McCarrison began to do research on the endemic goiter that was common throughout his post. Finding that eight villages had a goiter problem and one did not, he was soon able to discover the relationship of goiter to an iodine deficiency.

McCarrison related the remarkable health and longevity to the quality of the Hunza diet. A summary review of Hunza was published in *Studies in Deficiency Diseases* (1921):

My own experience provides an example of a race unsurpassed in perfection of physique and in freedom from disease in general, whose sole food consists to this day of grains, vegetables and fruit with a certain amount of milk, and butter, and goat's meat only on feast days. I refer to the people of the state of Hunza, situated in the extreme northernmost point of India...When the severe nature of the winter in that part of the Himalayas (Karakorum) is considered, and the fact that their housing accommodations and conservancy arrangements are of the most primitive, it becomes obvious that the enforced restriction to the unsophisticated food stuffs of nature is compatible with long life, continued vigor, and perfect physique.

In his classic nutritional study McCarrison used 1,189 laboratory weanling rats which he divided into three diet groups:

Group 1 - These rats were fed a typical Hunza diet of whole-grain chapattis, butter, legumes, raw carrots, raw cabbage, whole milk, eggs, meat, water and they were exposed to sunlight daily.

When the rats reached the age of 27 months (the equivalent of 55 years in humans), they were killed and examined: the rats were free of overt disease, there had not been any early mortality; the rats were alert yet lived together without aggression.

Group 2 - These rats were fed a typical "Bengali" diet of white rice, legumes, vegetables, and spices. These rats soon developed diseases of the lungs, nose, ears, eyes, gastrointestinal tract, urinary system, reproductive system, skin, blood, lymphatic system, nervous system and heart. The Bengali fed rats also suffered from hair loss, muscular weakness, ulcers, boils, tooth loss and they became agitated and aggressive.

Group 3 - McCarrison fed his third group of rat pups a typical working class English diet of white bread, margarine, sugared tea, boiled vegetables, canned meat and cheap jams. These rats developed "diseases of the lungs, diseases of the stomach and intestines, and diseases of the nerves - diseases from which one in every three sick persons among the insured classes in England and Wales suffers. Additionally these rats were nervous and apt to bite their attendants; they lived unhappily together, and by the sixteenth day of the experiment they began to kill and eat the weaker ones among them."

The story of the Hunza began 2,300 years ago with Alexander the Great. Alexander was the first born son of King Philip of Masedonia. Legend has said that "the night before the consummation of Philip's marriage with Olympias, she dreamed that a thunderbolt fell upon her body and kindled a great fire whose divided flames dispersed themselves all about and were then extinguished."

Philip dreamed "that he sealed up his wife's body with a seal whose impression was the figure of a lion." Some of the alchemists and diviners interpreted Philip's dream as a warning to "look narrowly to his wife.;" however, Aristander of Telnessus assured Philip that the meaning of his dream was "that the queen was with child of a boy, who would one day prove as stout and courageous as a lion."

Alexander was born on the sixth of Hecatombaeon, which is called Lous by the Masedonians - the same day that the Temple of Diana at Ephesus was burned to the ground. The temple caught fire and was destroyed while its priestess was assisting at the birth of Alexander. All of the diviners in Ephesus ran to and fro beating their faces and predicting "that this day had brought forth something that would prove destructive and fatal to all Asia."

Following Philip's military victory and occupation of Potidea, "he received three messages simultaneously:

1) His commander Parmenio had overthrown the Illyrians in a Great battle;

2) his race horse had won the course at the Olympic Games;

3) and his wife Olympia had given birth to a son - Alexander!"

Philip was overjoyed and he was assured by the diviners "that a son whose birth coincided with three such successes could not fail to be invincible."

"Alexander was fair and of light color, passing into ruddiness in his face and upon his breast." From his early childhood Alexander was energetic and eager, he displayed a love of glory and pursued glory with an endless spirit. As a teenager, Alexander was very bold; when he was asked if he would compete in the Olympic Games, he replied, "I will if I might have kings to run against!"

While still a boy, Alexander entertained visiting royalty in the stead of his father. The visitors included the ambassadors of the king of Persia. Alexander asked, "What is the nature of the road to inner Asia, the character of your king, and how does he carry himself to his enemies? What forces is he able to bring into the field?" His forwardness and lofty purpose appeared early in his life and the visiting royalty "looked upon Philip's famed ability as nothing compared to that of his son Alexander."

Whenever Alexander heard that his father had conquered a town of importance or had won some notable victory, instead of being happy, Alexander would tell his companions, "father would anticipate everything and leave him and them no opportunities of performing illustrious actions."

A Thessalian horse trader brought King Philip a fiery war horse called Bucephalus, offering him at a price of thirteen talents. When Philip and his party went into the field to try him out, they found him so vicious and unmanageable that he reared up when they mounted him and would not so much as endure the voice of any of Philip's grooms. They were just about to lead Bucephalus away as totally useless and intractable, when Alexander said, "I could manage this horse, better than others do!"

"Do you reproach those who are older than yourself, as if you knew more and were better able to manage him than they? And what if you do not," said Philip, "what will you forfeit for your rashness?"

"I will pay the whole price of the horse," replied Alexander.

At this boy's answer, the king's entire company began to roar with laughter. As soon as wagers were settled, Alexander ran to Bucephalus, took hold of the bridle, and turned him directly into the sun (Alexander had observed the horse was shying from his own shadow).

Alexander let the horse move forward a little, still keeping the reins in hand, he stroked him gently; when the horse grew eager and fiery, "he let fall his upper garment softly and with one nimble leap securely mounted him; when he was seated, little by little he drew in the bridle and curbed him without either striking or spurring him.

Presently, when he found him free from all rebelliousness and only impatient for the course, he let him go at full speed, inciting him with a commanding voice and also urging with his heel."

King Philip and his court looked on, first in silence, then nervousness until, seeing him turn at the end of the course and return rejoicing and waving in triumph - they all burst into cheers and applause.

Philip, shedding tears of joy and pride, kissed Alexander as the boy dismounted and said, "Oh, my son, look for a kingdom equal to and worthy of thyself, for Macedonia is too little for thee!"

Philip now looked upon the instruction of Alexander to be of greater importance than to be entrusted to ordinary masters of music, poetry and typical school subjects, and to require as Sophocles stated, "The bridle and the rudder, too."

Philip sent for Aristotle, the most learned and most celebrated Greek philosopher and scholar of his time. Philip rewarded Aristotle with "a munificence proportionate with the private tutelage of his son, prince Alexander."

Aristotle taught Alexander his doctrine of morals and politics, herbal medicine, alchemy and abstract and profound theories only shared by philosophers amongst themselves. Alexander as a student had a feverish inclination to practice medicine; for whenever his friends were sick, he would "prescribe healing diets and medication (herbs and minerals) proper to their disease."

Alexander loved Aristotle no less than if he were his own father, "as he had received life from one, so the other had taught him to live well."

While in Asia, Alexander heard that Aristotle had publicly published several of the oral treatises normally reserved for communications between great thinkers and he was disturbed enough to write him a letter:

"Alexander to Aristotle, greeting,

You have not done well to publish
your books of oral doctrines; for what is
there now that we excel in, if those
things which we have been particularly
instructed in be laid open to all? For
my part, I assure you, I had rather excel
in the knowledge, of what is excellent,
than in the extent of my power and dominion,

Farewell!"

Later, while King Philip was absent on his extended expedition against the Byzantines, he left Alexander, now only 16 years old, "as his lieutenant in Macedonia committing the charge of his seal to him."

Alexander refused to sit idling away the time, so he declared war on the Maedi and reduced them to slaves after conquering their capital city by storm - not too surprising, Alexander renamed the conquered city Alexandropolis!

During the battle of Chaeronea, which Philip fought against the Greeks, Alexander was the first man in the charge against the fierce and sacred Thebams guards near the Cephisus River.

Despite King Philip's pride and love for his brave son,

they soon became enemies. The straw that broke the camel's back was the marriage of King Philip to Cleopatra, the child queen of Egypt. When Cleopatra's uncle Attalus, toasted the marriage and asked the gods for "a lawful successor to the kingdom," Alexander became furious and threw a cup at him shouting, "you villain; what am I then a bastard?" Philip, took to Attalus' defense, rose up from his bride's side and would have run Alexander through with a sword but in his drunken rage he slipped and fell to the floor. Being the young cock, Alexander couldn't resist mocking his father, "see there, the man who makes preparations to pass out of Europe into Asia, overturned in passing from one seat to another." Philip and Alexander were soon reconciled by Demaratus, a family friend.

The marriage between Philip and Cleopatra was not an affair of the heart or the product of lust for a flat-chested gangly pre-teenage girl, but rather a political treaty between Macedonia and Egypt - the Macedonians wanted and got exclusive rights to the highly mineralized wheat from the Nile flood plains, wheat that was legendary in providing strength and stamina to the armies that ate it - Macedonia needed this Egyptian wheat to support its armies for the coming invasion of Asia! The Egyptians wanted and got a peace treaty from the Macedonians exempting them from participating in the war with Asia and protection by the Macedonians from the Asian hordes. It was a marriage made at the bargain table.

However, the father and son reconciliation was short-lived. Pixodorus, viceroy of Caria, sent an emissary to make a match between his oldest daughter and Philip's son Arrhidaeus. Alexander's contemporaries and friends convinced him that Philip, by a political marriage and important alliance was going to transfer the Macedonian Kingdom to his brother Arrhidaeus.

Alexander, out of alarm, sent Thessalus as his own representative into Caria to urge Pixodorus to change his mind and offer his daughter into marriage to Alexander himself, so that Alexander might be his son-in-law. Pixodorus responded that Alexander's offer was much more favorable to him.

Philip, enraged at Alexander's offer, "chastised Alexander bitterly" for being unworthy of the power he was to inherit, as to marry a low Carian, who at best was a slave of a barbarous prince. Philip further wrote to the Corinthians to send Thessalus (Alexander's messenger) to him in chains; he also banished Alexander's closest friends for their part in the intrigue.

Soon after these terrible events, a Macedonian named Pausanias was stripped of his post and properties in Egypt by Cleopatra and her uncle Attalus. Pausanias, unable to get the decision overturned and himself reinstated by Philip, became enraged and assassinated Philip. The guilt for the murder of Philip was laid at the feet of Alexander's mother, Olympias, who was reported to have incited young Pausanias to revenge.

Some accusing fingers also pointed to Alexander, however, these suspicions were dispelled after he captured Pausanias and his conspirators and had them summarily executed. Alexander was now 20 years old.

Alexander inherited a troubled Macedonia, besieged on all sides with restless and dangerous enemies. The barbarians that had been conquered by Philip's armies were anxious to be governed by their own princes. Philip had also been victorious over the Greeks, however, he hadn't had time to consolidate his battlefield gains and win them over to the Macedonian law and culture all he had conquered before being assassinated.

Alexander's response was to declare war and he immediately invaded the heart of the barbarian territory as far east as the Danube River, conquering and overthrowing Syrmus, the king of the Tribillians.

The Tribillians revolted and became allies with the Athenians against Alexander. Alexander ordered his armies into a forced march through the pass of Thermopylae; he sent the following message to the Greek Demosthenes, "You called me a child when I was in the country of the Tribillians and a youth when I was in Thessaly - I will appear as a man before the walls of Athens."

When Alexander arrived at the walls of Thebes he only demanded the authors of the rebellion - Phoenix and Prothytes and declared a general amnesty to all who would submit to Macedonian law. The Thebans responded by demanding Philotas Antipater be surrendered to them and invited the Macedonian army to become Greeks. Alexander and his army immediately fell on Athens, sacked the city and burned it to the ground; then to terrify the people of Greece into submission he publicly executed 6,000 of the Theban leaders and sold 30,000 of the lesser members of the Athenian Court into slavery - only the priests and those who had historically been friends of the Macedonians were spared.

The ambassadors of Greece assembled at the Isthmus and voted to join their armies with Alexander's in his march against the Persians and to prove their allegiance, they voted Alexander their general of the allied armies.

Alexander's armies were actually the smaller of the forces in the alliance - he commanded 30,000 foot soldiers and 4,000 cavalry. After gaining a positive "You will be victorious" from the head priests of Athens, Alexander marched northeast towards Persia (Iran).

Darius, the great warlord king of Persia, had his armies camped at the eastern banks of the Granicus River - the Gateway to Asia. It seemed that Alexander would have to fight at the very entrance to Asia when he reached the western banks of the river in the evening. Parmenio, military advisor to Alexander urged him to wait until morning as dark was but moments away. Alexander immediately spurred his horse into the river and called his army to him:

"They advanced against whole showers of darts thrown from atop the almost sheer eastern bank. Despite his lack of prudence Alexander prevailed, he and 13 troops of cavalry gained the top of the bank where they engaged in hand to hand combat.

Alexander, easily recognized, was attacked from all sides, his cuirass was pierced by a javelin. Two Persion officers, Rhoesaces and Spithridates set on him at once, he dodged them and broke his spear striking at Rhoesaces so that he was forced to defend himself with a dagger; while engaged in this hand-to-hand combat, the other Persian officer, Spithridates rode his horse full tilt at Alexander and struck him such a blow on the helmet with his battle axe that he sheared off the plumed crest and the edge of the blade clipped off a large shock of blond hair. As Spithridates raised up in his stirrups to deliver a second and probably fatal blow, Alexander's lieutenant - the Black Clitus, pierced the Persian's body through and through with his spear at the same time as Alexander killed Rhoesaces with his dagger."

While the advance cavalry were engaged in the dangerous hand to hand combat, the Macedonian foot soldiers crossed the river and forming a great pincher advanced into the battle. When the Persian advance force turned and fled, they left 20,000 foot soldiers and 2,500 cavalry of their own dead on the river bank. Alexander had lost only 34, of whom five were foot soldiers and the balance cavalry.

The overwhelming victory at the Granicus River resulted in the surrender of Sardis, the capital of the Persian Maritime province as well as hundreds of other small towns and villages. Only the two cities of Halicarniossus and Miletus held out; Alexander destroyed them by force.

While Alexander was deciding what route to take into the heart of Persia, an ancient copper plate was washed up on the flooded banks of a spring near the city of Xanthus in Lycia. The inscription on the plate's edge stated, "the time will come when the Persian Empire would be destroyed by the Greecians." Enthused by this finding, Alexander took his armies to destroy Cilicia and Phoenicia and then along the seacoast to Pamphyia; normally this coastline was rugged and pounded by great waves and surf, but an unusually low low-tide allowed Alexander and his armies a speedy unhampered passage.

Alexander conquered the Pisidians and the Phrygians at their capital of Gordium, the home of the ancient Midas. Alexander came across the fabled chariot fastened to a pillar by braided cords made from a cherry tree. The legend stated, "Whosoever should untie this, for him was reserved the empire of the world." Alexander, unable to untie the knot, cut it through with his sword. He then advanced to Pophiagornia and Cappadocia, both of which he destroyed.

When Darius, king of Persia, heard that Memnon, his finest officer along with thousands of cavalry was killed in the battles, he decided to carry on the war with the Macedonians in the upper mountainous provinces of Asia. Darius marched from Susa very confident, number one because of his superiority of numbers which totaled 600,000 men and number two, in a dream he saw the Macedonian army on fire and Alexander waiting for him clad as the child he saw when he visited Philip's court ten years earlier.

Darius' confidence grew stronger as Alexander and his armies remained encamped in Cilicia so Alexander could recover from an illness - Darius mistook this delay as a sign of cowardice in Alexander.

A Macedonian general named Amyntas and two other generals married to Persian women were in contact with the Persian king Darius, giving him Alexander's proposed battle plans. When Amyntas learned that Darius was going to ambush Alexander in the mountain passes he advised the king to keep his larger army in the open plain, where his superior numbers could be brought to advantage. Darius, instead of heeding this advice, said he was afraid that Alexander would flee and escape to fight another day; however, Amyntas stated:

"That fear is needless, for assure yourself that far from avoiding you, he will make all the speed he can to meet you, and is now most likely on his march towards you!"

Amyntas' advice to Darius was to no avail, as Darius immediately marched into Cilicia at the same time as Alexander advanced into Syria to confront him. Passing one another in the night, they turned their armies around towards each other; Alexander took up position in the passes using the sea, the mountains and the Pinarus River to force Darius to split his forces. Not to allow himself to be outflanked by such a superior number, Alexander strung out his right flank much wider than his left flank and fought there himself in the forward where he was wounded in the thigh by an arrow. After putting the Persian army to flight, Alexander counted 110,000 dead of Darius' army - unfortunately Darius was not found amongst the dead.

Learning that Amyntas and his two fellow generals had Persian wives and had most probably given council to Darius regarding this last battle, Alexander sent members of his personal body guard to execute the three generals and their wives.

The generals in turn learned of the execution orders and thus forewarned were able to fight their way free and with their three wives, fled northeast following the Indus River and eventually crossing through the pass of Babusar and across the 3,000 foot deep chasm of the Hunza River.

The pass into Hunza is 13,700 foot high and is only passable during the three summer months. This was part of the trade route taken by Marco Polo on his return from Cathay in 1326; over the 3,000 foot deep Hunza River gorge via a suspended bridge made of goat hair.

The three generals and their wives formed the nucleus of a warrior tribe that initially flourished by preying on and raiding the trade routes and caravans that flowed from China to India and back again.

The Hunzas were not always known as Hunzas; up until the turn of the 20th century, the valley was known as the Kanjut and the people known as the Kanjuts. When Indian Girkis tried to invade Kanjut they gave the valley and the people in the name Hunza, because all of the people in the valley were allied and united as arrows in a quiver. In the Burushaski language (a mix of Masedonian and Persian) the name Hunza translates to "arrow."

The indigenous plant life of the Hunza Valley was rather limited. Ninety-nine percent of the valley was bare rock and the growing season limited to 45 days. Later, cultivated plants included barley, millet, wheat, buckwheat, potatoes, turnips, carrots, beans, peas, beans, pumpkins, tomatoes, melons, onions, garlic, cabbage, spinach, cauliflower, apricots, mulberries, walnuts, apples, plums, peaches, cherries and pears. Pomegranate trees are scattered throughout the valley.

The Hunzas consume milk, buttermilk, yogurt and butter (which they put into their tea and use as a cooking shortening). Hunza children are breast-fed until two years of age.

A large variety of indigenous wildlife (i.e.- ibex, or "Markhors," Marco Polo sheep, geese, ducks, pheasants and partridge) provided the early Hunza with meat (the Hunza do not eat pork because they are muslim).

The Hunza salt supply is mined from hills near the Shimshal and Muztagh Rivers and used in their tea and for cooking in its raw brown state (the color originates from the trace minerals included in the salt deposit when the seas dried up).

The 14 Hunza Practices

1) The Hunza diet includes grains (whole and sprouted), vegetables (raw or steamed), fruit (fruit is dried and reconstituted in water or diced and served in gelatin made from goat or mutton tendon and cartilage); meat at 2 - 4 pounds per week (i.e.- mutton, goat, yak, beef, poultry, eggs, brain, kidney, liver, etc.); dairy (i.e.- whole milk, soured milk, yogurt, cheese and butter as ghee) is a staple. Grape wine known as Pani (flavored with the oil of bitter apricot pits) is consumed daily.

2) Their farm soils are maintained by organic agricultural practices, "That which is taken from the soil is returned to the soil." Composting (including wood ash, and manure ash), plant debris, kitchen waste and animal and human waste is returned to the soil.

3) All Hunzas work seven days each week and 12 hours each day.

4) Fat sources include whole milk, butter, ghee, plant oils and animal fats (meat, skin, brain, eggs, etc.).

5) Relatively pollution free environment (no industrial or agricultural chemicals).

6) Daily consumption of salt by adding chunks of rock salt to their tea, cooking and as a condiment. Oftentimes their salt is "cut" with wood ash to salt at a ratio of 10:1.

7) No agricultural sprays or chemicals of any kind.

8) All children are breast-fed for 2(girls) to 4 (boys) years (no vaccinations or antibiotics). Recorded birth defects are

limited to two "mukhanas" or hermaphrodites in the 2,300 year history of Hunza.

9) All grains, vegetables and fruit are sun dried for storage.

10) Native herbs and spices are used for medicine, condiments and as foods - no western doctors or pharmaceuticals!

11) "Glacial milk" is the exclusive water source used for drinking and irrigation purposes (the fields are flooded, when the water soaks into the soil a thick layer of mineral silt or "rock flour" is left on the surface of the field - this silt is hoed or plowed into the soil before planting).

12) Cooking oils originate from plant oils (apricot), ghee (clarified butter) and animal fat (tallow, chicken, yak, beef, etc.).

13) Locally grown whole grains are used for their chapatti breads rather than purchased processed flours.

14) The Hunzas eat 1,880 to 2,000 calories each day, except for the three months of "starvation spring" when they only eat two to three meals per week.

The Hunza remained unvanquished until 1891 when the British Empire (to open trade routes) conquered and pacified the Hunzas by installing an Ismali ruler known as the Mir.

The average annual precipitation in Hunza is less than two inches and the surrounding mountains, the Karakorum Range is only 300 miles long, and the mountains are bare, naked and metallic gray looking.

Mount Rakaposhi, 25,500 foot high, overlooks the 8,500 foot high Hunza Valley along with more than 60 summits higher than, 22,000 feet. Mount Rakaposhi is one of the most difficult mountains on to climb - it took 23 attempts to conquer the summit of Rakaposhi! The first 22 attempts failed but a British expedition in 1958 finally succeeded in scaling the nearly sheer face.

Maps refer to this Karakorum Range at the junction of many countries as the Pamirs - the Afghanistan Pamir; the Russian Pamir; the Chinese Pamir, etc.

Pamir translated from the Persian language becomes "Roof of the World." Tibet is often called "Roof of the World," however, Lhasa is at an elevation of only 13,000 feet and is surrounded by summits only 18,000 feet high or less.

A few miles above the junction of the pearl gray waters of the Hunza River and the Gilgit River in a village called Secundersbad; it is here that the Hunza Valley begins; the Hunza Valley follows the Hunza River up to its sources beyond Misgar, almost on the Chinese border where it springs from glacial torrents spewing from under the 5,000 square mile Ultar Glacier.

The Hunza Valley is barely 200 miles long. When the original generals from Alexander's army arrived in the Hunza Valley, there were no naturally fertile valleys in Hunza as compared with the Willamette Valley in Oregon. The Hunza Valley was originally bare rock, the manufactured "soil" only being carried basket by basket up the 3,000 foot gorge walls and placed in hand crafted stone terraces that were designed to level and increase the growing surfaces.

This man made soil is continuously replaced again by hand from the mineral laden silt dredged up by hand from the bed of the Hunza River 3,000 feet below, irrigation with Glacial Milk (laden with a suspended colloidal mineral silt)and fertilized with wood ash (plant mineral) containing compost.

Then there was the problem of water in the barren "safe haven." Fortunately, one of the Macedonian generals was a military engineer. He was able to locate a year round source of water roaring from under the Ultar Glacier 50 miles away.

The Ultar Glacier originates on the 25,500 foot high Mount Rakaposhi. He was able to design and construct a gravity propelled aquaduct which carried water for drinking and irrigation.

The water originating from under the millions of tons of ice grinding on the parent rock of Mount Rakaposhi was so rich with minerals that it was bluish white, so white that the original people called it "Glacial Milk." For generation after generation, crop after crop and year after year for more than 2,300 years the Hunza people have drunk and irrigated their terraced fields with "Glacial Milk," unwittingly assuring their people of an optimal intake of the more than 60 minerals in the "Glacial Milk" of the Ultar Glacier truely the "land of milk and honey"!

Except for the polar glaciers, the Karakorum Range has the largest collection of glaciers in the world. Millions of tons of glacial ice (in some places hundreds or thousands of feet thick) grind four inches of living mountain rock into a fine "rock flour" each year, which is carried in suspension as "Glacial Milk." No rock, no mineral, no metal, no alchemy is resistant enough to be exempt from the grinding forces of these millions of tons of ice!

The "Glacial Milk" ejaculates from under the glaciers in great white water "nullahs." Thousands of glacial nullahs merge and join the Hunza River, very quickly the Hunza River joins the Gilget River; the two great glacial rivers now married join the Indus River - this now thundering river carries a colloidal suspension of all of the mineral building blocks of the Karakorum Range.

All of the minerals known are found in these mountains. "'Tis this wealth of solvent minerals in liquid form that is guided by means of conduits to the stone-terraced fields of the valleys of Hunza and allowed to soak and penetrate into their soil."

There are sister mountain ranges paralleling the Karakorums - the Hindukush (translates to "the Hindu killers") and the Himalayas have most of the worlds tallest mountains; yet their "Glacial Milks" are not as complete or as dense with minerals as the "Glacial Milk" from the Ultar Glacier that feeds and nourishes the Hunza Valley.

Glacial Milk is a mixed liquid, a solution of ionically dissolved elements and a suspension of finely ground rock dust (rock flour) shaved and ground from the living parent rock of the mountain by glacial friction. The suspended minerals in the Glacial Milk are referred to as "metallic colloidal minerals." The average particle size of these colloid particles is 7,000 times smaller than a red blood cell - so small, that they can only be visualized by an electron microscope.

The individual elements in "Glacial Milk" are not found in their separate pure atomic form, but rather they are found in aggregations or "mini-alloys" to form suspended solute particles.

The presence of these aggregate particles (ranging in size from one hundred thousandth to one ten millionth of a centimeter in diameter) are only detected by chemical analysis or the electron microscope.

The raw rock inorganic colloids cannot passively commute through semi-permeable membranes and therefore produce little or no osmotic pressure, depression of the freezing point of water (unlike a salt solution) or elevation of the boiling point. These molecular mini-alloys or aggregates carry a uniform negative charge.

Plants - wild forms and crops such as grains, vegetables, fruits and nuts actively take up these inorganic metallic colloids and convert them into intracellular (within the cell) organic plant colloids - these organic plant colloids are the form of minerals found in and used by all living cells of plants, animals and humans.

Organic colloidal minerals derived from plants are up to 98% available to humans as compared to as little as 8 to 12% availability of metallic minerals.

It is the eating of the plants rich in organic colloidal minerals, that is the secret of health and longevity of the cultures we have called the "age beaters!!!"

The serendipitous irrigation of their terraced fields with the common denominator of a highly mineralized "Glacial Milk" and the fertilization of their fields with an organic compost rich with the recycled colloidal plant minerals found in wood ashes from their heating and cooking fires is the secret of the Hunzas's long and fruitful lives.

Hunza Recipes*

The Hunzakuts use apricot oil for cooking; extra-virgin olive can be used as a substitute.

Chapattis -

Hunzakuts eat these flat breads with meals, especially stew, spinach and dahl.

5 cups whole-grain flour (wheat, rye, millet, buckwheat)
Water at room temperature.
Olive oil or apricot oil

1. Mix the flour and a small amount of water (enough so that the flour mixes with the water without becoming sticky) to make dough, and knead for 5 minutes.

2. Take a small handful of dough and mold into a sphere. Roll out with a rolling pin to make a small disc. Slap the dough from hand to hand to increase the diameter and make it thinner.

3. Heat a heavy-bottomed frying pan or griddle, then, cook the chapatti for a few moments on each side. Lubricate pan with the oil if necessary. Makes 5 chapattis.

Daudo: Lamb, Feta and Pasta Stew

8 - 10 oz lamb, cut into small chunks
1 onion, whole
3 bay leaves
3 Tblsp extra-virgin olive oil
1 onion, chopped fine
3 cloves garlic, chopped
1 rib celery, chopped small
6 - 8 tomatoes, chopped small
2 Tblsp tomato puree
4 oz pasta (can use chapattis cut into small strips)
2 tsp oregano or mixed herbs
5 oz feta cheese
Sea salt and black pepper (ground) to taste

1. Boil the lamb in a pan of water with the whole onion and bay leaves for about an hour, to create stock. Put the meat aside and keep the stock. Remove the fat from the surface of the stock.

2. Gently heat the olive oil in a heavy-bottomed saucepan over a low flame - if necessary, add 2 Tblsp of stock to keep the temperature low. Gently cook the onion, garlic and celery in the olive oil until soft, but prevent browning. Add the meat and cook for a few minutes, then add the tomatoes with the tomato puree and gently cook for 5 - 10 minutes.

3. Put in enough stock so that the liquid level is about an inch above the solids. Simmer with the lid on for about an hour. Add more juice if necessary (or a glass of red wine).

4. Add the pasta and cook until it is al dente.

5. Add the oregano or mixed herbs.

6. Serve with the feta cheese crumbled over the top. Serves 2 - 3.

Dhal with Lemon and Cilantro

7 oz lentils
1 large onion shredded
2 Tblsp extra-virgin olive oil
3 Tomatoes, chopped very small
2 Tblsp tomato paste
2 - 3 fresh green chilis, chopped small
2 tsp garam masala or curry powder
sea salt
2 lemons
1 bunch cilantro, chopped
brown bread or brown rice

1. Wash the lentils well. Put them in a pan with 2 cups water, bring to a boil, and cook for about 15 minutes, until soft but not mushy.

2. At the same time, use a heavy-bottomed pan to gently cook the onion in the olive oil, until soft and starting to turn yellow. Add the tomatoes, tomato paste, and chilis, and cook until soft. Add extra tomato paste and/or water to make the dhal more liquid.

3. When the lentils are cooked, add them to the mixture and simmer for 5 minutes.

4. Squeeze in the juice of 1 - 2 lemons to taste.

5. Add the cilantro at the last minute and stir in. Crumble chapatti into the dhal or add brown rice. Serves 2.

Sultan coq: fruit and nut bar

7 oz apricot kernels or almonds
7 oz walnuts
7 oz dried mulberries or golden raisins
2 Tblsp water

1. In a coffee grinder, grind the apricot kernels or almonds and walnuts, then add the dried mulberries or raisins and grind.

2. Put in a bowl and fold together with water to make a thick paste. Roll the paste into golf ball sized lumps, then shape into small cookies or pancakes.

---

* *Sally Beare. 50 Secrets of the World's Longest Living People. 2006*
** *This ingredient is not part of the Hunza diet.*

"The Okinawan lifestyle (and diet), not genes is the primary reason for their extraordinary health and longevity."

Dr. B. J. Willcox, Dr. D. C. Willcox
& Dr. M. Suzuki
The Okinawa Program

"Sea water is water only in the sense that water is the dominant compound. It is a most complex liquid, containing about 3.5 per cent of dissolved inorganic compounds. Kelp, growing in the sea, converts these inorganic compounds (minerals) into organic form."

D. C. Jarvis, M.D.
Folk Medicine

Okinawa

Originally, Okinawa was the Kingdom of the Ryukyus; the 161 island archipelago is now a prefecture, or state of Japan, 1,000 miles from Tokyo. In the United States Okinawa is principally known for its part in WWII.

The Battle of Okinawa, the "typhoon of steel," was one of the longest and bloodiest of the WWII Pacific Theater where some 70,000 U.S. marines, sailors and soldiers were killed or wounded and 150,000 Okinawan civilians died - it was the only battle fought on what was considered Japanese home territory.

As of 1996, Okinawans (the Hawaiians of Japan), according to the WHO, were the longest lived people of the industrialized world. The centenarians of Okinawa have been studied more intensely than any other long lived peoples on Earth.

A 25 year long study, The *Okinawa Program,* was launched by the identical twin Willcox brothers. Bradley J. Willcox, who received his M.D. from Harvard School of Medicine and his twin brother, D. Craig Willcox, received his Ph.D. in pharmacy along with Makoto Suzuki, M.D., PhD., a cardiologist from Okinawa International University conducted the Okinawa Centenarian Study.

In Okinawa, individuals generally have a very high life expectancy of 78 years for men and 86 years for women and what is considered to be the greatest number of disability-free years of 72.3 men and 77.7 years for women.

Okinawans have a documented rate of centenarians at 5/10,000.

The Okinawan lifestyle (and diet), not genes is the primary reason for their extraordinary health and longevity. The Okinawan diet contains an average of 1,500 calories and consists of boiled pork, chicken, eggs, dried minnows, miso and fish soup, tofu, many types of garden and sea vegetables, sea weed, kelp, onions, garlic, daikon, greens, purple sweet potatoes, bitter melon and tubers grown in their own gardens; antioxidant rich tumeric tea, green tea and awamori (sake - rice wine) are the daily drinks.

Teaism

According to Kakuzo Okakura:

The historical isolation of Japan from the rest of the world, so conducive to introspection, has been highly favorable to the development of "Teaism." Our home and habits, costume and cuisine, porcelain, lacquer, painting - our very literature - all have been subject to its influence. No student of Japanese (or Okinawan) culture could ever ignore its presence. It has permeated the elegance of nonle boudoirs, and entered the abode of the humble. Our peasants have learned to arrange flowers, our meanest labourrer to offer his salutation to the rocks and waters. In our common parlance we speak of the man "with no tea" in him, when he is insusceptible to the seriocomic interests of the personal drama. Again we stigmatise the untamed asthete who, regardless of the mundane tragedy, runs riot in the springtide of emancipated emotions, as one "with too much tea" in him.

The Okinawan centenarians show a "greater appetite" for mineral rich garden vegetables and dairy products than the general population.

Seaweed

Sea water is a complex-water; universally around the world analysis of sea water reveal that it contains 3.5% dissolved inorganic salts and minerals. The oceans are located in the lowest levels of the earth's surface and are therefore the catch basin into which mineral substances of every kind have been drained by the many moving forces of nature.

The various elements and minerals, carried by wind and water, as soon as they arrive in the oceans, join in the great milling of chemical changes, reacting, dissolving, precipitating, re-dissolving, being integrated into living organisms (plants and animals), travel and move through the seasonal life cycles and then are set free again.

It is not a secret that every known reaction occurs in the oceans, as they are stirred and mixed by wind, perennial currents, frozen and thawed, exposed to light including entire spectrums of intensities and colors.

The current chemical composition of the ocean is the accumulation of millions of years of time and natural forces - all things found in the earth ultimately finds their way into the sea.

Chemists have realized, for centuries that, in the great oceans there are dissolved all of the naturally occurring elements and minerals. It is estimated that each cubic mile of ocean contains 200,000,000 tons of elemental and mineral compounds.

Kelp and algae growing in the sea takes up these inorganic salts and converts them into useable organic forms. When used as fertilizer (either as dried kelp or kelp ash) or added directly to the diet as a vegetable, kelp is a significant source of dietary plant minerals.

Seaweed, a staple Okinawan sea vegetable, is a generic term for more than 2,500 varieties of aquatic plants that grow in bodies of fresh and salt water. In common terms "sea weed" is placed in groups according to color - i.e. - brown, red, green, and blue-green.

Kombu is a form of kelp, it is classified as a brown seaweed that is found in abundance in the cold sea surrounding the northern Japanese island of Hokkaido. Kombu has been very popular in Okinawa since the early 1800s, when it was first gathered and brought to southern China. Kelp is very popular with Okinawans and they eat approximately three times the quantities that the Japanese eat. It tastes like pasta mixed with seafood.

Nori is classified as red seaweed, however, it looks black when dried. This seaweed is typically used to wrap sushi and rice balls, and as a seasoning for salads, soups and noodles. Okinawans eat nori with breakfast as flat strips mixed with rice. The Irish and Welsh eat nori as "laver" which is used to make flat cakes.

Hijiki is a form of black seaweed that is served in short bitter-tasting strips. Okinawans typically eat hijiki simmered with vegetables and soybeans.

Wakame is a form of kelp that tastes like spinach lasagna. It is commonly put in soups, salads and buckwheat noodles (soba).

General Analysis of Sea Kelp

Content	Percent
Moisture	6.00
Protein (crude)	7.50
Fiber (crude)	7.20
Nitrogen free extract	45.28
Fat (ether extract)	0.34
Ash (plant minerals)	33.68

George W. Cavanaugh, Agricultural Chemistry, Cornell

General Composition of Kelp Ash

Mineral Elements	Percent
Calcium	1.00
Phosphorus	0.34
Magnesium	0.74
Sodium	4.00
Potassium	12.00
Chlorine	13.37
Sulfur	1.00
Iron	0.04
Iodine	0.19
Trace elements (total)	1.00

Spectrographic Qualitative Analysis of Kelp Ash

Element	Percent
Sodium	> 10.0
Potassium	> 10.0
Calcium	> 10.0
Iron	0.1
Aluminum	0.1
Magnesium	0.1
Strontium	0.1
Silicon	0.01 - 0.1
Manganese	0.01 - 0.1
Copper	0.001 - 0.01
Tin	0.001 - 0.01
Lead	0.001 - 0.01
Vanadium	0.001
Zinc	0.001
Titanium	0.0001 - 0.001
Chromium	0.0001 - 0.001
Barium	0.0001 - 0.001
Silver	0.0001

Bitter melon, or Goya chample (*Momordica charantia*), is a staple in the Okinawan diet which we ate a lot of while visiting Okinawa. Goya or bitter melon, which looks like a cucumber with warts, is thought to have been brought to the Ryukyu Kingdom from old China during the Ming and Manchu dynasties. It is thought to have been used as a food staple from around 1100 A.D. and as an added benefit it is known to support healthy blood sugar levels in diabetics.

In 2003, a small group of our associates went to Okinawa with us to determine the Okinawan's health and longevity secrets and where these exceedingly long lived people obtained their nutritional minerals.

We first went to the Department of Agriculture and learned that the soil of the entire 800 mile long Okinawa archipelago of 161 islands was made up of red, yellow or black clay - very similar to the red sandy clay that is characteristic of the American state of Georgia.

In 1605, Sokan Noguni, an Okinawan returned home from a visit to China with a sweet potato. It was the perfect tuber for Okinawa's rocky soil. Soon the sweet potato was grown all over the island and by 1902, it provided 80% of the total caloric intake of the people.

The Okinawan's eventually erected a statue of Noguni, who is respectfully referred to as Lord Sokan, the Imo (sweet potato) King.

Many large studies, including the 25 year long Okinawa project, were conducted in an attempt to determine their secret of longevity. Because of the detailed completeness of the questions in these studies, we felt we didn't need to again ask questions on diet, religion, exercise and professions that had been asked over and over again - we took the information in these studies to be correct. We decided that we were going to ask only one question - "what did you do with the wood ashes from your heating and cooking fires?"

We visited many of the Okinawa "old ones," and shared traditional meals of boiled pork, steamed sea vegetables, bitter melon, sweet potatoes and squash with them. Drink included green tea and rice wine.

We asked old men in their 90s and many over the age of 100 years, "what did you do with the wood ashes from your cooking and heating fires?" The old men replied, "I don't know." We asked the same question of Okinawa women over the age of 90 and 100 years of age, and they replied, "Everyone knows that, we put the wood ashes into our gardens and rice paddies to fertilize our rice, vegetables and fruit."

And then the lady centenarians shared something we hadn't thought of, "We also added rice straw ashes to our noodle dough and rice as we cooked them because it added a wonderful yellow color and enhanced the flavor." Culinary ashes (plant minerals) were part of the Okinawa secret!

The last thing we learned from the Okinawa old ones and centenarians was that, "Each morning, an ash merchant would appear and buy our excess ashes to sell to restaurants and farmers."

During the Edo period (1603 - 1867) of Japan, rice straw was used to make a variety of products including sandals, hats, mats and rope. The manufacture of products from rice straw was a common cottage industry that was developed to supplement the meager Japanese cash income.

The old and used straw items were burned as fuel in the kitchen ovens and heating stoves - farmers and "ash traders" purchased or traded for the ash which was then resold for fertilizer. In this way, almost all of the 10 million tons of the annual production of rice straw ash was returned to the soil.

A recent comparison of the mineral content of the bones from the modern Japanese and the 3,000 year old bones from ancient Japanese monks showed that the ancient bones contained a wider variety of minerals and a greater amount of each mineral - a testimony to the value of wood and rice straw ashes for fertilizer and for "culinary ashes."

Okinawa Recipes*

Dashi

2 strips kombu seaweed
1 large pinch of bonito (dried fish) flakes
3/4 Tblsp soy sauce

1. Boil the kombu for 3 - 4 minutes in a small pan of water (1/2 pint). Remove from the heat.

2. Add the bonito flakes and return to the heat. Remove from heat just as water begins to boil.

3. Allow to stand for 5 minutes, or until bonito flakes sink. Strain and keep the liquid. Discard the solids (these solids can be used to produce a second batch).

4. Add the soy sauce. Serves 2 - 3.

Pork Noodles with Dashi

4 oz cooked pork slices or salmon
1 Tablsp olive oil
1/2 clove garlic
1 Tblsp dashi
1 - 2 tsp soy sauce
3/4 tsp sake or sweet white wine
1 cup stock (pork, or vegetable if using salmon)
4 oz Asian noodles, buckwheat udon
3 stalks green onions, chopped very fine

1. If using pork, boil the meat in about a pint of water for 25

minutes. Skim the fat off of the top of the water and keep the rest of the liquid to use as stock.

2. Heat the oil in a wok or frying pan. Add the garlic and cook gently for a minute or so, but prevent browning - bring down the cooking temperature by adding a Tblsp of stock.

3. Add the pork or salmon and stir for just a few seconds.

4. Add the dashi, soy, sake and stock and bring to a boil.

5. Add the noodles and heat.

6. Garnish with the onion and serve. Serves 1 - 2.

Pork and Vegetable Soup with Sake

11 oz pork
11 oz pork liver
Sake or awamori
3 potatoes, diced
1 carrot, diced
1 - 2 spring onions, cut into thin "matchsticks."
1 Tblsp miso
1 - 2 tsp chopped ginger

1. Cut the meat into small pieces and marinate in a bowl of sake or awamori for 20 minutes

2. Boil the meat in a pan of water, just covering the meat. Skim fat from the top of the soup as it appears.

3. After 15 - 20 minutes, add the potatoes and carrots, then, continue cooking for about 10 minutes, until the potatoes and carrots are soft but not overcooked.

4. Remove from heat and stir in the miso.

5. Garnish with the spring onions, and serve soup with a glass of warm sake. Serves 4.

Rice with Seaweed

1 1/2 cups brown rice
2 strips kombu seaweed/hijiki seaweed
1 onion, chopped small
1 clove garlic, chopped small
1 Tblsp extra-virgin olive oil
1 tsp sesame oil
1 Tblsp soy sauce

1. Wash and cook rice.

2. If using kombu seaweed, boil for 20 minutes, then cut into matchstick-size strips. If using hijiki seaweed, soak for 15 minutes in warm water, then drain.

3. Gently cook the onion and garlic in the olive oil for about 10 minutes, or until onions are just turning yellow, add the cooked rice and stir, then add the seaweed.

4. Add the sesame oil and the soy sauce, stir for a few moments. Serves 2.

**Sally Beare: 50 Secrets of the World's Longest Living People. 2006.*
***This is not part of the Okinawa diet.*

Part 4

The Currency of the Age Beaters

"A critical examination of the lifestyles and eating habits of the centenarians of the world's Blue Zones quickly reveals the simple and universal common threads that have produced and can predictably and repeatedly reproduce 100 year old humans regardless of genetic make up, gender, ethnic, religious or national origin."

Dr. Joel D. Wallach & Dr. Ma Lan

Chapter 12

"I want to prove that the boundaries (of age) set up by the gods are not unbreakable."

Gilgamesh, King of Sumaria
Clay Tablets, 5000 B.C.

The Common Threads of Anti-Aging

The aging process starts the moment you are conceived and continues unabated, progressing forward at varying speeds, and degrees at an hourly, daily, weekly and annual rate until the ultimate end of the process - death.

There is an accumulated knowledge, however, that will allow each of us to prevent and slow the aging process so that we can successfully reach beyond 100 years of age in a beautiful, healthful and functional way.

While there are genetic upper limits to human longevity, all humans certainly and predictably have the genetic potential, the genetic equipment and the genetic capacity to live well beyond 100! The only reason that all humans don't achieve or reach their genetic potential for longevity beyond 100 years is that: 1) consciously or unconsciously, they omit essential pieces of the anti-aging circuitry in their daily lives necessary to fulfill this potential; and/or 2) they ignorantly or proactively take pleasure in consciously stepping on land mines.

While the percentage of hundred year olds currently varies from country to country (Blue Zones), all humans can easily reach 100 years of age by simply following certain known and predictable physiological laws.

These physiological laws for longevity are as unforgiving and predictable as gravity. If you step off of the roof of a third story house without a ladder, the law of gravity will surely take you suddenly and rudely to the ground. If you are unaware of, or simply ignore the physiological requirements to live to be 100, you will surely not make it to 100 years of age even if you have "good genes."

On the other hand, if everyone in your family died at 35 years of age and you accurately fulfill your physiological requirements for longevity and you avoid the land mines, you can easily make it healthfully to 100.

Centenarian Common Threads

A critical examination of the lifestyles and eating habits of the centenarians of the world's Blue Zones quickly reveals the simple and universal common threads that have produced and can predictably and repeatedly reproduce 100 year old humans regardless of genetic makeup, gender, ethnic, religious or national origin.

The omission of any one or any part of the four longevity pieces will result in catastrophic failure:

Antioxidants:

Daily consumption of antioxidant rich food and drink is a universal feature of those living in Blue Zones and in particular centenarians. These potent carbon compounds quench or neutralize free radicals that attack our cells, cell walls, mitochondria and physiological processes and increase our risk of cardiovascular disease, cancer, Alzheimer's disease and other dementias, cataracts, diabetes and aggressively speed up the process and damage of aging itself.

A universally agreed upon method of predicting the antioxidant power and free radical neutralizing value of foods, drink and supplements is the Oxygen Radical Absorbance Capacity or ORAC value - based on current studies, we believe that the optimal total daily intake of ORAC points to reach the age of 100 years is 20,000 to 25,000 per day.

In 2007, scientists with the USDA published an updated list of ORAC values for 277 foods commonly consumed by the U.S. population (fruits, vegetables, nuts, seeds, spices, grains, drinks, etc.).

ORAC is a method of measuring antioxidant capacities of various foods. It was developed by scientists at the National Institute on Aging, a division of the National Institute of Health (NIH) in Baltimore, Maryland and Tufts University, Boston, Massachusetts.

The ORAC analysis, which utilizes Florescein as the florescent probe, provides a measure of the scavenging capacity of antioxidants against the peroxyl radical, which is one of the most common reactive oxygen species (ROS) found in the body.

In 2008, the U. S. Department of Agriculture (USDA) listed a database of the ORAC values. Correlation between the high antioxidant capacity of fruits and vegetables, and the positive impact of diets high in fruits and vegetables, is well accepted and universally known to play an important role in the Free-radical theory of aging.

In many countries, of North America, Europe, Asia, Central and South America and their Blue Zones, the daily consumption of a wide variety of vegetables, fruit, dark berries, chocolate, wine, coffee and tea are the universal rich cultural sources of antioxidants.

In the "Blue Zones" of the world, large quantities of vitamin C, Beta carotene, flavanols, lycopenes, leutenes, proanthocyanins, resveratrols, catechens (EGCGs) and polyphenols are found in dark fruits and berries, yellow and red vegetables, cocoa, red wine, green tea or coffee - these are the antioxidants that have universally been found to be consumed daily in the Blue Zones and are known to protect the centenarians.

The ORAC Value of Common Foods and Drink of Centenarians

Food/Juice	ORAC Value/Serving
Cloves, ground	314,446
Cinnamon	267,536
Sorghum, black	100,800
Aronia Black chokeberry	16,062
Small Red Bean	13,727
Wild blueberry	13,427
Red kidney bean	13,259
Peppermint	13,978
Pinto bean	11,864
Cranberry	8,983
Artichoke hearts	7,904

Acai	1,842
Raspberry	6,058
Strawberry	5,938
Red Delicious apple	5,900
Granny Smith apple	5,381
Pecan	17,940
Sweet cherry	4,873
Black plum	4,844
Russet potato	4,649
Black bean	4,181
Plum	4,118
Baby food, (peaches)	6,257
Baby food, (apple/blueberry)	4,822
Baby food, (applesauce-strained)	4,123
Baby food, (bananas)	2,658
Gala apple	3,903
Wine, red (Merlot)	3,873
Wine, red (Cabernet Suavignon)	5,034
Wine, rose	1,005
Wine, white	392
Raisins	2,830
Avocado, raw	1,933
Kale	1,770

Noni juice	398
Mangosteen juice	498
Wolfberry (Gogi) juice	363
Almonds	4,282
Hazelnuts (filberts)	9,275
Acai berry juice	1,842
Kiwi	1,159
Lentils, raw	7,282
Prune juice	7,291
Prune	5,770
Blueberry juice	9,019
Pomagranate juice (100%)	2,341
Chocolate (dark liquid)/juice blend	3,000
Dark chocolate pieces	3,040
Sweet potato, baked	2,115
Green tea, brewed	1,128
Mangos, raw	988
Oranges, navel	1,785
Pears, raw	1,911
Pomagranate/Blueberry	962

On the surface when one searches for the common threads or the single basis of the longevity success of the various cultures found in the "Blue Zones" of the world, one comes up empty handed - everything seems unrelated, desperate and foundationless and therefore to the "expert" gerontologists, claims and recipes seem quite unscientific, mythical and unimportant.

However, when one examines categories of longevity constants instead of looking for one single "magic pill" or the waters of a "fountain of youth" in a particular country the answer becomes obvious!

The answer, the secrets of health, longevity and even immortality are hidden in plain view - it's only a matter of knowing the basic "language of immortality" to then be able to translate all of the different "dialects of immortality" into a single universal language!

One of the unimpeachable ingredients in the universal formula for health, longevity and immortality is antioxidants. Like children, we can argue, "mine is better than yours," however, the successful centenarians in the "Blue Zones" consume multiple forms and sources of antioxidants daily. Some variations of seasonal consumption are based on growing seasons and therefore seasonal availability, however, the daily consumption of multiple antioxidants is a constant (20,000 to 25,000 ORAC points/day).

Antioxidants of the "Blue Zones"

Country	Antioxidant
Azerbaijan	Red Wine
	Vodka
	Tea
	Fruit
	Vegetables

Sardinia	Red Wine Tea Fruit Vegetables
Nycoya, Costa Rica	Fruit Vegetables Chocolate Wine Coffee
Hunza	Red Wine Tea Fruit Vegetables
Okinawa	Rice wine Green tea Kelp Sweet potatoes Vegetables
Bama, China	"Snake" wine Green tea Sweet potatoes Fruit Vegetables

Vilcabamba	Chocolate Chili pepper Red wine Fruit Vegetables
Titicaca	Chocolate Chili pepper Red wine Fruit Vegetables
Italy	Red wine Garlic Chili Pepper Fruit Vegetables
Greece	Red wine Fruit Vegetables Garlic
USA (Mormon, Adventist)	Berries (dark) Green leafy vegetables Yellow/red vegetables Fruit

Wine & Beer

"Alcohol has existed longer than all human memory. It has outlived generations, nations, epochs and ages. It is part of us, and that is fortunate indeed. For although alcohol will always be the master of some, for most of us it will continue to be the servant of man."

National Institute on Alcohol Abuse and Alcoholism

Wine is simply fermented grape (*Vitis vinifera*) juice, with an alcohol content of 5.5 to 14 percent (grape spirits can be added to wines in order to raise the alcohol content to 15 to 22 percent). The first evidence for the consumption and production of wine goes back more than 10,000 years ago. Wine frequently appears as a finished product in Egyptian pictographs circa 4,000 B.C.

Brewing as an art, dates from the beginning of civilization in ancient Egypt, many Egyptian gods were gods of a family or were local diaties, however, Osiris, the god of wine was worshiped throughout Egypt. The Egyptians believed that Osiris in addition to creating wine also invented beer. The Egyptians considered beer as a necessity of life and as a result was brewed in every home "on an everyday basis."

Both beer and wine were deified and offered to the gods whose hieroglyph was a winepress. The ancient Egyptians brewed at least 17 varieties of beer and 24 varieties of wine.

The Egyptians used alcoholic beverages for pleasure, nutrition, medicine, ritual, renumeration and funerary purposes. The wine and beer placed in tombs were to be used by the dead during their journey into the "after-life."

The earliest wines are thought to have been made from fermented berries or honey in the wild grape regions of the Middle East.

Recorded in the Old Testament (Genesis 9:20), Noah planted a vineyard on Mt. Ararat in what is now eastern Turkey.

It is recorded in writings from Sumer, that beer and wine were used for "medicinal" purposes as early as 2,000 B.C.

In 1952, Neolithic (Stone Age - 10,000 B.C.) beer jugs were discovered, and it is theorized that beer probably preceded bread as a staple.

Beer was the beverage of choice amongst the Babylonians, and as early as 2,700 B.C. they worshipped a wine goddess and other wine deities. Babylonians regularly used both beer and wine as offerings to their gods. In 1,750 B.C., the great Code of Hammurabi devoted considerable attention to the rules of "fair commerce" in alcohol (beer and wine).

A variety of alcoholic beverages have been used in China since prehistoric times. In China, wine and beer were considered a spiritual food rather than a food for the physical body. Extensive documentary evidence attests to the role that alcohol played in the ancient Chinese religious life.

In ancient China, people always drank wine and beer when holding a memorial ceremony, offering sacrifices to gods or their ancestors, pledging resolution before going into battle, celebrating victory, before feuding and official executions, for taking an oath of allegiance, while attending ceremonies of birth, marriage, reunions, departures, death, and festival banguets.

A Chinese imperial edict in 1,116 B.C. makes it clear that the use of alcohol in moderation was believed to be prescribed by heaven. The consumption of alcohol was clearly beneficial to the Chinese treasury. During the time of Marco Polo, wine and beer drinking was very common and very popular and the alcohol tax was one of the treasury's largest sources of revenue.

Laws against making wine and beer in China were inacted and repealed 41 times between 1,100 B.C. and 1,400 A.D. A writer recorded in 650 B.C. that "People will not do without beer. To prohibit it and (attempt) to secure total abstinence from it is beyond the power even of sages. Hence, therefore, we have warnings on the abuse of it."

The art of wine making only reached the Hellenic

peninsula in approximately 2,000 B.C.; the first alcoholic beverage to obtain wide-spread popularity in what is now Greece was "mead," a fermented beverage made from honey and water. By 1,700 B.C., winemaking became commonplace in Greece and over the next 1,000 years wine became important in hospitality, it was used for medicinal purposes, and it became an integral part of daily meals.

As a beverage, wine was consumed in many ways - warm or chilled, straight or mixed with water, plain or with added spices.

The Greeks are considered the most temperate of ancient cultures. This restriction of drunkenness is thought to result from Grecian societal rules that stress moderation in the consumption of alcohol, their praise of temperant behavior, their habit of diluting wine with water and avoidance of excess.

Instances of habitual intoxication amongst the Greeks was rare, however, they were not against drunkenness at banquents and festivals.

An exception to the Greek record of temperance was the cult of Dionysus, whose members believed that drunkenness would bring them spiritually closer to their gods.

The Greek "Symposium," a gathering of men for an evening of conversation, entertainment and drinking usually ended in drunkenness. There are no records in ancient Greece that mass drunkenness was a problem, however, in 425 B.C., warnings against intemperance by foreigners, particularly at Symposia became more frequent.

Xenophon (431-351 B.C.) and Plato (429-347 B.C.) both lauded the moderate use of wine as beneficial to health, longevity and happiness. Hippocrates (460-370 B. C.) identified and wrote of the many medicinal properties of wine, which had a long history of being prescribed for its therapeutic value.

The Hebrews were introduced to wine during their enslavement in Egypt. When Moses took them to Canaan (1,200 B. C.) they lamented leaving behind the wines of Egypt (Numbers 20:5); however, the Hebrews found vineyards to be abundantly available in their new land.

With the advent of Christianity and its gradual displacement of the previously predominant religions, the drinking habits of Europe were directly affected by the content of the New Testament. Jesus used wine and approved of its moderate use and consumption. Paul considered wine to be a creation of God and therefore inherently good, he recommended its use for medicinal purposes, while at the same time condemned drunkenness.

The spread of Christianity and viticulture in Western Europe occurred simultaneously. St. Martin of Tours was actively involved in preaching the gospel and planting vineyards.

The period between the fall of Rome and the beginning of the High Renaissance, the Middle Ages (1500 A.D.), is known for rapid development of human culture. In the Middle Ages, mead, rustic beers, and wild fruit wines became commonly available and popular, particularly among the Celtics, Anglo-Saxons, Germans and Scandinavians, while wines remained the favorite beverage in the Romance countries (Italy, Spain and France).

After the Roman Empire collapsed, monistaries became the centers of brewing beer and winemaking. Rustic beers continued to be brewed in the common home, whereas the professional and commercial brewing techniques where developed and closely guarded by the monks.

The monistaries kept the art of viticulture alive. With their greater resources, security and stability, they were able to develop and improve the quality of their vineyards. Throughout the time of the Middle Ages, the finest vineyards were owned and managed by the monistaries, and "vinum theologium" or wine of the church was considered to be the finest of all wines. In addition to fermenting the quantity of wine necessary to celebrate the mass, the monasteries also produced large volumes of wine for commercial trade to support the maintenance and expansion of the monastic movement.

Common Wines of the World

Wine	Grape Variety

Cabernet Sauvignon Black grape

This is the most well known black grape variety in the world. It is the most important Bordeaux variety and has also been successful in the New World. The grapes are high in tannins, so these wines age well, especially if aged in oak barrels. At their best, these wines are rich in color, aroma and depth and have a long lasting flavor of black currants.

Chardonnay White grapes

Without a doubt, the most popular white wine/white grape variety. It is the variety used to produce the classic white Burgundy and one of the three varieties of white grapes used to make Champagne. Wines from this grape are typically dry, and light with a crisp apple-like flavor to a full-bodied buttery flavor depending upon the method of production.

Chenin Blanc White grapes

This grape is characteristically a high acid variety that requires a high level of sunlight to ripen, otherwise the wines become tart. The main growing regions for Chenin Blanc include Loire, New Zealand and South Africa. The wines range from very dry to sweet and sparkling; the successful dry wines are fresh and fruity and sweet wines are well-balanced and honeyed.

Gamay Red grapes

Beaujolais wine, fermented from the Gamay grape, is of enormous commercial value in Burgundy, where it is the grape that accounts for more than half of all wine produced. Characteristically, these wines are uncomplicated, light, fruity reds intended for quaffing when young and fresh. These wines have a distinctive intense pear aroma and raspberry flavor, which is the result of the production methods. Most high grade Beaujolais can be aged.

Gewurztraminer Pale pink grape

The very aromatic wines fermented from these spicey pink grapes are full-bodied white wines that can be dry or sweet. These wines have a low acidity and a high alcohol content (greater than 13%). The best of this category of white wines come from Alsace. Because of its exotic perfume and intense litchi flavor, Gewurztraminer is one of the few wines that fits well with spicy foods.

Grenache Black grape

When fermented by itself, the Grenache black grape produces a warm, fruity flavored wine with a high alcohol content and an aroma of freshly ground black pepper. These grapes are low in tannins, and as a result they are often blended with high tannic acid grapes such as Cabernet sauvignon or Syrah. The primary growing areas of the Grenache grape are southern France, Australia, California and Spain.

Merlot Black grape

The Merlot grape is the most commonly planted black grape variety of Bordeaux, where it is frequently blended with Cabernet sauvignon. Unblended Merlot are usually soft and easy-drinking wines, with flavors ranging from plums to fruitcake. Cabernet sauvignon lends "backbone" to Merlot, which is lower in tannins and acidity, yet brings a richness and smoothness to the Merlot which would otherwise be perceived as harsh.

Pinot Noir Red grape

This is the grape that is used to make red Burgundy wines. Yields are not high, which makes it challenging and expensive to produce. Pinot noir grapes make a pale-colored, light to medium-bodied red wine that has a strawberry or raspberry aroma. The highest quality Pinot noir are made in Burgundy and they have the reputation of being "the most sumptuous reds in the world." New Zealand and Oregon in the U.S. produce good Pinot noir wines. The Pinot noir is also the main grape variety used to produce high quality champagne.

Riesling White grapes

This classic German grape variety makes many of the finest white wines in the world - they range from very dry to very sweet. The Riesling wines are light in body and low in alcohol, yet strongly flavored and "very long-lived." Fantastic, very sweet white wines are typically made from Riesling grapes that have been subjected to "noble rot."

("Noble rot" - an overgrowth of the fungus, *Botrytis cinerea,* causes a shriveling and dehydration of the grapes, however, this condition causes an increase in sweetness. The finest examples of very sweet dessert wines made from botrytized grapes are produced in Bordeaux and Germany. "Noble rot" affects Riesling, Sauvignon blanc, Chenin blanc, Semillon, and Gewurztraminer grapes in a positive way.)

Sauvignon Blanc White grape

Wines produced from this grape are typically very dry, fresh white wines that should be consumed young. They are easily recognized by their intense taste and aromas that are those of green grass and gooseberries. Sancerre and Pouilly Fume', from the Loire, are the best known Sauvignon blancs, however, New Zealand is known to produce a good Sauvignon blanc.

Semillon White grape

This very utilitarian white grape makes a wide range of white wines, from dry to very sweet - good Semillon wines are made in Australia and Bordeaux. It is typically blended, usually with Sauvignon blanc and Chardonnay. Dry and blended Semillon wines are best consumed when they are young, however, many of the sweeter wines will improve with age. Semillon is at its best when infested with "noble rot," which produces some of the most well known dessert wines such as Sauternes and Barsac.

Syrah (Shiraz) Red grape

Referred to as Shiraz, in Australia (sparkling version) and South Africa the Syrah grape produces a dark, full-bodied, heavy, red wine with great potential longevity, especially when oak aged. They contain a considerable level of tannic acid and are best consumed when three years old with food. Mature Shiraz wines have aromas of black currant, cedar and mixed spice. Syrah is commonly grown in the Rhone Valley.

Zinfandel Black grape

Thought of as California's own grape variety, Zinfandel produces wines that range from light and elegant (white or rose) to massive tannic reds - the grape's berry-like aroma and taste always comes through. The best Zinfandels are those that are rich and darkly colored with a short oaking - these wines are at their peak when they are five years old.

Distillation of alcohol was one of the more important discoveries during the Middle Ages. Albertus Magnus (1193-1280 A.D.) was the first individual to clearly describe the process for the distillation of spirits. Details of the new art soon spread amongst the monks, physicians and alchemists, who were looking to distilled alcohol as a cure for human ailments. Distilled beverages were originally called *aqua vitae* or "water of life" - later they were called brandy. The term brandy was derived from the Dutch word "brandewijn" which translates to burnt or distilled wine.

Wine Consumption by Country in 2002

Rank	Country	Amount (Liters)
1	Italy	54
2	France	47
3	Switzerland	42
4	Austria	36
5	Denmark	32
6	Belgium	30
7	Germany	26
8	Australia	21
9	United Kingdom	20
10	Netherlands	20
11	New Zealand	19
12	Sweden	16
13	Ireland	13
14	Norway	11
15	Japan	10
16	Canada	10
17	Finland	10
18	United States	7

Global Market Information Database (2002)

The Bubonic Plague which began in the 14th century reduced European village populations by as much as 82%. Reaction to the unstoppable varied from "processions of flagellants who mobbed city and village streets, hoping, by the pains they inflicted on themselves and upon each other, to take the edge off the plagues they attributed to God's wrath over human folly," to a dramatic increase in the consumption of alcohol, in hopes of protecting themselves.

In Bavaria, beer consumption is believed to have risen to 300 liters per capita per year (compared with the 150 liters consumed today) and in Florence, wine consumption reached ten barrels per capita per year.

The consumption of distilled spirits which was originally used exclusively for medicinal purposes increased significantly.

With the end of the Middle Ages, the popularity of beer spread to England, France and Scotland. Beer brewers were soon officially recognized as a guild in England, and the adulteration of beer and wine became a crime punishable by death.

The early Modern Period was a time of increasing prosperity and wealth. Towns and cities sprouted up all over Europe, grew in size and numbers, new territories were "discovered" and colonized and world trade developed.

In the 16th century, the consumption of alcoholic beverages reached 100 liters per person per year in Valladoid, Spain; Polish peasants consumed about three liters of beer per day. In Coventry, the average weekly consumption of beer and ale was 17 pints per person per week (three pints per week today), Swedish beer consumption reached what is thought to be 40 times what it is today, English sailors were issued one gallon of beer per day, while English soldiers were issued two thirds of a gallon, in Denmark adult laborers and sailors consumed one gallon per day.

In 1668, Dom Perignon, a wine-master from a French abbey, created a sparkling champagne. He employed extra-thick glass bottles to contain the pressure, created a new and efficient cork and created the art of sparkling champagne. It would take another 100 years before the drink became popular.

Distilled Spirits

The original grain spirit, "whiskey," was first distilled in Ireland, whiskey was widely consumed in Scotland. It was in the 17th century that Franciscus Sylvius (aka Fraz de la Boe), a professor of medicine at the University of Leyden, distilled spirits from grain.

Distilled spirits were typically flavored with juniper berries. The flavored beverage was known as junever, a Dutch word which translates to "juniper." The French changed the name to genievre, which the English changed to "geneva," which was then shortened to "gin."

Gin was originally used for medicinal purposes, however, in 1690, the English passed "An Act for Encouraging the Distillation of Brandy and Spirits from corn," and within four years the annual production of distilled spirits, the majority of which was gin, reached more than one million gallons.

The 17th century colonialists from Virginia, carried on the European belief that alcoholic drink was a "natural food" and was good when consumed in moderation. Beer came with the original colonists, who believed "it was essential to their well being."

The Puritan minister Increase Mather preached in favor of alcohol and also preached against its abuse: "Drink is in itself a good creature of God, and to to be received with thankfulness, but the abuse of drink is from Satan; the wine is from God, but the Drunkard is from the Devil." At that time the first distillery was established in the colonies on what is now Staten Island, the production of hops began in Massachusetts, and both brewing and distilling were supported by legislation in Maryland.

Rum, originally produced in the West Indies by Europeans, is produced by distilling fermented molasses; by 1657, a rum distillery was operating in Boston. The Boston distillery became so successful that in only one generation the production of rum became colonial New England's biggest and most successful industry.

The English government began to actively promote gin distillation to use surplus grain and raise revenue through taxation. Suported by public policy, cheap gin began to flood the market as there was no negativity attached to excessive drinking and at the same time the growing numbers of poor in London sought relief from the harsh realities of big city life by drinking large quantities of gin - the result was the appearance of the "Gin Epidemic."

Resveratrol (phytoalexin)

Another important function of alcoholic beverages has been for therapeutic and medicinal purposes. In 1928, Johanna Brandt, a South African healer wrote a book entitled the *Grape Cure*, a collection of diseases, including cancer, heart disease and diabetes, that would benefit from the consumption of dark red grapes - there was something in those red grapes! Brandt, however, was considered a charleton by local medical associations and they chased her out of the United States.

The French consume more fat per person than any other culture in the world, yet they rank third on everyone's charts on health and longevity out of 193 nations. American physicians call this amazing phenomina the "French Paradox."

It is generally agreed throughout the scientific world that resveratrol, the anti-aging substance found in red wines are the basis for the "Grape Cure" and the "French Paradox."

USDA Analysis of Wine

Red Wine: for a 3.5 oz glass of red wine (103 g); 91 g of water, 9.6 g alcohol, 0.3 g ash (minerals), 0.2 g protein, 1.8 g of "Carbohydrate by difference," and 74 calories.

White Wine: for a 3.5 oz glass of white wine (103 g); 91.5 g of water, 9.5 g of alcohol, 0.2 g of ash (minerals), 0.1 g of protein, 0.8 g of "Carbohydrate by difference," and 70 calories.

Blush Wine: for a 3.5 oz glass of blush wine (103 g); 91.5 g of water, 9.6 g of alcohol, 0.2 g of ash (minerals), 0.2 g protein, 1.4 g of "Carbohydrate by difference," and 73 calories.

Resveratrol Content of Wine

Beverage	Resveratrol (mg/Liter)
Red wine (Global)	1.98 - 7.13
Red wine (Spanish)	1.92 - 12.59
Red wine (Tuscan)	0.3 - 2.1
Red Grape juice (Spanish)	1.14 - 8.69
Rose wines (Spanish)	0.43 - 3.52
Pinot Noir	0.40 - 2.0
White wines (Spanish)	0.05 - 1.80

Resveratrol Content of Selected Foods

Food	Serving Size	Total Resveratrol (mg)
Peanuts (raw)	1 C/ 146 g	0.01 - 0.26
Peanuts (boiled)	1 C/ 180 g	0.32 - 1.28
Peanut butter	1 C/ 258 g	0.04 - 0.13
Red grapes	1 C/ 160 g	0.24 - 1.25

Modern research reveals that the moderate consumption of red wine is preferable to complete abstenence. Red wine is known to reduce vascular inflammation and the risk of coronary heart disease and cancer, a plethora of degenerative diseases and to significantly increase longevity in yeast, worms, flies, fish, small mammalian vertebrates (including primates) and fish.

A 16-year study of 13,000 people in Denmark revealed that a daily glass of red wine could significantly reduce the risk of thrombotic stroke by 32%.

Resveratrol (trans-3, 4′, 5-trihydroxystilbene), is a fat soluble, powerful and naturally occurring polyphenol antioxidant, and it is found in varying amounts in wine. In general red wines contain more resveratrol than white wines do.

Grapes and wine grown in humid environments produce more resveratrol than wines grown in more arid environments. The theory for this phenomena is that grapes grown in humid environments produce more resveratrol in order to repell damaging fungi.

Resveratrol appears to function in animals and humans by activating a family of enzymes called sirtuins (Sir-2) - these proteins are involved in the same anti-aging effects as a Calorie Restricted diet.

Resveratrol can be found in the skins, seeds; notable grape varieties that contain high levels of resveratrol are muscadine grapes, Pinot noir grapes and Concord grapes.

Resveratrol is also found in the Japanese Knotweed (*Polygonum cuspidatum*), blueberries and peanuts.

In a study, which appeared in the November 11, 2005, issue of the *Journal of Biological Chemistry*, investigators demonstrated that resveratrol significantly lowers the levels of secreted and intracellular amyloid-beta (Abeta) peptides produced from different cell lines.

Several epidemiological studies indicate that the moderate consumption of wine is associated with a lower incidence of Alzheimer's disease.

The October 30, 2006 edition of the *Wall Street Journal* reported that studies on the red wine compound resveratrol extend animal lifespans by as much as 40%. Resveratrol was also considered for its potential life extending properties in an article related to Calorie Restricted diets in the October 31, 2006 edition of *The New York Times* - the scientific journal *Nature* published the original article that was quoted by both newspapers.

The study conducted on mice by Harvard Medical School and the National Institute of Aging researchers, finds that resveratrol negates the negative effects of a high-fat, high-calorie diet, a finding which experts are calling remarkable. In the study, one-year-old mice were randomly split into three groups, a control group fed a standard mouse pellet diet, a group fed a high-fat (60% fat), high calorie diet, and a group fed the same high-fat, high-calorie diet plus resveratrol. Within six months both groups of mice on he experimental diets had become obese. However, after a year, the mice which were also receiving the resveratrol were healthier, they did not develop the insulin resistance, heart disease or liver damage that their counterparts did. In addition the mice getting the resveratrol had a 31% lower risk of death.

Coffee

Coffee (*Coffea arabica*) has been consumed for more than 1,000 years as a health drink, central nervous system stimulant, physical stimulant, as an energizer and to increase one's metabolic rate. Today, approximately 60% of Americans drink a significant quantity of coffee daily.

Different types of coffee are preferred in different parts of the world. Arabica coffee is produced mostly in South and Central America, particularly in Brazil, Columbia, Mexico and Guatemala, while "robusta" coffee is produced mostly in African countries including the Ivory Coast, Uganda, Angola, etc. In the United States, Columbian and Central American coffees are preferred over Brazilian and African coffees. The March 1981 issue of *National Geographic* concluded that the world's annual coffee bean harvest would make 3,644,000,000 cubic feet of liquid coffee, a volume equal to the Mississippi's outflow for one and one half hours.

History of Coffee

There are several accounts that describe the discovery of the benefits of coffee. A favorite account tells of the legendary Sufi mystic Shaikh ash-Shadhili traveling through Ethiopia and that he noticed goats with great energy, whereupon he tried eating the berries that the goats were eating and he personally experienced the same increase in energy.

The second legend involves Kaldi, a goat herder from Caffa, Ethiopia, who told his friends about a strange "dancing" behavior in his goats after they consumed a particular plant. He noticed that his goats became hyperactive and jumpy (a behavior he described as dancing) after eating the red cherries from a shiny green plant when they changed pastures. He tried a few of the berries himself and was soon as hyperactive as his goats.

The story goes on that a local monk happened by and chastised Kaldi for "partaking of the devil's fruit." The monk soon realized, however, that the berries from the shiny green plant could help him stay awake longer and that he could then pray for several more hours each day.

Omar, an Arabian, and his followers were banished from a town for petty crimes and directed out to the desert where it was predicted that they would die of thirst and starvation. As a last resort, Omar and his friends boiled and ate the berries from the shiny green plant.

Omar and his band of friends not only survived, but they became folk legends and their survival was considered a religious sign by the local residents of the town called Mocha. Locally the previously humble plant was named after the town and became "mocha!"

The coffee plant is a native of the African nation of Ethiopia, however, through merchants and their use of traditional trade routes coffee was transplanted to Arabia where it became a significant and initially monopolized trade good. It is believed that the name coffee comes specifically from the Kingdom of Kaffa in Ethiopia.

Prior to 1000 A.D., the people of the Galla tribe of Ethiopia traditionally ground up the coffee berry, wrapped the ground up coffee bean in animal fat and used it as a source of energy on long trips or raids on neighboring tribes.

Arab merchants brought the energy laden beans back to their home countries and started coffee plantations about 1000 A.D. They called the boiled drink, "qahwa" which translates to "that which prevents sleep" or "qahhwat al-bun" which translates to "wine of the bean."

The first scientific writings on coffee appear as "Bunchum" in the writings of the 10th century Persian physician Razi. The most important of the early writers on coffee was Abd al-Qadir al-Jazin, who in 1857 compiled a history on coffee, including the legal controversies of coffee entitled Umdat al Safwa fi hill al-qahwa." He reported that Sheikh Jamal-al-Din al-Dhabhani, mufti of Aden, was the first to adopt the use of coffee (circa 1454).

The Turks were the first people to use coffee as a drink and that is why Turkish coffee is so highly prized by coffee experts yet today. The Turks often added spices such as cloves, cinnamon, cardamom and anise to the beverage to create unique flavors.

The export of the coffee plant outside of the Muslim nations was deemed to be a crime by governments and the world wide distribution of coffee was actually started as an illegal enterprise. An Arab by the name of Baba Budan smuggled the beans to Mysore, India and started a coffee plantation.

Coffee was introduced to Constantinople in 1453 by the Ottoman Turks who called the brew "kahve." The world's first "coffee shop" called Kiva Han opened there in 1475. At the same time Turkish law allowed that a woman could divorce her husband if he failed to provide her with her daily coffee.

In 1511, Khair Beg, a corrupt governor of Mecca, attempted to ban coffee because he feared that, "The brew's influence would kindle opposition to his power." Orthodox imams at a theological court in Mecca also banned the drink. The popularity of coffee, however, resulted in the bans being overturned by an order of the local Ottoman Turkish sultan Selim 1. He declared that, "Coffee and its use was sacred" and had the governor executed in 1524.

According to Leonhard Rauwolf's account, coffee became available in England in 1583, largely through the efforts of the British East India Company and the Dutch East India Company.

The first English coffee house was opened in St Michael's Alley in Cornhill. The proprietor was Pasqua Rose'e, a servant of Daniel Ewards. Edwards was a trader in Turkish goods who imported the coffee and financed Rose'e to set up the coffee house. The popularity of coffee houses spread rapidly throughout Europe and America and by 1675, there were more than 3,000 coffee houses in England alone!

In 1598, the word "coffee" entered the English language from the Italian word caffe'.

In 1600, coffee was introduced to the western world by Italian merchants.

In the early days of the introduction of coffee to the Christian world, the drink was believed to be "the devil's drink" and there were calls to ban the Muslim brew. Pope Clement VIII heard this complaint and decided to taste the coffee brew before he declared coffee drinking a sin. He enjoyed the coffee so much that in 1600 he baptized the drink and declared, "Coffee is so delicious it would be a pity to let the infidels have exclusive use of the drink."

In 1607, Captain John Smith introduces coffee to North America during the founding of the colony of Virginia at the village of Jamestown.

In 1645, the first coffee house opens in Itay. The busy trade between the merchants of Venice and the Muslims of North Africa, Egypt and East Africa introduced a broad variety of African goods. The merchants of Venice then decided to sell coffee to the wealthy of the city because they could charge a high price for the exotic drink.

In 1652, the first coffee house opens in England. Coffee houses quickly multiplied and became popular gathering places for people of all ranks of life, where discussions and the great debates of the day took place. The price of a cup of coffee was a penny, as a result coffee houses became known as "penny universities."

Antoine Galland (1646-1715) had translated the 1587 writings of Abd al-Qadir al-Jazin on the history of coffee for the French Royal Library and described the Muslim connection with coffee, tea and chocolate. He said, "We are indebted to the great (Arab) physicians for introducing coffee to the modern world through their writings, as well as sugar, tea and chocolate."

By 1668 coffee replaced beer as the universal breakfast drink in New York. In the same year Edward Lloyd's coffee house opens in England and is frequented by merchants and maritime insurance agents. The coffee house ultimately becomes Lloyd's of London, the most well known insurance company in the world.

In 1669, Soleiman Agha, Ambassador from Sultan Mehmed IV arrived in Paris with his entourage bringing with him a large supply of coffee beans. They treated their high ranking guests with coffee to drink and "by May of 1670, drinking coffee in side walk cafes was a custom in Paris."

In 1672, the first coffee house opened in Paris.

In 1675, Turkish forces surrounded the city of Vienna and threatened Austria itself. Franz Georg Kolschitzky, a Viennese citizen, of Polish extract (Franciszek Jerzy Kulczycki), who lived in Turkey, broke through the Turkish lines with a relief force and saved the city. In their haste, the fleeing Turks left behind many things including sacks of "dry black fodder" which Kolschitzky recognized as coffee. He claimed the coffee as his and promptly establishes central Europe's first coffee house in 1683. He invented the habit of filtering out the "grounds," sweetening the coffee with sugar and adding milk to the warm drink.

In 1690, the Dutch merchants smuggle live coffee plants out of the port city of Mocha to Ceylon and their East Indian colony of Java (the source of the drink's nickname) and they become the first people in the west to cultivate coffee commercially.

In 1713, the Dutch mistakenly provide Louis XIV of France with a live coffee bush. In 1723, Gabriel Mathieu do Clieu, a French naval officer, steels a coffee bush seedling and delivers it to Martinique. Within 50 years an official survey lists 19 million coffee trees in Martinique and over time 90% of the world's coffee production comes from the descendants of the single stolen plant!

In 1721 the first Berlin coffee house opens in Germany.

In 1727 the Brazillian coffee industry starts up when Lt. Colonel Francisco del Melo Palheta is dispatched by Brazil to arbitrate a border dispute between the French and the Dutch colonies in Guiana. He settles the dispute and he establishes a secret relationship with the wife of the French Governor.

Officially the French government closely held the cultivation secrets of coffee to prevent other nations from establishing competing coffee exports, however, when his lady bid him farewell, she sent Palheta off with a bouquet in which she had hid live plants and beans of coffee.

In 1732 Johann Sebastian Bach composes his famous Kaffe-Kantate. He wrote the piece partly as an ode to coffee and partly as a slap at the movement in Germany to keep women from drinking coffee. The cantata includes the aria, Ah! How sweet coffee tastes! Lovelier than a thousand kisses, than muscatel wine! I must have my coffee."

In December 1773, the "Boston Tea Party" makes drinking coffee a patriotic duty in America and countries that supported the fledgling nation.

In 1775, Frederick the Great of Prussia, attempted to block the import of green coffee, however, as Prussia's wealth was drained as citizens continued to buy the foreign beverage he relented and finally allowed the importation of green coffee.

By the 1800s, Brazil's coffee harvests changed coffee from an indulgence of the elite to a drink of the masses. Brazil relied heavily on slave labor from Africa to operate their coffee plantations until the abolition of Brazilian slavery in 1888. Brazil continued to be the largest coffee producer until the 19th and early 20th centuries when Columbia, Guatemala, Indonesia and Vietnam jumped into the coffee market. In the 21st century Vietnam ranked second only to Brazil in coffee production!

In 1886, Joel Cheek, originally a wholesale grocer, named his particular coffee blend "Maxwell House" after his hotel in Nashville, TN where his brew was featured as a hot drink.

In the early 1900s, the afternoon coffee gatherings of women in Germany become known as "KaffeeKlatsch" to describe the gossip sessions - the term was later used to describe gatherings of relaxed conversation where coffee was served.

In 1900 the Hills brothers begin packing and selling roast coffee in vacuum cans which resulted in the end of local roasting shops and the coffee mills.

In 1901 the first soluble "instant" coffee is invented and marketed by Satori Kato, a Japanese-American chemist from Chicago.

In 1903 Ludwig Roselius, a German coffee importer, donated a supply of damaged coffee beans to inventors who perfected the process of removing caffeine from the coffee beans without damaging the flavor. Roselius marketed the "decaffeinated" coffee under the brand name of "Sanka." The brand name of Sanka was not introduced into the United States until 1923.

In 1906 an English chemist by the name of George Constant Washington, notices a fine dust forming on the spout of his silver coffee carafe. After some time he perfects an instant coffee, which he mass-produces and markets under the brand name of "Red E Coffee."

By 1907, in less than a century, Brazil produces 97% of the world's coffee harvest!

In 1920 prohibition is voted into law, causing coffee sales to skyrocket!

In 1938, Brazil engages the Nestle Company to come up with a way to economically use their coffee surpluses. Nestle scientists create freeze-dried coffee and they market it in Switzerland as Nescafe.

By 1940 the United States imports 70% of the world's coffee crop!

In 1942 American GIs are issued Maxwell House coffee in their meal ration packages, while back in America widespread coffee hoarding and black market selling leads to coffee rationing by the government.

In 1946, Achilles Gaggia, an Italian, perfects the first espresso machine. Cappuccino is named for its color's resemblance to the color of the robes of the monks of the Capuchin order.

In 1969, one week before the Woodstock concert, the "Manson Family" murders coffee heiress Abigail Folger as she visits with her friend Sharon Tate at the home of the movie producer Roman Polanski.

In 1971, Starbucks (named for the first mate in Melvile's *Moby Dick*) opens its first coffee bean store in Seattle's Pike Place public market. In 1983, Howard Schultz, who started as a coffee bean salesman for Starbucks, visited Milan, Italy and fell in love with the environment of the "espresso bar." "It was about conversation. About community. About human connection. And fine coffee was the link. I thought. You know, we could do this in Seattle," says Schultz.

In April of 1984, Schultz set up a small espresso bar in the rear corner of the coffee bean store and offered "caffe latte" which created a marketing frenzy over the fresh-roasted whole bean coffee. Within days there were long lines on the sidewalk outside of the coffee bean store! He left Starbucks and opened his own espresso bar, which he called Il Giornale (The Daily). Two years later he bought out Starbucks and by 2008 he opened 8,500 stores world wide.

In mid-2008, Schultz was forced to close 600 Starbucks stores in the U.S. and two thirds of his Australian stores because of a widespread financial crisis - job transfers out of the U.S. to China, India and Mexico and a resultant housing mortgage collapse.

It was about 200 years ago that we learned that the "buzz" we got from coffee and tea was produced by the same phytochemical substance. The buzz was in fact produced by an alkaloid (caffeine) that is found universally in the leaves, seeds and the fruit of coffee, tea, cacao, kola and as many as 60 other plant species. This "wonder drug" was prescribed for human energy enhancement as far back as 500 B.C. by Lao-tzu, the spiritual leader who created Taoism.

In 1820 coffee shops flourished throughout Western Europe. At this time, Friedlieb Ferdinand Runge, a German chemist isolated and purified the active ingredient of coffee - caffeine or "something found in coffee." In 1838, plant chemists discovered that the buzz ingredient in tea was the same phytochemical as Runge's caffeine. Before the end of the 19th century caffeine would be found in kola nuts and cacao.

It was not an accident that coffee and tea became popular in Europe just as the Industrial Revolution was launched. The universal use of caffeinated drinks replaced the popular consumption of beer and paved the way for humans to move from the subsistence farm to the factory!

The act of boiling water to make coffee or tea reduced the incidence of water borne disease in the factory's employees and the caffeine prevented accidents by keeping them from falling asleep and falling into the machinery. Truly, coffee and tea greased the rails into the Industrial Revolution.

Caffeine, like other "drugs" has a significant impact on mental and physical performance. Numerous studies have shown that caffeine is analeptic (it stimulates the central nervous system) and ergogenic (improves energy levels and physical performance); it improves reaction speed, combats fatigue, improves performance in driving, flying, solving simple math problems and improves data entry accuracy.

In 2006 a significant study was released that showed the high antioxidant content of coffee (i.e. polyphenols, catechins, epicatechins, etc.) could reduce the risk of diabetes, heart disease and rheumatoid arthritis, and more specifically the caffeine in coffee was linked to relieving post workout pain and facilitating healthy fat metabolism.

Twenty-five years ago, lattes and cappuccinos were typically found in the coffee houses of New York, San Francisco and Seattle - now they are being offered in the humble fastfood environment including McDonald's, Jack in the Box and Dunkin' Donuts.

According to a National Coffee Association Study, the daily consumption of coffee in the United States for the year 2007 surpassed that of sodas for the first time in more than 15 years, with 57% of Americans drinking coffee every day compared to 51% for sodas. The United States imported 1.39 million tons of coffee in 2005.

In May of 2007 McDonald's began offering its McCafes' versions of lattes, cappuccinos and mochas at its stores in southern California and Michigan. McDonalds expects to "provide a latte at the highest quality but at an awesome price." McDonald's McCafe recently received a higher rating than Starbucks in a *Consumer Reports* taste test! Starbucks retaliated by offering hot breakfast sandwiches - an egg McMuffin with ingredients such as Havarti cheese, Black Forest ham and baby spinach.

Tea - "The Elixir of Immortality"

The tea plant (*Camella sinensis* or *Thea sinensis*), a native of southern China, was known from very early times to Chinese botanists and as a medicine to Traditional Chinese Medicine. It is written of by various names including Tou, Tseh, Chung, Kha and Ming, and was highly revered for its ability to relieve fatigue, delighting the soul, strengthening the will and repairing eyesight.

Tea could be administered as a drink internally, but as frequently it was applied topically as a paste to alleviate arthritis pains. The Taoists claimed it as an important ingredient of the "Elixir of Immortality." The Budhists used tea extensively to prevent drowsiness during their long hours of meditation.

By the 4th and 5th centuries, Tea became a favorite drink of the people of the Yangtse-Kiang Valley. It was during this time that the modern name, Cha was coined as a corruption of the more classic Tou.

Emperors rewarded ministers with rare blends of tea leaves for special services rendered. The leaves were steamed, crushed in a mortar, made into a cake, and boiled together with rice, ginger, salt, orange peel, spices, milk and sometimes onions. These customs of tea preparation remain today in Tibet and Mongolia. The use of lemon slices with tea was introduced by the Russians.

Luwuh, a poet, recognized in the Tea-service the "same harmony and order which reigned through all things." In his classic writings, the "Chaking" (*The Holy Scripture of Tea*), he formulated the Code of Tea. Since his writings, Luwuh continues to be "worshipped as the tutelary god of the Chinese tea merchants."

The "Chaking" is made up of three volumes and ten chapters. In the first chapter Luwuh discuses the nature of the tea plant, in the second he describes the tools required for the gathering of the leaves, in the third he talks about how to select the finest tea leaves. According to Luwuh, the best quality leaves must have "creases like the leathern boot of the Tartar horsemen, curl like the dew-lap of a mighty bullock, unfold like a mist rising out of a ravine, gleams like a lake touched by a zephyr, and be wet and soft like fine earth newly swept by rain."

The fourth chapter is devoted to the enumeration and description of the 24 members of the tea tools and equipment, starting with the tripod brazier and concluding with the bamboo cabinet for stowing the utensils.

Luwuh favored Taoist symbolism which also influenced the art of Chinese porcelain making. The Celestial porcelain had its beginnings in an attempt to produce the exotic and the exquisite shade of jade, resulting, in the Tang dynasty, in the blue glaze of the south, and the white glaze of the north. Luwuh believed the blue as the ideal color for the tea-cup, as it lent additional greenness to the tea; whereas the white imparted a pinkish and "distasteful result;" the result was not good because he used cake-tea.

Sometime later the tea-masters of Sung favored the powdered tea, they preferred heavy bowls of blue-black and dark brown colors. The Mings used steeped tea and preffered the lighter bowls of white porcelain.

In the fifth chapter Luwuh reveals the methods of making tea. He eliminated all ingredients except salt. He devoted much space to the choice of water and to the degree the water was boiled. Luwuh preferred mountain spring water, with river and spring water coming in second and third. He described 3 stages of boiling:

The first boil is when the little bubbles like the eye of fishes swim on the surface;

the second boil is when the bubbles are like crystal beads rolling in a fountain;

the third boil is when the billows surge wildly in the kettle.

The cake-tea is typically roasted before the fire until it becomes soft "like a baby's arm" and is shredded into powder between two pieces of paper. Salt is added to the first boil, the tea in the second. At the third boil, a dipperful of cold water is added to the kettle "to settle the tea and revive the youth of the water." The tea was then served and consumed.

The tea-room does not pretend to be other than a mere cottage - The simplicity and purism of the tea-room - Symbolism in the construction of the tea-room - The system of its decoration - A sanctuary from the vexations of the outer world.

The tea-room (the Sukiya) does not pretend to be other than a mere cottage - a straw hut, as it is usually referred to. The original characters, for the Sukiya, ment - the "Abode of Fancy." It is an Abode of Fancy in that it is built to welcome a creative impulse. It is an Abode of Vacancy as it is without decoration.

It is an Abode of the Unsymmetrical as it is designed for the witnessing of the Imperfect, leaving something unfinished on purpose to invite mental activity to create the completion. To the western eye the extreme Japanese simplistic interior of the tea-room appears barren.

The first free standing tea-room was the brain-child of Senno-Soyeki, generally known as Rikiu, the greatest and most revered of all tea-masters created and perfected the formalities of the Tea-ceremony. The dimensions of the tea-room had been determined earlier by Jowo, a highly regarded 15th century tea-master. The original tea-rooms consisted of a small portion of the drawing-room partitioned off by screens for the purpose of the tea-gathering. The portion partitioned off was referred to as the Kakoi or enclosure, a name that is still used to describe tea-rooms that are built into a private home. The Sukiya refers to the tea-room itself, it classically is designed to comfortably seat five or less people, symbolizing the thought "more than Graces and less than the Muses," an anteroom (midsuya) where the tea utensils are washed and arranged before being brought into the tea-room, a portico (machiai) in which the guests congregate until they are invited to enter the room, and a garden path (roji) which connects the machiai with the tea-room. The tea-room is in itself unimpressive in appearance. It is smaller than the smallest of Japanese houses, and the materials used in its construction are purposely intended to give the idea of "refined poverty." A good tea-room will cost more than a typical mansion!

Green tea (*Camella sinensis* or *Thea sinensis*) and black tea both originate from the same plant and differ only in the preparation. Green tea is dried for a short period of time and heated sooner than black tea to prevent fermentation (China and Japan). Black tea comes from India, Sri Lanka, Kenya, Indonesia, Turkey, Pakistan, Malawi and Argentina. In the 21st century tea is a $750 million cash crop in India's eastern state of Assam alone. Historically there is thought to be three stages in the evolution of tea.

The three stages of the evolution of Tea:

The Boiled Tea, the Whipped Tea, and the Steeped Tea, representative of the Tang, the Sung and the Ming dynasties of China - Luwuh, the first apostle of tea - the Tea - ideals of the three dynasties - To the latter-day Chinese Tea is a deliscious beverage, but not an ideal - In Japan, Tea is a religion of the art of life.

As of 2007, China consumes 700,000 tons of tea each year.

Green tea contains xanthines, caffeine, theobromine, tannins, polyphenols, catechins, flavonoids, oils and fats and vitamin C. The catechins in green tea are the antioxidants credited with significant anti-cancer activity (can reduce risk of cancer by as much as 90%). Catechins are 100 times more potent than vitamin C and 25 times more potent than vitamin E in neutralizing free radicals.

Over thousands of years human cultures have designed rituals to enhance the pleasure when they consume their favorite beverage. Frequently, the preparation ritual or ceremony has evolved to the point that it adds significant value to the drink. T. R. Reid says, "In Japan's austerely elegant chanoyu, or tea ceremony, the simple surroundings of the tearoom, the soft rustle of kimono across tatami floor, the spare beauty of a hand-molded brown cup, matter as much as the tea itself." The earliest record of tea in European writings is said to be found in the statement of an Arabian traveler, that after the year 879 A.D. the main sources of revenue in Canton were the duties on salt and tea. Marco Polo records the deposition of a Chinese minister of finance in 1285 A.D. for his arbitrary augmentation of the tea-taxes. It was at the period of the Great Discoveries that the European people began to know more about the extreme Orient.

At the end of the 16th century the Hollanders brought the news that a pleasant drink was made in the East from the leaves of a bush. The travelers Giovanni Batista Ramusio (1559), L.

Almeida (1576), Maffeno (1588), Tareira (1610), also mentioned tea. In the last-named year, ships of the Dutch East India Company brought the first tea into Europe. It was known in France in 1636, and reached Russia in 1638. England welcomed tea in 1650 and generally spoke of it as "That excellent and by all physicians approved China drink, called by the Chineans Tcha, and by other nations Tay, alias Tee."

Like many good things found in the world, the mystique and marketing of tea generated opposition. Henry Saville (1678) denounced drinking tea as a "filthy custom." Jonas Hanway (Essay on Tea, 1756) said that, "men seemed to lose their stature and comeliness, women their beauty through the use of tea." Its cost in its first introduction to the west (15 or 16 shillings a pound) prevented popular consumption and made it "regalia for high treatments and entertainments, presents being made thereof to princes and grandees."

The coffee houses of London in the second half of the 18th century became tea-houses, the haunts of writers and artists such as Addison and Steele who "beguiled themselves over their dish of tea." Tea quickly became a necessity of life and as a result - taxable.

In 1711, the *Spectator*, stated, "I would therefore in a particular manner recommend these my speculations to all well-regulated families that set apart an hour every morning for tea, bread and butter; and would earnestly advise them for their good to order this paper to be punctually served up and to be looked upon as a part of the tea-equipage."

Samuel Johnson described himself as "a hardened and shameless tea-drinker, who for twenty years diluted his meals with only the infusion of the fascinating plant; who, with tea, amused the evening, with tea solaced the midnight, and with tea welcomed the morning."

Colonial America accepted the King of England's oppression until he imposed a 3% tax on tea. The American Revolution against England began with Samuel Adams and a loyal band of revolutionaries (Sons of Liberty) dressing as

Indians and throwing imported English tea into the Boston Harbor as a protest.

The "Boston Tea Party" began when the British Parliament passed the Tea Act in 1773 in hopes of forcing the colonies to purchase tea directly from Great Britain's failing East India Company rather than from colonial importers, who often sold smuggled tea purchased from Holland through the Dutch East India Company.

The new law was seen by Americans as an attempt by Great Britain to undercut local merchants in order to reward a London monopoly, and a tea boycott soon spread throughout the colonies. However, a boycott seemed too passive a strategy for Boston's Samuel Adams.

On December 16, 1773 Adams led a wild meeting that was sponsored by the Sons of Liberty at Boston's Old South Church. A crowd of more than 8,000 people attended and filled the hall and the crowd soon spilled out onto the street. Adams, who was a charismatic speaker, whipped the crowd into hysteria, and urged the crowd to defy the British by throwing the officially approved tea into the Boston Harbor.

At a signal from Adams, dozens of members of the Sons of Liberty appeared from the back of the church made up as Mohawk warriors. They led the screaming crowd to the wharf, where H.M.S. Dartmouth, Eleanor and Beaver were tied up. They then boarded the vessels and proceeded to throw 342 large bales of British tea overboard!

Adams was commited to have a political victory without causing a bloody response from the British. He convinced the rebels to restrain themselves, "No violence or you'll hurt the cause!" As one patriot wrote, "We were surrounded by British armed ships, but no attempt was made to resist us."

The Boston Tea Party energized and galvanized the entire population of the American Colonies. Parliament countered by passing five laws that the Americans quickly labeled the "Intolerable Acts," which closed Boston Harbor, established martial law, and effectively abolished local and state government in Boston and the entire state of Massachusetts.

Though the Intolerable Acts only directly affected Massachusetts, the severity of these five laws united the colonials everywhere, and caused them to quickly organize a Continental Congress.

At that moment the colonials moved from the cry, "No taxation without representation," to "Give me liberty or give me death!"

After hearing of the events in Boston, King George III predicted, "The die is now cast. The Colonies must either submit or triumph."

Chocolate

The Spanish first found the Mayans drinking a beverage considerably different from what we usually think of as hot chocolate.

The Maya preferably consumed hot chocolate thick and foamy. While standing, the Maya poured the chocolate beverage from a spouted pot into another vessel on the ground. The act of pouring over a distance, combined with the fatty cacao butter, produced a thick head of rich, dark, chocolate foam - the most revered part of the drink. The scientific name for the cacao tree is, *Theobroma cacao*, or "food of the gods."

In 1981, a team of archaeologists from the University of Texas at Austin, discovered 14 spouted drinking vessels used by the ancient Mayan civilization dating back from about 900 B.C. to A.D. 1300. The origin of chocolate use goes back to the Olmec civilization which preceded the Maya. The Olmec, or "rubber people," were the first culture in the Western Hemisphere to relish chocolate.

In modern times, chocolate is thought of as an

indulgence, as something that overweight and obese people gorge themselves on - yet, chocolate can be one of the great natural herbal weight control products ever known to man.

Studies published in the *Journal of the American College of Nutrition*, reported that chocolate does not raise cholesterol or increase LDL.

In a 2003 issue of the journal, *Hypertension*, it was reported that the flavanoids in cacao could help increase blood flow to the heart, brain, hands and legs.

An article in the *Journal of Agriculture and Food Chemistry*, reported that cacao has a higher antioxidant rating than tea or red wine.

When people crave chocolate, they are really mineral deficient (pica, munchies, etc.). In fact, bitter, dark unsweetened chocolate has a very low glycemic index because up to 70% of the chocolate's calories come from fat, and fat does not raise blood sugar.

Cacao butter, the fat in chocolate, is comprised of stearic acid (34%), palmitic acid (20%) and oleic acid (30%). Both stearic and palmitic acids are saturated fats; oleic acid is a mono-saturated fat that is also found in olive oil.

Cacao powder is made when the fat, or "Cocoa butter," is pressed out of the "liquor" - most cocoa powders have little or no fat.

Chemistry of Chocolate

Chocolate is a rich source of cocoagin, caffeine, theobromine, flavanol and flavonoids. These compounds have thermogenic (energy generating) properties and antioxidant properties that make bitter chocolate a great energy generator, a great weight loss product and a super free radical neutralizing herb.

Dozens of scientific studies have found that chocolate is rich with a broad range of phytonutrients. The class of phytonutrients, known as polyphenols, are one of dark chocolate's most important chemical constituents. These phytochemicals include some of the most potent antioxidant and anti-inflammatory compounds that occur in nature. Polyphenols occur as flavonoids or bioflavanoids, phenolic acids, simple phenols, phenylpropanoids, quinines, stilbenes and xanthones.

Flavanoids make up two-thirds of the polyphenol family of phytochemicals. Flavanoids typically cause the the plant (cocoa, green tea, etc.) to have a bitter taste - "bitter" chocolate. Chocolate, with a dark color and bitter taste, has a significant level of clinically useful antioxidants.

Anthocyanins are an extremely valuable subgroup of flavonoids that provide extra nutritional benefits. Anthocyanins provide anti-inflammatory and antioxidant features and also supports the body's ability to metabolize sugar. Supporting healthy metabolism and healthy blood sugar levels lowers the risks of developing type II diabetes and obesity. Anthocyanins are able to support healthy blood sugar levels and efficiently neutralize free radicals.

Anthocyanins are unusual in that they prevent and repair free radical damage to small blood vessels. Damage to blood vessel's walls (inflammation) is the direct cause of atherosclerosis, coronary thrombosis and stroke. Anthocyanins can block histamine response, reduce the affects of allergic reactions, inflammation and irritation. Several studies showed that anthocyanins can stop the inflammation associated with arthritis, gastric ulcers, diabetes and cardiovascular disease.

Catechins and epicatechins are phytonutrients that add to chocolate's disease relieving arsenal. Studies show that catechins and epicatechins prevent the creation of carcinogens, and they initiate and support the body's inherent "detoxification" and defense processes. Many investigators believe that epicatechins should be listed as a third category of vitamins: i. e. - 1) fat soluble; 2) water soluble; 3) flavanols/ catechins.

Many additional categories of polyphenols and phytonutrients are found in chocolate. Dozens of significant and well respected studies have shown that the antioxidant nutrients found in chocolate can lead to a longer, more energetic and fuller life!

An important phytochemical found in chocolate is phenylethylamine (PEA), this neurotransmitter stimulates the body's pleasure centers. Large quantities of PEA are associated with feelings of excitement, attraction and sexual pleasure. It is the affects of the PEA in chocolate that has caused chocolate to be given as a traditional seductive gift for Valentine's Day, anniversaries and to get out of the "dog house."

Anandaminde is another neurotransmitter found in chocolate. This phytochemical targets the same brain structures that are targeted by the active ingredient in marijuana - THC.

The cardiovascular benefits of dark chocolate are considerably higher than those attributed to green tea, red wine and other whole food antioxidants.

A team of researchers from the Harvard School of Public Health reviewed 136 studies on the relationship of chocolate and cocoa to cardiovascular health. The study included research ranging from lab tests to human studies. The research team concluded that chocolate is a major source of flavanoids (epicatechins, catechins and procyanidins) and determined that "the primary fat in chocolate (stearic acid) did not have adverse effects on blood vessels, cholesterol or overall cardiovascular health" because it is metabolized differently than other types of saturated fats.

The Harvard study also concluded that regular chocolate intake can lower blood pressure, decrease vascular inflammation, decreased rates of thrombosis, increased levels of HDL and lowered levels of LDL, improved vascular endothelial function and health, increased nitric acid production and increased activity of prostacyclins, which support the relaxation of blood vessels.

Research performed jointly by a team from the University of California, Davis and Tufts University, and published in 2005 in *The American Journal of Clinical Nutrition*, demonstrated that the proanthocyanin and flavanol content of cocoa demonstrated significant antioxidant properties and the ability to protect the heart and vascular systems. According to Dr. Carl Keen, "These nutrients have been shown to affect numerous intracellular signaling cascades, and to influence the cardiovascular system by enhancing vascular function and decreasing platelet activity."

A 2006 study completed by a team of researchers from the University of California-Davis and the University of Dusseldorf, Germany determined that the compound epicatechin found in cocoa is directly linked to improved circulation and other hallmarks of healthy cardiovascular function. The researchers stated that, "The results of the study provide direct proof that epicatechin is responsible for the beneficial vascular effects observed after the consumption of certain flavanol-rich cocoa (foods)."

Crucial to this study were volunteers from the Panamanian tribe of Indians called the Kuna. High blood pressure and other negative signs of cardiovascular disease are rare amongst the island-dwelling Kuna, who are also known to consume large amounts (3 to 4 cups per day) of chocolate in the form of a traditional beverage.

Further studies showed that the Kuna who migrated to urban environments, and consequently consume less cocoa, do not enjoy the same level of cardiovascular health.

When the Kuna returned again to a high consumption level of cocoa, the researchers found that the risk factors for cardiovascular disease were reduced significantly.

The well respected investigators Mary and Marguerite Engler completed a study that elucidated the mechanism of how chocolate improves the health of the endothelial lining of blood vessels. In their studies, 21 subjects were given either a high-flavanoid dark chocolate or a low-flavanoid dark chocolate every day for two weeks. The results indicated that those individuals eating the high-flavanoid dark chocolate had a significantly higher endothelial (vascular lining) function than those consuming the low-flavanoid chocolate.

Chocolate Tasting

There are many ways to evaluate chocolate; one is by the percentage of chocolate in the product; the country of origin; another is by the ORAC value; and yet another is by taste.

Evaluating and choosing chocolate by taste is done much in the same manner as evaluating and choosing a good wine. Taste is defined by categories: "Chocolatey," "Fruity," "Nutty," "Earthy," "Floral," and "Citrus."

Calorie Restricted Diets

Calorie Restricted diets (without malnutrition), universally known to increase the life span of all laboratory, pet and farm animals, is a common thread found amongst centenarians in history and currently amongst centenarians in all Blue Zones.

In most cases the caloric levels fall between 1,250 and 1,800 calories per day, with those performing more physical labor consuming the higher calorie levels.

Mineral-rich Diets

Mineral rich diets, found universally in all Blue Zones, are an absolute requirement to reach the centenarian club. In all cases, the Blue Zones have multiple sources rich in a wide spectrum of minerals.

A high protein, low carbohydrate diet is relatively forgiving of a low vitamin intake, but unforgiving of a low mineral diet.

Sources of Nutritional Minerals in the Blue Zones

Glacial Milk

River silt

Rock dust

Wood ashes (universal)

Kelp ashes

Sea weed ashes

Rice straw ashes

Peat moss ashes

Manure ashes

Land Mines

Land mines that will certainly prevent you from reaching 100 years of age include smoking, drinking excess alcohol, using street or prescription drugs, not getting second medical opinions, eating fried foods (trans fatty acids), eating burnt or well-done meats (heterocyclic amines), consuming sugar and large quantities of super-heated carbohydrates (acrylamides), indulging in dangerous high-risk behaviors (DUI, mountain climbing alone, exercise without supplementing, prescription drugs, prescription polypharmacy, etc.).

One of the unintended benefits of the Blues Zones is that they are remote and have little or no access to doctors, pharmaceuticals, commercial French fries, fried chicken, fried fish, fried shrimp, fried clams, high fructose corn syrup, soft drinks, white flour, etc.

Looking Good

Avoiding the land mines includes not "doing yourself in" as a result of unintended consequences. Included in the timeless and endless quest for a "fountain of youth" is a passion for beauty - to many, "beauty" is a significant aspect of and an outward sign of "youth."

Gray hair, wrinkles, blemishes, sagging facial and body parts and lack of energy are universally interpreted as the inevitable signals and outward signs of decline, aging and the harbingers of a shortened life and impending death.

Over thousands of years great and powerful leaders have left no stone unturned and have spent vast sums of money, rivaling the expenditures of the Crusades and the construction of monuments (pyramids) looking for endless youth and immortality to no avail.

Even when Columbus convinced the Queen of Spain to fund his exploration for a westerly route to the "West Indies," riches and plunder for Spain, her personal interest was in having the accountant (Ponce de Leon) of the mission to look for a "Fountain of Youth" and a source of immortality.

Even in the 21st century longevity "experts" give little hope for a simple cost effective method of healthfully extending life and "looking good until the end."

It is therefore, not too surprising that a great deal of personal energy, time and money is spent by the average person in the pursuit of beauty, youth and longevity. Great pain ("plastic surgery," chemical peels, BoTox, etc.) and risks of injury (infections, misadventure, malpractice, etc.) and death (gastric bypass surgery, liposuction, etc.) are braved in this endless quest of beauty, youth and longevity.

We believe that it is worth learning how to use and apply non-invasive anti-aging vitamin-mineral supplements, non-surgical facelifts, non-chemical peels, phyto-hormones (i.e. phyto-estrogens, phyto-progesterones, HGH, thyroid support, adrenal support, etc.) and beauty products and non-toxic cosmetics safely.

Chapter 13

"The true remedies were pure air, sunlight, abstentiousness, rest, exercise, proper diet, pure water, and faith in the healing power of God"

Helen White
Battle Creek Sanitarium, 1863

Religious Dietary Practices

All human cultures have developed dietary laws, many of which are attached to their religious beliefs. It is of interest to note that just about all gerontologists highlight a deep abiding religious faith as a common feature of people who live beyond 100 years of age.

There are dietary taboos from ancient times that prevent the consumption of certain foods that are perceived as dangerous or sinful. Across the global spectrum of man's history is his observation that he is dependant upon nature and therefore God for food and life.

In some religions, a prohibition on the consumption of stimulating drinks (i.e. coffee, tea, cocoa, alcohol, etc.), certain meats (i.e. predators, carrion eaters, vultures, hyenas, garbage eaters, catfish, crab, shrimp, those that are not cud-chewers, pigs, etc.) and methods of cooking have demonstrated over long periods of time to be beneficial for reducing the risk of degenerative diseases and for extending life spans.

In other cases some religions, such as the Seventh-day Adventists and Mormons, have proactively encouraged the consumption of fruit and vegetables (i.e. antioxidants, etc.), a practice which has been shown to reduce the risk of degenerative diseases and extend life spans.

Many religions require their members to avoid gluttony (one of the seven "deadly sins") and eat sparingly, eating only for their minimal requirements and then in addition require fasting, all of such practices encourage a Calorie Restricted diet.

There are religions that espouse some form of meat restriction (eat meat "sparingly") or some form of "vegetarianism" - some are as old as Hinduism and Jainism and some as new as Seventh-day Adventism and Mormonism. There are the strict orthodox dietary laws of Judaism and a spin-off of those dietary laws which became an integral practice of Mohammedanism.

There are dietary laws that are professed by early religious practice that separate people from people and caste from caste.

In the collection and diversity of Christian faiths there are the days of feasting and the days of fasting (abstinence and self-denial) and the Sacrament of the Lord's Supper. There is Christ's direct instruction to his disciples to mention bread in their prayers.

It is therefore not too far out of line to say that "in the beginning God created diet."

"And the Lord God commanded the man, saying, Of every tree of the garden thou mayest freely eat;

But of the tree of knowledge of good and evil, thou shalt not eat of it; for in the day that thou eatest thereof thou shalt surely die."

The Concept of Forbidden Fruit

The forbidden fruit, as it is called, is commonly romanticized as a sexual prohibition, however, early Bible interpretation and some modern religious groups, particularly the Mormons, believe that the prohibition was just as the Bible says it was - a food unsuited for man's body in its newly created and immortal state. And, when the first man and woman, who were made in the image of God, first ate "the forbidden fruit," their bodies fell vulnerable to disease, decay and death.

It was, therefore, through diet, that humanity, gained the knowledge of good and evil and of the dire consequences of bad choices, of cause and effect.

This direct interpretation of the Book of Genesis has been part of Judaic and Christian law for centuries and is thought to be the basis of the German proverb, "man ist was man isst!" - "man is what he eats."

The concept that, certain foods are unclean and dangerous, thus making the body an unfit abode for the spirit has long been a touchstone of religious belief that persists even yet today.

The religious concept that grains, vegetables and fruit are good is widespread even today. In the Sinai Desert, where the Israelites wandered for 40 years, manna filled a huge gap in the subsistence diet of the Children of Israel. There are two forms of manna, one that "rained from heaven" and one that "sprang from the ground."

The manna that sprang from the heavens appears to have been a mix of flower and tree pollen, the manna that sprang from the ground is a lichen of the genus *Lecanora spp.* that grew on the ground and rocks in large patches and is said to taste like honey on a cracker.

Fertility and Food

Fertility ceremonies and myth related to the harvest season and the Earth's bounty were an integral part of the ancient religion and mythology of Sumer. According to the Epic of Gilgamesh, which is believed to be the oldest writing existing in recorded history, it seems sprang full-grown upon the earth, like Athena from the head of Zeus, around 3500 B.C.).

Therefore, even before the story of the Creation was written down in Genesis, the abundance of the earth was celebrated in legend and interwoven with worship - and food and diet as part of religion has been in the historical record ever since.

Fasting and Health

Along with the gratitude to God and the Earth for abundance, there has always been the consideration and practice of asceticism (one who led an austere life of self denial) to prove to God that the practitioner loved Him.

The practice of fasting or severely restricting one's diet in order to "subdue the flesh and strengthen the soul" is also as old as religion. There were sects among the Jews who made abstinence part of their doctrine -the Essenes.

Before Christ began his ministry he retired to the desert wilderness, fasted and prayed for 40 days and overcame his temptations that were offered by the devil.

Paul, in his first epistle to the Corinthians, drew a parallel between the athlete's life and the Christian life. The word *ascetic* is derived from the Greek word for exercise, and was intended to transmit the concept of the strict health regimen and diet of the athlete. Asceticism has been espoused as a tool to fight the war against the deadly sins of gluttony, envy, pride, sloth, covetousness, anger and lust.

The early Anchorite Christians purposely wandered in the deserts of the Middle East and Africa looking for a pure life that would be pleasing to God and they ate only what the desert provided (a very severely Calorie Restricted diet).

Catholics observe the rules of abstinence during Lent, the Muslims fast during Ramadan, the Mormons fast the first Sunday of each month.

In China, the diet and fasting of Taoism play a role, with certain foods and herbs supplying the vital energy for specific organs. According to the Tao, the heart is related to fire, the lungs to metal, the kidneys to water and foods that nourish these organs include poultry, vegetables and fish.

In Confucianism, dietary laws were connected to ancestor worship, and when one was making a sacrifice to their ancestor's spirits they took great care to ensure that their diet was ritually proper.

The Hindus and Jainists of India proscribed meat because of their belief of the transmigration (reincarnation) of souls. No living creature could be killed for meat as the soul inhabiting the creature might have once been or might eventually be the soul of a man.

The Jainists were so strict that they carefully inspected fruit and vegetables before they would eat them to ensure that they did not have any insects or grubs on them - some went to the extreme to wear masks to prevent the inhalation of small flying insects.

Buddhism, which began in India and spread throughout Asia, had strict laws prohibiting the killing of animals but held no prohibition on eating them. The only time that Buddhist's prohibit the consumption of meat is during ritual feasts and celebratory fasting.

Strong or Stimulant Drinks

The prohibition of alcoholic beverages is one of the five precepts of the Middle View in Buddhism and the concept of the Middle View led to the ethic of moderation in eating (Calorie Restricted diet) and to the ethic that is against suicide through fasting.

In Islam, "strong drink" (distilled liquor) is unequivocally forbidden, however, wine is reluctantly permitted - there is "sinfulness in wine but also some utility." The Koran concludes that the sinfulness of wine outweighs the usefulness of wine.

The Children of Israel were more liberal regarding strong drink. In their early scriptures describing the Promised Land "flowing with milk (Glacial Milk) and honey (verdant fields and abundant orchards)," they were appreciative for the bounty of nature, however, they were also strict regarding their dietary laws.

The dietary strictures in Leviticus and Deuteronomy are simple and direct: No meat of predators, either birds or beasts; no animals that do not have a cloven hoof, and even if they do have a cloven hoof they must also chew the cud. No seafood that does not have fins and scales. No reptiles. Only certain insects could be consumed; and absolutely no consumption of blood. Later, came the Talmud and the "hedge about the Law" which became the most strict and the most complex of all dietary laws in history.

Amish

The Amish (Pennsylvania Dutch) are members of the original Dutch Reform Church, a conservative Christian sect who have opted out of the American Social Security System, Medicare and private insurance and have since their beginnings in the 15th century looked to themselves for health care and self insurance.

The Amish operate today as 18th century farmers and have rejected electricity and other modern conveniences and still use wood to heat their homes and cook their meals. Wood ashes (plant minerals) are an important byproduct of daily living for the Amish; they use the wood ash (plant minerals) added to compost as fertilizer in their gardens.

The Amish employ horses to get around in buggies and wagons; they use horses to pull and power farm implements.

The Amish are born in their homes and die in their homes. The use herbs, nutritional supplements, homeopathic remedies, acupuncture, chiropractors, naturopathic physicians and midwives as health professionals - they have for the most part opted out of the modern medical system and they take care of their elderly in their own homes.

Mormon

The state of Utah is 70% Mormon and is the healthiest state and the longest lived peoples in America. According to the National Center for Health Statistics, Utah has the lowest death rate from virtually all the common degenerative diseases.

Joseph Smith was killed by a mob in 1844, not long before the Mormons escaped Nauvoo; however, by that time Smith had compiled his book of his visions and revelations and this book became the Doctrine and the Covenants of the Mormon faith.

Literally driven by mobs from the Illinois city of Nauvoo, the Mormons made their epic migration west so they could live isolated from the rest of the world.

The Mormon religion (Latter Day Saints of Jesus Christ) is a relatively new American religion. Their beliefs say the Mormon religion began in 1820 near the small town of Manchester, New York - a boy of 14 named Joseph Smith sought help in prayer because he was bewildered by the religious upheavals and rivalries of the times. "God the Father and Jesus Christ appeared to him and told him not to become involved with any existing denomination."

Joseph waited three years for further enlightenment and then according to the *Book of Mormon*, "A messenger from God appeared, a man named Moroni who had once lived on the North American continent and whose ancestors had escaped from Jerusalem before the Babylonian captivity.

Moroni related the story of a historical record to Joseph, that Moroni's father, a man named Mormon, had given to him to hide before he and his people were killed by their bitter enemy from the same branch of Isreal - the American Indians.

Moroni told Joseph Smith where the record was hidden and how it was to be translated. In modern times, the Book of Mormon and the Bible, together, form the core scriptures of the Church of Jesus Christ of Latter-day Saints."

In 1800, a bounty was placed on the heads of Mormons by the Governor of Missouri; this event precipitated a legendary mass migration of Mormons from Nauvoo, Illinois, east of the Mississippi River westward to Salt Lake City, Utah.

The Mormons live an average of 10 years longer than the average American. A common and consistent thread that is the touchstone of the Mormon religion is their dietary laws. The 89th Section of the Doctrine and Covenants, the Word of Wisdom was revealed on February 27, 1833 - this section gives Mormons their basic laws of diet and health:

"For, behold, the beasts of the field and the fowls of the air, and that which cometh of the earth, is ordained for the use of man for food and for raiment, and that he might have in abundance."

Doctrine and Covenants 49:18,19

The Mormons are very faithful in avoiding "stimulant drinks" which includes alcoholic drinks, caffeine (coffee, tea, soft drinks, energy drinks, energy herbs, stimulating herbs, etc.), they restrict calories and limit meat intake to a secondary position behind the consumption of grains and vegetables.

As a group the Mormons tend to live a smoke free lifestyle that is based on strong parenting beliefs.

According to Brigham Young, Smith's successor as president of the Mormon Church, Smith was conducting a class for members of the priesthood. This class was held in a small room above the kitchen of Smith's home and the room was frequently clouded with large volumes of tobacco smoke. To Smith, the atmosphere in the room was unseemly, so one day he left the room, "inquired of the Lord" and received the Word of Wisdom.

Essentially, the instructions, which were given "not by commandment or constraint, but by revelation and the word of wisdom," were in keeping with the traditional Christian attitude, that all foods are for man. The prohibitions are for non-foods - tobacco, alcohol and "hot drinks" which were interpreted to mean drinks containing harmful drugs, such as tea, coffee, caffeine containing "soft" drinks and chocolate.

The remainder of the revelation was a proactive statement regarding nutrition and the prudent consumption and storage of food:

Every herb in its season and every fruit in its season to be used with prudence and thanksgiving.

Flesh of beasts and fowl to be used sparingly. "And it is pleasing unto me that they should not be used, only in times of winter, or of cold, or famine."

All grain is good for man and all plant food "whether

in the ground or above the ground" - wheat for man; corn for the ox; oats for the horse; rye for the fowls and swine; and barley for all useful animals and for mild drinks.

It is a precept of the Mormons to be prepared. Every church or "ward," has a "bishop's storehouse" from which members can draw on in time of need.

Mormons eat for the sake of their physical and spiritual health and they fast for the same reason. It is traditional for the Mormon to fast on the first Sunday of each month and give the price of two Sunday meals to help the needy.

Mormon Health and Longevity

The average lifespan of Mormons is 10 years longer than that of the average American. Dr. James E. Enstrom, of the School of Public Health, University of California at Los Angeles, examined a 1965 study done by the California State Department of Health that showed Mormons in Alameda County, across the bay from San Francisco, have a total mortality rate of only 55% of the adult population of the county as a whole. The original sample was small, 111 Mormons in a total of 6,928 people, however, the data reinforced statistics from other sources.

When Dr. Enstrom reviewed data which the U.S. Cancer Institute had gleaned from the U.S. Census and state mortality records, he learned that areas of Utah that are heavily Mormon have lower death rates than areas with a lower percentage of Mormons.

In one area in particular - Utah County, just south of Salt Lake City, where Provo is, there is a Mormon population of 85% compared to 70% for all of Utah. And Utah County's cancer-death rate is lower than the state's as a whole and only 65% as high as the U.S. as a whole.

Enstrom then examined the cancer death rate among California's 400,000 Mormons using membership information and names of those who had died, and mortality records, showing the cause of death (supplied by the state of California); the data revealed that California Mormons have a cancer death rate of only slightly more than half (55%) of the U.S. cancer death rate.

Seventh Day Adventist

The Seventh Day Adventist, are a relatively young American religion, who pursue a strict vegetarian diet.
No religious movement, ancient or modern, has put greater emphasis on diet and nutrition than the Seventh-day Adventist church - on the average the Adventists live eight to ten years longer than the average American.

Long before nutrition reached the level of a science, Ellen G. White was teaching Seventh-day Adventists in the basic concepts of healthy living. In addition to denouncing the use of alcohol and addictive drugs (i.e. tobacco, alcohol, pharmaceuticals, street drugs, etc.) she insisted on a "well-balanced diet" before the phrase was coined.

More than 70 years ago White stated that tobacco is "a slow, insidious, but most malignant poison." She also emphasized the avoidance of preserved meats and refined foods, particularly white flour and sugar - she was one of the first natural food enthusiasts.

In the early part of the 1800s, in numerous parts of the Christian world, there was a sudden awareness of the second coming of Christ - the leaders of many established churches became caught up in the new Reformation.

One of the believers of imminent second coming of Christ (Adventists) was William Miller. After a serious study of biblical prophecy, Miller concluded that Christ would return to earth on October 22, 1844. Despite their disappointment when the appointed day came and went, many of the "Millerites" remained faithful and continued to meet in small groups and study the Bible and pray.

Among these loyal Millerites was a young woman named Ellen Harmon. In December of 1844 at an Adventist meeting in Portland, Maine Harmon had her first vision.

Ellen Harmon (became Mrs. James White) became the guiding force of the Seventh-day Adventist Church - it was only a few weeks later that she saw the famous vision of the last days of the world that showed her "the only hope of mankind - obedience to the commandments of God."

During her vision there was a special emphasis on the Fourth Commandment, to keep the Sabbath day holy, and it was shown to the young woman that the Sabbath was the seventh day, not the first, so in 1861 the church formally adopted these two primary beliefs into its name. Her books have sold in the tens of millions, making her one of the best-selling and most prolific authors of all time. Just one book, *Steps to Christ,* has sold more than 10 million copies and has been translated into 80 languages.

White inspired and directed the begining of a vast network of missions, schools and colleges, hospitals, clinics and dispensaries in all parts of the globe, including the well known school of medicine at Loma Linda University, 60 miles east of Los Angeles.

In 1863, Ellen White saw the vision that still forms the core of the Adventist diet and health programs. The event is often referred to as the "Otsego vision" because it came in the home of some Adventists whom she was visiting in Otsego, Michigan:

"It is wrong to eat merely to gratify the appetite, but no indifference should be manifested regarding the quality of the food, or the manner of its preparation. If the food eaten is not relished, the body will not be so well nourished. The food should be carefully chosen and prepared with intelligence and skill."

"Here is a suggestion for all whose work is sedentary or chiefly mental; let those who have sufficient moral courage and self control try it: At each meal take only two or three kinds of simple food, and eat no more than is required to satisfy hunger. Take active exercise every day, and see if you do not receive benefit."

"For use in bread making, the superfine flour is not the best. Its use is neither healthful nor economical. Fine-flour bread is lacking nutritive elements to be found in bread made from the whole wheat. It is a frequent cause of constipation and other unhealthful conditions."

"Those who eat flesh are but eating grains and vegetables at second hand; for the animal receives from these things the nutrition that produces growth. The life that was in the grains and vegetables passes into the eater. We receive it by eating the flesh of the animal. How much better to get it direct, by eating the food that God provided for our use!"

In the same year of 1863, the headquarters of the church was established in Battle Creek, Michigan, and it was there that the first Adventist medical institution was established. At first it was called the Western Health Reform Institute, and then simply the Battle Creek Sanitarium and then affectionately the "San."

Basically the Adventists follow the instructions in Leviticus concerning clean and unclean food. Pork is forbidden, as is shellfish, and the flesh of predators. Adventists also abstain totally from the use of alcohol, tobacco and harmful drugs, including coffee and tea - many believers do not eat meat and those who do eat it only "sparingly."

White became suspicious of the widespread and careless use of "poisonous drugs" by the doctors of the day - at the Battle Creek Sanitarium the "true remedies" were "pure air, sunlight, abstentiousness, rest, exercise, proper diet, pure water and faith in the healing power of God."

By 1903, when the church headquarters was moved to Washington, D.C., the sanitarium, was the largest and best equipped health institution in the world. Its medical superintendent was Dr. John Harvey Kellogg, and it was he and his brother, W. K. Kellogg, who gave the world cornflakes - W. K. Kellogg started the prepared breakfast cereal industry.

Immortality

The answer, the secrets of health, longevity and even immortality are hidden in plain view - its only a matter of knowing the basic "language of immortality" to then be able to translate all of the different "dialects of immortality" into a single universal language!

References

Aetios of Amida: The Gynaecology and Obstetrics of the VIth Century A.D. (Translated from the Latin edition of Cosonariores, 1542, by J.V.Ricci).

Agatston, A.: The South Beach Diet. Random House New york. 2003.

Ahrens, L.H.: Distribution of the Elements in Our Planet. McGraw-Hill. New York.1965.

Alexander, C.: If the Stones Could Speak. National Geographic. 34 - 59. June, 2008.

Anon: Basic Guide to Canine Nutrition. White Plaines, New York. Gaines Dog Research Center. 1965.

Anon: Daily Nutrient Requirements of Pigs. Pub.1192. Nat. Acad. Sci. Nat. Res. Council. 1964. pp 12-14.

Anon: Nutrient Requirements of Beef Cattle. Nat. Acad. Sci. NRC. Pub. 1137.1963.

Anon: Nutrient Requirements of Horses. In: Nutrient Requirements of Domestic Animals. 2nd Ed. Nat. Acad. Sci. Nat. Res. Council. Pub.1401. 1966.

Anon: 25 ways to look ten years younger. OK. 42 - 45. June 9, 2008.

Asensi, M., Medina, I., Ortega, A., et al: "Inhibition of cancer growth by resveratrol is related to its low bioavailability." Free Radic. Biol. Med. 33 (3):387 - 98. August 2002.

Atkins. R. C.: Dr. Atkins' New Diet Revolution. Avon Books. New York. 2002.

Awika, J.M., et al: Screening methods to measure antioxidant activity of sorghum (Sorghum bicolor) and sorghum products. J. Agric. Food Chem., 51:6657 - 6662. 2003.

Bacchiocca, M., Biagiotti, E. and Ninfali, P.: Nutritional and technological reasons for evaluating the antioxidant capacity of vegetable products. Ital. J. Food Sci. 2006, 18:209-217.

Bailey, F. L.: Navajo Foods and Cooking Methods. Am. Anthro. 42:270-90. 1940.

Banik, A. E.: Hunza Land. Whitehorn Publishing Company. Long Beach, CA. 1961.

Barinaga, M.: How Long is the Human Life Span? Science. 254:936-938. 2008.

Barrows, Jr., C.H. and Kokkman, G.C.: Diet and Life Extension in Animal Model Systems. Age. 1:31.1978.

Baur, J. Pearson, K. et al: Resveratrol improves health and increases survival of mice on a high-calorie diet. Nature. 2006. 10.1038.

Bazzarre, T. L.,et al.: Chronic Disease Risk Factors in Vitamin/Mineral Supplement Users and Non-users in a Farm Population. J. Am. Coll. Nutr. 10:3.1991. pp247-257.

Bear, F. E.: Chemistry of the Soil. 2 ed. Chapman and Hill. London. 1964.

Beare, S.: 50 Secrets of the World's Longest Living People. Marlowe & Company. New York. 2003.

Berg, B. N.: Nutrition and Longevity in the Rat.I. Food Intake in Relation to Size, Health and Fertility. July, 1960. J. Nutr. (71).p242-254.

Berg, B.N. and Simms, H.S.: Nutrition and Longevity in the Rat.II. Longevity and Onset of Disease with Different Levels of Food Intake. J. Nutr. 71:255-263. July, 1960.

Berry, R.: The Vegetarians. Autumn Press. Brookline, MA. 1978.

Bland, J.: Diagnostic Usefulness of Trace Elements in Human Hair. Northwest Diagnostic Services. Bellvue, WA. 1981.

Bland, J.: Hair Tissue Mineral Analysis: An Emergent Diagnostic Technique. Bellvue-Redmond Medical Laboratories. WA. 1979.

Boezo, M.H.: De Pica. Sm. Leipsig.1638.

Bondy, P. K. and Rosenberg, L. E.: Metabolic Control and Disease. (8th ed.). W. B. Saunders Co. Philadelphia. 1974.

Brizzee, K. R. and Ordy, J.M.: Age Pigment, Cell Loss and Hippocampal Function. Mechanisms of Aging and Development. 9:143.1979.

Buettner, D.: The Blue Zone. National Geographic. Washington, D.C. 2008.

Buettner, D.: Living Healthy to 100. AARP Magazine. 57 - 59. May/June, 2008.

Cardarelli, N. F.: Tin as a Vital Nutrient: Implications in Cancer Prophylaxis and other Physiological Processes. CRC-Press. Boca Raton, FL.1986.

Carlander, O.: Aetiology of Pica. Lancet. 277:569.1959.

Carlisle, E.M.: In Vivo Requirements for Silicon in Articular Cartilage and Connective Tissue Formation in the Chick. J.Nutr. 106:478.1976.

Carlson, A.H. and Hallzel, F.: Apparent Prolongation of the Life Span of Rats by Intermittent Fasting. J. Nutr. 31:363.1946.

Chan, F.I., et al.: Selenium Deficiency and Keshan Disease. Chinese J Med. June 1979.

Christensen, N. K.: Juniper Ash as a Source of Calcium in the Navajo diet. J. Am. Diet Assoc. 98(3) 333-334. March 1998.

Cook, J.: Diet and Your Religion. Woodbridge Press Publishing Company. Santa Barbara, CA. 1976.

Cooper, M.: Pica: A Survey of the Historical Literature as Well as Reports from the Fields of Veterinary Medicine and Anthropology, the Present Study of Pica I Young Children, and a Discussion of it's Paediatric and Physiological Implications. Charles Thomas. Springfield, IL. 1957.

Corliss, R. and Lemonick, M. D.: How to Live to be 100. Time. New York. August 30, 2004.

Crabb, C.: The Nutrients are Blowing in the Wind. U.S. News & World Report. October, 1991. p66.

Deeming, S. and McDermid, A.M.: Hair Analysis of Trace Elements in Hunan Subjects as Influenced by Age, Sex and Contraceptive Drugs. Am. J. Clin. Nutr.31:1175.1978.

Denton, D.: The Hunger for Salt: An Anthropological, Physiological and Medical Analysis. Springer-Verlag. Berlin. Heidelberg. New York. 1982.

Diamond, J.: Guns, Germs and Steel. W. W. Norton & Company. New York. 1997.

Diamond, J.: Collapse. Viking. New York. 2005.

Diaz, F., et al.: Comparative Performances of Baby Pigs Fed Infant and Baby Pig Diets. J. Nutr. May,1959. pp131-140.

Easton, J.: Human Longevity: Recording the Name, Age, Place of Residence and Year of the Deceased of 1712 Persons Who Attained a Century and Upwards from AD 66 to 1799, Comprising a Period of 1733 years with Anecdotes of the most Remarkable. London. 1799.

Eaton, S.B., et al.: The Paleolithic Prescription: A Program of Diet & Exercise and a Design For Living. Harper & Row, Publishers. New York. Cambridge. 1988.

Edwards, C.H. et al.: Odd Dietary Practices of Women. J. Am. Diet. Assoc.30:976.1954.

Edwards, C.H., et al.: Clay and Corn Starch Eating Women. J.Am. Diet. Assoc. 35:810.1959.

Edwards, C. H., et al.: Effects of Clay and Corn Starch Intake on Women and Their Infants. J. Am. Diet. Assoc. 44:109.1964.

Elliott, P. J. and Jirousek, M.: "Sirtuins: Novel targets for metabolic disease." Current Opinion in Investigational Drugs. 9 (4):1472-4472. 2008.

Erten, J., et al.: Hair Zinc in Healthy and Malnourished Children. Am. J. Clin. Nutr. 32:570. 1979.

Fixx, J. E.: The Complete Book of Running. Random House, Inc. New York. 1977.

Freese, B.: Coal. Penguin Books. London. 2003.

Freund, H. et al: Chromium deficiency during total parenteral nutrition. JAMA. 241(5): 496-8. 1979.

Ferguson, J.H. and Keaton, A.G.: Studies of Diets of Pregnant Women in Mississippi: Ingestion of Clay and Laundry Starch. New Orleans Med. Surg. J. 102:460.1950.

Galdston, I.(ed.): Human Nutrition: Historic and Scientific. The New York Academy of Medicine. International Universities Press, Inc. New York. 1960.

Geargakas, D.: The Methuselah Factors. Simon and Schuster. New York. 1980.

Gershoff, S. N., et al.: Trace Minerals in Human and Rat Hair. Am. J. Clin. Nutr. 30:868. 1977.

Gescher, A.J., Steward, W.P.: Relationship between mechanisms, bioavailability, and preclinical chemopreventive efficacy of resveratrol: a conundrum. Cancer Epidemiol Biomarkers Prev. 2003; 12(10):953-957.

Ghen, M. J.(ed): The Advanced Guide to Longevity Medicine. Partners in Wellness and Mitchell J. Ghen. Atlanta, GA. 2001.

Giroud, A.: Nutrition of the Embryo. Fed. Proc. 27:163-184.1968.

Goldstein, M. and Beall, C.: The Remote World of Tibet's Nomads. Nat. Geo. 175:6. June,1989.pp752-781.

Green, H. H.: Perverted Appetites. Physiol. Rev.5:336.1925.

Grenoble, P.B.: Pritikin People. Berkley Books.New York.1986.

Gu, L., House, S. E., Wu, X, Ou, B and Prior, R,L.: Procyanidin and catachin contents and antioxidant capacity of cocoa and chocolate products. J. Agric. Food Chem. 2006, 54:4057-4061.

Gutelius, M.F., et al.: Nutritional Studies of Children with Pica.II. Treatment of Pica with Iron Given Intramuscularly. Paediatrics. 29:1018.1962.

Hambridge, K.M. and Rodgerson, D.O.: Comparison of Hair Chromium Levels of Multiparous and Parous Women. Am. J. Obstet, Gynec.103:320.1969.

Hanson, D. J.: History of Alcohol and Drinking Around the World. Google 2007.

Harman, D.: Free Radical Theory of Aging: Nutritional Implications. Age. 1:145.1978.

Harman, D.: Free Radical Theory of Aging: Origin of Life, Evolution and Aging. Age.3:100.1980.

Harman, D.and Eddy, D.E.: Free Radical Theory of Aging: Effect of Adding Antioxidants to Maternal Mouse Diets on Lifespan of the Offspring. Age.1:162.1978.

Harrington,A.: The Immortalists. Random House. New York. 1969.

Harris, M.: Cannibals and Kings. Vintage Books. New York. 1977.

Hayflick, L.: The Cellular Basis for Biological Aging. In: Handbook of the Biology of Aging. (ed. C.E.Finch and L. Hayflick). Van Nostrand Reinhold.1977.

Heaney,R.P. and Barger-Lux, J.: Low Calcium Intake: The Culprit in Many Human Diseases. Feedstuffs.July,1994.pp14-17.

Hendrikkson,P, Krook, L. and Larsen, B.: Mechanism of Bone Resorption in a Case of Human Periodontal Disease. Svensk. Tandl.Tidskn. 62:323.1969.

Herbert, V.: Nutrition Cultism. George F. Stickley Company. Philadelphia,PA.1980.

Hisanaga, A.,et al.: Variation of Trace Metals in Ancient and contemporary Japanese Bones. Bio. Trace Ele. Res. 22:221-231.1989.

Hoekstra, W.O.: Biochemical Function of Selenium and its Relationship to Vitamin E. Fed. Proc. 34:2083. 1975.

Howard, Sir Albert: The Soil and Health: A Study of Organic Agriculture. Schocken Books. New York. 1972.

Isaacson, W.: Benjamin Franklin. Simon & Schuster Paperbacks. New York. June 2003.

Isaacson, W.: Einstein. Simon & Schuster. New York. 2007.

James, W.P.T., et al.: Calcium Binding by Dietary Fibre. Lancet.1:638.1978.

Jarvis, D.C.: Folk Medicine. Henry Holt and Company. 1958.

Jeejeebhoy, K. N. et al: Chromium deficiency, glucose tolerance, and neuropathy reversed by chromium supplementation, in a patient receiving long-term total parenteral nutrition. Am J Clin Nutr.30(4): 531-38. 1977.

Jensen, B.: Health & Long Life. Bernard Jensen Enterprises. Escondido, CA. 1975.

Josephson, M.: Edison. McGraw-Hill. 1959.

Kahlenberg, L. and Class, J.O.: The Presence of Aluminum in Animal and Plant Tissues. J.Biol.Chem.83:261.1929.

Katsuhiko, Yokoi, et al.: Effect of Dietary Tin Deficiency on Growth and Mineral Status in Rats. Biol. Trace Ele. Res. The Humana Press, Inc. 24:223. 1990.

Kaufmann, K.: Silica: The Amazing Gel. Burnaby, B.C. Canada. Alive Books. 1992.

Kern, F.: Normal Plasma Cholesterol in an 88 Year Old Man Who Eats 25 Eggs a Day. New Eng.J.Med. March,1991. pp896-899.

Kitchen, H., et al.: Hemoglobin Polymorphism:Its Relation to Sickling of Erythrocytes in White-tailed Deer. Science.144:1237-1239. June, 1964.

Klevay, L.: Hair as a Biopsy Material. Arch. Intern. Med.138:1127.1978.

Klug, A. and Rhodes, D.: Zinc Fingers: A Novel Protein Motif for Nucleic Acid Recognition. In: Trends in Biochemical Sciences. 12:464. Dec. 1987.

Krause, M. and Mahan, L. K.: Food, Nutrition and Diet Therapy. (7th ed.). W.B. Saunders Company. Philadelphia. 1984.

Kruglinski. S.: West's World. DISCOVER. Summer. 2008. pp 82-85.

Kulczycki, L. L. and Schauf, V.: Cystic Fibrosis in Blacks in Washington, D.C. Am. J. Dis. Child. 127:64.1974.

Kurlansky, M.: Salt: A World History. Penguin Books. London. 2002.

Lagouge, M., Argmann, C., Gerhart-Hines, Z., et al: "Resveratrol improves mitochondrial function and protects against metabolic disease by activating SIRTI and PGC-1alpha." Cell.127 (6): 1109 -22. 2006.

Lanzkowsky, P.: Investigation into the Aetiology and Treatment of Pica. Arch.Dis. Child.34:140.1959.

Leaf, A.: Every Day is a Gift when you are Over 100. Nat. Geo.143:1. January, 1973. pp92-119.

LeConte, J.: Observations on Geophagia. South. Med. Surg. J.1:417.1846.

Liu, R.K. and Walford,R.L.: The Effect of Lowered Body Temperature on Lifespan and Immune and Non-Immune Processes. Gerontologica.18:363.1972.

Long, V.M., et al.: Manganese Metabolism in College Men Consuming Vegetarian Diets.J.Nutr.85:132-138.March,1965.
Mann, C. C.: Our Good Earth. National Geographic. September 2008. pp 80 - 111.

Marambaud,P., Zhao, H. and Davies,P.: Resveratrol promotes clearance of Alzheimer's disease amyloid-beta peptides. J. Biol Chem. Nov. 2005.11:280 (45): 377-82.

Marden, L.: Titicaca: Abode of the Sun. Nat. Geo. 139:2. February,1971. pp 272-291.

Marek, A. C.: Live Longer and Healthier. Smart Money. 51 - 57. June 2008.

Maron, B. J., et al.: Sudden Death in Hypertrophic Cardiomyopathy: A Profile of 78 patients. Circulation. 65:1388. 1982.

Maron, B. J., et al.: Sudden Death in Young Athletes. Circulation. 62:218.1979.

Maugh,T.: Hair: A Diagnostic Tool to Compliment Blood, Serum and Urine. Science.202:1271.1978.

McCarry, J.: High Road to Hunza. Nat. Geo. March,1994. pp 114-134.

McDonald, R. and Marshole, S.R.: Value of Iron Therapy in Pica. Paediatrics.84:558.1964.

McGlothin, P. and Averill, M.: The CR Way. Harper Collins. New York. 2008.

McKay, C.M., et al.: The Effect of Retarded Growth Upon the Length of Life Span and Upon the Ultimate Body Size. July,

1935. J.Nutr.pp63-79.

McNeill, J.H.: Biological Effects of Vanadium. The University of British Columbia, Vancouver, B.C. June 16, 1993.

Mergiletus, A.F.: Pica: Doctoral Thesis in Medicine. Submitted to Academia Patria. 1701.

Mertz, W.: Chromium occurrence and function in a biological system. Physiol. Rev. 49: 163-230. 1969.

Mertz, W.(ed):Trace Elements in Human and Animal Nutrition. Academic Press,Inc. New York.1987.

Mertz, W. and Schwarz, K.: Chromium (III) and the glucose tolerance factor. Arch. Biochem. Biophys. 85:292-5. 1959.

Michaud, S. and Michaud, R.: Trek to Lofty Hunza and Beyond. Nat. Geo. November,1975. 148:5.pp644-669.

Miller, K.B., et al: Antioxidant activity and polyphenol and procyanidin contents of selected commercially available cocoa-containing and chocolate products in the United States. J. Agric. Food Chem. 2006, 54:4062-4068.

Murray, M. and Lyon, M.: How to Prevent and Treat Diabetes with Natural Medicine. Riverhead Books. New York. 2003.

Nash, J. M.: Cracking the Fat Riddle. Time. September 2, 2003.

Newman, C.: Why are we so fat? National Geographic. August 2004.

Nielsen, F.H.: Vanadium. In: Trace Elements in Human and Animal Nutrition. Vol. 1. 5th ed (Mertz, W. ed.) 1987.

Nielson, F.H.: New Essential Trace Elements for the Life Sciences. Biol.Trace Ele. Res.199.1990.pp599-611.

Ninfali, P. et al: Antioxidant capacity of vegetables, spices and dressings relevant to nutrition. Brit. J. Nutr. 2005, 93:257-266.

Olmstead, L. Schrauzer, G. N., et al.: Selenium Supplementation of Symptomatic Human Immunodeficiency Virus Infected Patients. Biol. Trace Ele. Research. Humana Press, Inc. 20:59. 1989.

Olshansky,S.J., et al.: In Search of Methuselah: Estimating the Upper Limits to Human Longevity. Science.250:634-640. November,1990.

Oppenheimer, E.H. and Esterly, J. R.: Pathology of Cystic Fibrosis. Review of the Literature and Comparison with 146 Autopsied Cases. In: Perspectives in Pediatric Pathology. Vol. 2. Yearbook Medical Pub., Inc. Chicago. 1975. pp 241-278.

Parr, R.M., et al.: Minor and Trace Elements in Human Milk from Guatemala, Hungary, Nigeria, Phillipines, Sweden and Zaire. Bio.Trace Ele.Res.29:51-75.1991.

Pauling, L.: How to Live Longer and Feel Better. W.H. Freeman and Co. New York. 1986.

Pearson, D. and Shaw,S.: Life Extension. Warner Books, Inc. New York.1982.

Porter, R.: Greatest Benefit. W.W. Norton & Company. New York. 1997.

Reynolds, R.D., et al.:Pagophagia and Iron Deficiency Anemia. Ann.Inter.Med.69:435.1968.

Rhodes, D. and Klug, A.: Zinc Fingers. Scientific American. February 1993. p56.

Sandberg, A-S, et al.: The Effect of Wheat Bran on the Absorption of Minerals in the Small Intestine. Br.J.Nutr.48:185.1982.

Schrauzer, G. N., et al.: Lithium in Scalp Hair of Adults, Students and Violent Criminals. Biol. Trace. Ele.Res. 34:161.1992.

Schrauzer, G. N., et al.: Lithium in Drinking Water and the Incidences of Crimes, Suicides, and Arrests Related to Drug Addictions. Biol. Trace. Ele. Res. 25:105.1990.

Schrauzer, G.N.: Selenium in Nutritional Cancer Prophylaxis: An Update. Vitamins, Nutrition and Cancer. Karger. Basel. Pp240-250. 1984.

Schrauzer,G.N.: Selenium: Mechanistic Aspects of Anticarcinogenic Action. Biol. Trace Ele. Res. The Humana Press, Inc. 33:51. 1992.

Schrauzer, G.N., et al.: Effect of Simulated American, Bulgarian, and Japanese Human Diets and of Selenium Supplementation on the Incidence of Virally Induced Mammary Tumors in Female Mice. Biol. Trace Ele. Res. The Humana Press, Inc. 20:169.1989.

Schrauzer, G.N., et al.: Cancer Mortality Correlation Studies-III:Statistical Associations with Dietary Selenium Intakes. Bioinorganic Chem. 7:23.1977.

Schrauzer, G.N., et al.: Selenium in the Blood of Japanese and American Women with and Without Breast Cancer and Fibrocystic Disease. Jpn. J. Cancer Res. 76:374. May 1985.

Schwarz, K.: Essentiality and Metabolic Functions of Selenium. Med.Clin.North Am. 60:745-758. July,1976.

Schwarz, K. and Foltz, C.M.: Selenium as an integral part of Factor 3 Against Dietary Necrotic Liver Degeneration. J.Am. Chem. Soc. 19:3292.1959.

Senturia, B.D.: Results of Treatment of Chronic Arthritis and Rhuematoid Conditions with Colloidal Sulphur. J.Bone Joint Surg.16:119-125.1934.

Sheehan, G.: Dr. Sheehan on Running. Bantam Books. New York. 1978.

Sheehan, G.: Medical Advice for Runners. World Publications. Mountain View, CA. 1978.

Shu-Yu Yu, et el.: A Preliminary Report on the Intervention Trials of Primary Liver Cancer in High-Risk Populations with Nutritional Supplementation of Selenium in China. Biol. Trace Ele. Res. The Humana Press, Inc. 29:289.1991.

Shu-Yu Yu, et al.: Chemoprevention Trial of Human Hepatitis with Selenium Supplementation in China. Biol. Trace Ele. Res. The Humana Press, Inc. 20:15.1989.

Sinclair, D. A., et al: "Calorie Restriction Promotes Mammalian Cell Survival by Inducing the SIRTI Deacetylase." Science. 305 (July 16, 2004):309-392.

Somers, S.: 365 Ways to Change Your Life. Crown Publishers. New York. 1999

Somers, S.: AGELESS. Crown Publishers. New York. 2006

Spezioli, M., et al.: Gallium Distribution in Human Brain Areas. Biol. Trace Ele. Res. 22:9.1989.

Stevenson, T.: 101 Essential Tips: WINE. DK. London, New York. 2003.

Stwertka, A.: A Guide to the Elements. 2nd Ed. Oxford University Press. Oxford. 2002.

Suzuki, F., et al.: Ability of Sera From Mice Treated with Ge-132, an Organic Germanium Compound, to Inhibit Experimental Murine Ascites Tumours. Br.J. Cancer. 52:757.1985.

Taggart,N.:Food Habits in Pregnancy. Proc.Nutr.Soc. 20:35.1961.

Tang, R-H, et al.: Stimulation of Proliferation of *Tetrahymena pyriformis* by Trace Rare Earths. Biol. Trace Ele. Res. 7:95.1985.

Tarpy, C.: Place of the Standing Stones. National Geographic. New York. May 2004. pp 66-79.

Taylor, R.:Hunza Health Secrets. Prentice Hall, Inc. New Jersey.1966.

Thomas, W.J.: The Longevity of Man, It's Facts and It's Fiction. London.J.Murray.1873.

Tobe, J.: Hunza: Adventures in a Land of Paradise. George J.McLeod.Ltd.Ontario.1960.

Tus, H. et al,: Keshan Disease as it Relates to Selenium Status. Chin J. Med. 1979.

Tus, H. et al.: Selenium in the Heart of China. Lancet. 27 Oct. 1979. p899.

Underwood, E.J.: Trace Elements in Human and Animal Nutrition. Academic Press. New York and London.1962.

Valenzano, D.R., et al: Resveratrol prolongs life span and retards the onset of age-related markers in a short-lived vertebrate. Cur. Biol. 2006. Feb. 7;16 (3):296-300.

Van Vleet, E. J., et al.: Hepatos Dietetia and Mulberry Heart Disease Associated with Selenium Deficiency in Indiana Swine. J. Am.Vet.Med. Assoc. 157:1208.1970.

Voorhees, E. B.: Fertilizers. The MacMillan Company. New York. 1926.

Walford, R.L.: The Immunological Theory of Aging. Munkagaard. Copenhagen. 1969.

Walford, R.L.: Maximum Lifespan. W.W.Norton & Company. New York.London.1983.

Walford, R.L.: The 120 Year Diet. Simon and Schuster. New York. 1986.

Wallach,J.D.:Goitrogenic Hypothyroidism in Feeder Lambs. VM/SAC. 60:1051-1053. 1965.

Wallach, J.D.: Degenerative Arthritis in a Black Rhino. JAVMA.151:887-889.1967.

Wallach, J.D.: Nutritional Diseases of Exotic Animals. JAVMA.157:5883-599. September, 1970.

Wallach,J.D.: The Nutrition and Feeding of Captive Ruminants in Zoos. In: Church, D.C.:Digestive Physiology and Nutrition of Ruminants. Corvallis. Oregon State University Press. Vol.3.1972.pp292-307.

Wallach, J. D.: Cystic Fibrosis: A proposal of Etiology and Pathogenesis. Workshop on Model Systems for the Study of Cystic Fibrosis. May 25-26, 1978. N.I.H., Bethesda, MD.

Wallach, J. D. and Boever, Wm.: Diseases of Exotic Animals. W. B. Saunders Company. Philadelphia. 1983.

Wallach, J.D. and Flieg, G.M.: Nutritional Secondary Hyperparathyroidism in Captive Birds. JAVMA. 155:1046.1969.

Wallach, J. D. and Garmaise, B.: Cystic Fibrosis: A Perinatal Manifestation of Selenium Deficiency. 13th Annual Conference on Trace Substances in Environmental Health. June 4-7, 1979. University of Missouri, Columbia, MO.

Wallach,J.D. and Hoessle,C.: Fibrous Osteodystrophy in Green Iguanas. JAVMA. 153:863-865. 1968.

Wallach, J.D. and Hoessle, C.: Steatitis in Captive Crocodilians. JAVMA. 153:845-847. 1968.

Wallach, J.D., Hoessle, C. and Bennet,J.: Hypoglycemic Shock in Captive Alligators. JAVMA. 151:893-896. 1967.

Wallach, J. D. and Ma, L.: Black Gene Lies. Wellness Publications, LLC. Bonita, CA. 2007.

Wallach, J. D. and Ma, L.: Dead Doctors Don't Lie. Wellness Publications, LLC. Bonita, CA. 1999.

Wallach, J. D. and Ma, L.: Energy Crisis. Wellness Publications, LLC. Bonita, CA. 2007.

Wallach, J. D. and Ma, L.: God Bless America. Wellness Publications, LLC. Bonita, CA. 2002.

Wallach, J. D. and Ma, L.: HELL'S KITCHEN. Wellness Publications, LLC. Bonita, CA. 2005.

Wallach, J. D. and Ma, L.: Let's Play Doctor! Wellness Publications, LLC. Bonita, CA. 1989.

Wallach, J. D. and Ma, L.: Let's Play Herbal doctor. Wellness Publications, LLC. Bonita, CA. 2001.

Wallach, J. D. and Ma, L.: Passport to Aromatherapy. Wellness Publications, LLC. Bonita, CA. 2005.

Wallach, J. D. and Ma, L.: RARE EARTHS: forbidden cures. Wellness Publications, LLC. Bonita, CA. 1994.

Wallach, J. D., Ma, L., Yu, W. H., Gu, B. Q., Yu, F. T. and Goddard, R. F.: Common Denominators in the Etiology and Pathology of Visceral Lesions of Cystic Fibrosis and Keshan Disease. Biol. Trace Ele. Res. Humana Press, Inc. 24:189. 1990.

Wallach, J.D. and Middleton, C.C.: Naturally Occuring Atherosclerosis in Aoudads (*Amotragus Lervia, Pallas*). Acta Zool. Pathol. Antverpiensia. 50:45-54.1970.

Wallach, J.D. and Wallach, J.E.: Rhino Express.Vantage Press. New York.1978.

Weil, A.: Healthy Aging. Anchor Books. New York. 2005.

Werbach, M.R.: Nutritional Influences on Illness. Third Line Press, Inc. Tarzana, CA.1987.

Werbach, M.R.: Nutritional Influences on Mental Illness. Third Line Press, Inc. Tarzana, CA.1991.

Willcox, B. J., Willcox, D. and Suzuki, M.: The OKINAWA PROGRAM. Clarkson Potter/Publishers. New York. 2001.

Williams, R.J.: Nutrition Against Disease. Pitman. New York.1971.

Willius, F.A. and Smith, H.L.: Further Observations on the Heart in Old Age. A Post Mortem Study of 381 Patients Aged 70 Years or More. Am. Heart Jour.8:170.1932.

Wolf, G.: "Calorie Restriction Increases Life Span: A Molecular Mechanism." Nutrition Reviews.64.2 (Feb. 2006): 89-92.

Wolfe, W. S., Weber, C. W. and Arviso, K. D.: Use and Nutrient Composition of Traditional Navajo Foods. Ecology Food Nutr. 17: 323-44. 1985.

Yu,S.Y., et al.: Selenium Chemoprevention of Liver Cancer in Animals and Possible Human Applications. BioTrace Ele. Res.15:1988.pp231-241.

Zhang, W.E. et al.: Effects of Traces of Rare Earth Elements on the Protozoan Blepherisma and on Mice. Biol. Trace Ele. Res. 17:81-90. 1988.

INDEX

A

B

C

D

E

F

G

H

I

J

K

L

M

N

O

P

Q

R

S

T

U

V

W

X

Y

Z

Let's Play Doctor

The Book That "Orthodox" Doctors Couldn't Kill - "How to" maximize your genetic potential for health and longevity.

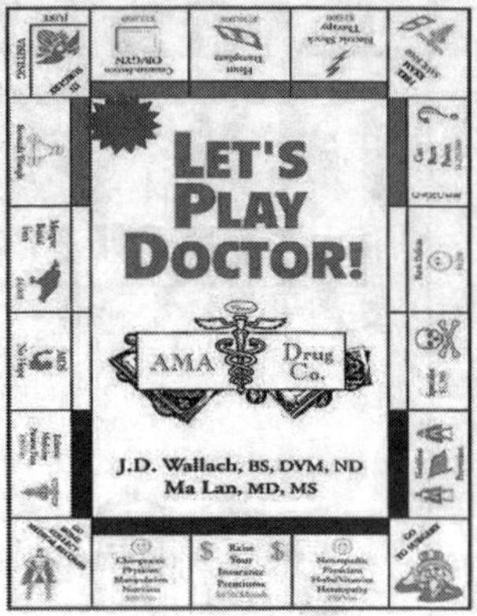

- Become your own primary health care provider
- Learn The Alternative Healing Arts
- Establish your own Health Clinic
- Establish a Home Pharmacy
- Home Surgery

$14.95 - 10 or more $8.00 each

Rare Earths Forbidden Cures

Their Secrets of Health and Longevity

The definitive home reference on minerals, mineral deficiencies and their relationship to:

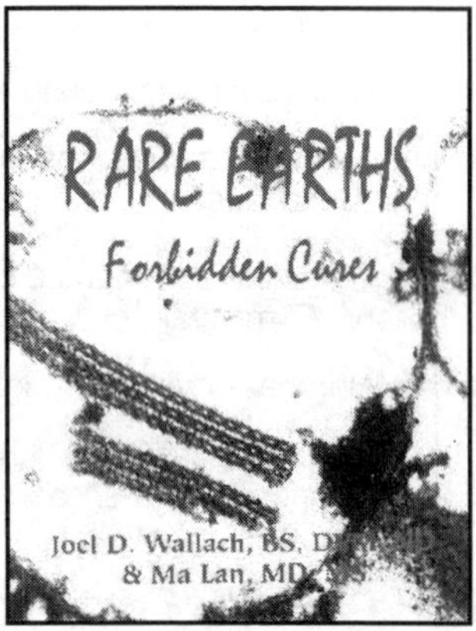

* Degenerative Diseases
* Learning Disabilities
* Criminal Behavior
* Birth Defects
* Addition
* Food Binges
* Depression
* Infertility and More!

$19.95 - 10 or more $12.00 each

1-800-755-4656
www.drjwallach.com

PASSPORT TO AROMATHERAPY

Essential oils or "essences" are highly concentrated volatile oils extracted from aromatic plants

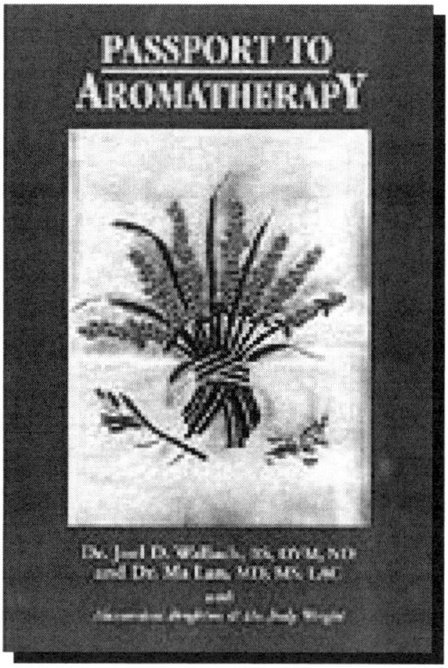

- Essential oils are legendary for their anti-microbial properties

- Essential oils are legendary for uplifting the emotions

$14.95 - 10 or more $8.00 each

Learn more about essential oils from this book

1-800-755-4656
www.drjwallach.com

BLACK GENE LIES

This book is a landmark expose that shows that the diseases of the black population in America, that the medical community attributes to a terrible "Black Gene", are in fact caused by regional and cultural eating habits and nutritional deficiencies of trace elements that are easily, safely and economically overcome by the use of simple nutritional supplement programs and herbal remedies

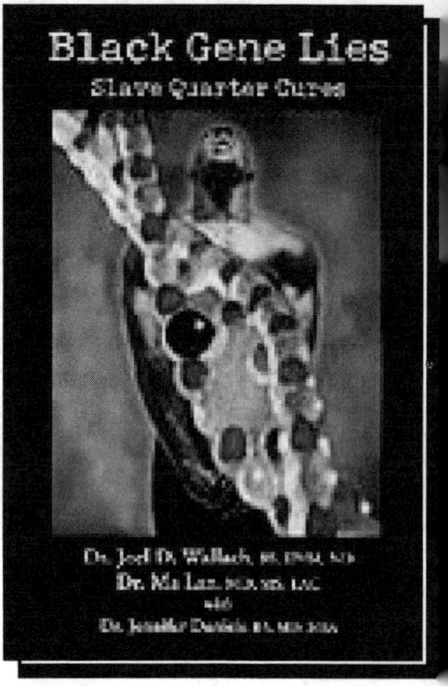

$19.95 - 10 or more $12.00 each

1-800-755-4656
www.drjwallach.com

GOD BLESS AMERICA!

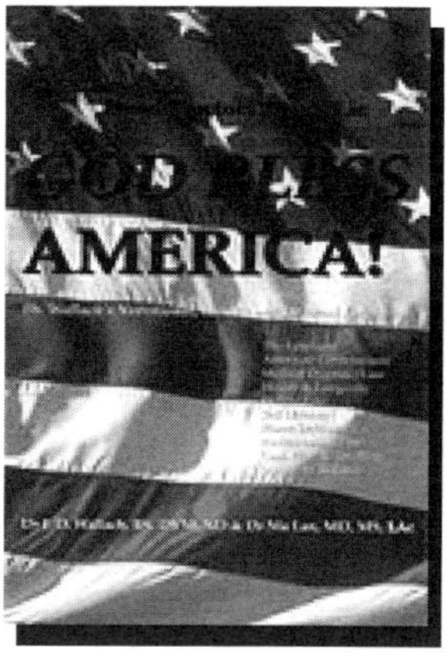

- The epiphany
- American centenarians
- Medical dogmas/lies
- Health and longevity
- Weight loss
- Home defense and
- anti-terrorism plan
  Cash flow and tax plan
- Longevity recipes

$14.95 - 10 or more $8.00 each

WALLach $treet for kids

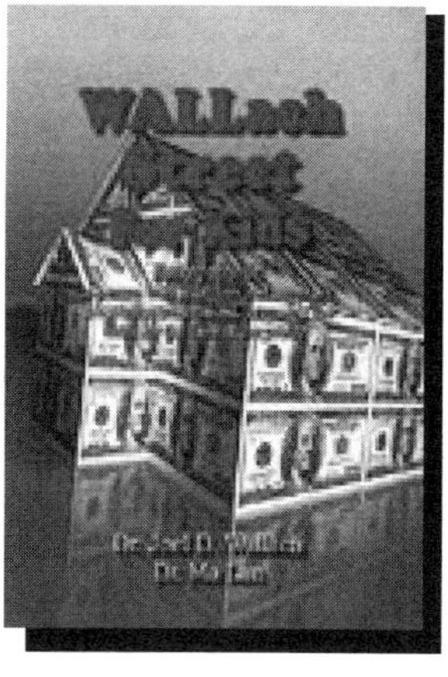

his book is about entrepreneurship, money and business r the purpose of educating entrepreneurial kids, teens and ung adults opportunities to find a "good jobs" in a chang- g global economy, the obvious direction for entrepreneurs to own their business. Ownership is the true measure of wer of business

$19.95 - 10 or more $12.00 each

1-800-755-4656
www.drjwallach.com

Audio CDs

CD001	Dead Doctors Don't Lie	The origiinal tape that started it all
CD002	DDDL in Chinese, Korean,Spanish,Japanese	
CD003	Trust me, I am a Doctor	Dr.Wallach's 1996 health lecture series
CD004	Good Doctor, Bad Doctor	Dr.Wallach's 1997 health lecture series
CD005	Live Doctors Do Lie	
CD006	Medical Dogmas & Lies	Dr.Wallach's 2000 health lecture series
CD007	Medical Milking Machine	Dr.Wallach's 2000 health lecture series
CD008	What's Up Doc II	Health Products Information
CD009	Women,Athletes and Children	Menopause, ADHD and Athletes,2003
CD010	Medical Mouse Trap	Dr.Wallach's lecture on Doctor's continue educti
CD011	The Best of Dead Doctors Don't Lie	combination of DDDL I,II and III
CD012	Lucky Mo	Children's musical story
CD013	Hell's Kitchen	Dr.Wallach's 2004 health lecture series
CD014	God's Recipe	Health alternative to Ritalin
CD015	$10 Path to Financial Freedom	How to get your Youngevity products for free
CD016	Ferret Fat Pak 101	Weight loss product
CD017	Live Free or Die	Jonathan Emord
CD018	Healthier and Longer Life	
CD020	Dial MD for Murder	Dr.Wallach's 2004 health lecture series
CD030	Truth is Forever	Christian Songs by Dee Stocks
CD031	HE Has the Power to Heal	Christian Songs by Dee Stocks
CD033	WBA and Youngevity Opportunity	Dr.Wallach interviewed by Leroy MacMath -Athl physical and financial health
CD034	Black Gene Lies I	interviewed by Herbalist Dirk Twine - the top kil diseases of African American
CD035	Black Gene Lies II	Dr.Wallach's lecture at World Changers Men's fellowship in Atlanta, GA
CD037	Tomato Warning	narration by Richard Dennis
CD046	Dead Athletes Don't Lie	
CD047	H5N1 Bird Flu	Dr.Ma Lan
CD048	Deadly Recipe	
CD056	Until Death Do Us Part	Outline information of Dr.Wallach's lectures
CD057	Energy Crisis	History on energy boost
CD058	Get your ACT together	Steve Wallach
CD059	New Best of DDDL	With 25 questions and answers
CD060	Tru Chocolate	Dr.Wallach , Sandy Elsberg and Elaine Lagatta

order 1-10: $3.00/each, 11-20: $2.00/each, 50 and more: $1.00/each
personalized CD label is available for minimum of 50 CD order.

Other CDs

CD028	Selenium	Dr.Gerhard Schrauzer
CD028	Seeing is believing	Dr.Pugh
CD032	Quality,Quality	Richard Renton
CD039	Beyond Juice	Ken Cole
CD051	Foundation for Success	Richard Stocks
CD052	Three Health Freedom Warriors	Dr.Wallach, Martin Luther King III,Jonathan Emo
CD053	Juice Cures	Jay Kordich

DVDs

		order 1-9	order 10
DVD001	Let's Talk Minerals	$12.95	$7.00
DVD002	Have You Heard	$12.95	$7.00
DVD005	Is It Possible to Reverse Aging (HGH)	$10.00	$7.00
DVD006	This Land Is Leached Land	$12.95	$8.00
DVD007	Take it Off, Keep it Off	$12.95	$8.00
DVD008	Undoing of Disease	$12.95	$8.00
DVD009	Live Long and Prosper	$12.95	$8.00
DVD012	Mineral Story	$12.95	$8.00
DVD013	Y factor	$10.00	$7.00
DVD014	Dead Doctors Don't Lie	$12.95	8.00
DVD015	Mineral Basics	$12.95	$8.00
DVD016	Health Confidence (Creflo Dollar's Church)	$25.00	$14.00

PERSONALIZED CD

1) Minimum Order: 50/per title
2) Title: any title
3) Price: $1.00/per CD
4) Set-up fee: none

LISTEN TO DR.WALLACH'S RADIO SHOW

Talk to Dr.Wallach live on Weekdays on his Radio Programs:

"Dead Doctors Don't Lie"

Toll free 888-379-2552

Priority line: 831-685-1080

Live 12:00 noon - 1:00 pm Pacific Time

"Let's Play Doctor"

Toll free: 877-912-7529

Live 1:00 pm - 2:00 pm Pacific Time

Listen to Dr.Wallach's radio show on line

www.kscoradio.com

click on: "pod cast"

click on: "Dead Doctors Don't Lie"